Disaster Victim Identification in the 21st Century

Published and forthcoming titles in the Forensic Science in Focus series

Published

The Global Practice of Forensic Science
Douglas H. Ubelaker (Editor)

Forensic Chemistry: Fundamentals and Applications
Jay A. Siegel (Editor)

Forensic Microbiology
David O. Carter, Jeffrey K. Tomberlin, M. Eric Benbow and Jessica L. Metcalf (Editors)

Forensic Anthropology: Theoretical Framework and Scientific Basis
Clifford Boyd and Donna Boyd (Editors)

The Future of Forensic Science
Daniel A. Martell (Editor)

Forensic Anthropology and the U.S. Judicial System
Laura C. Fulginiti, Alison Galloway and Kristen Hartnett-McCann (Editors)

Forensic Science and Humanitarian Action: Interacting with the Dead and the Living
Roberto C. Parra, Sara C. Zapico and Douglas H. Ubelaker (Editors)

Disaster Victim Identification in the 21st Century: A US Perspective
John A Williams and Victor W Weedn (Editors)

Forthcoming

Anthropology of Violent Death: Theoretical Foundations for Forensic Humanitarian Action
Roberto C. Parra and Douglas H. Ubelaker (Editors)

The Forensic Evaluation of Burnt Human Remains
Sarah Ellingham, Joe Adserias Garriga, Sara C. Zapico and Douglas H. Ubelaker (Editors)

Artificial Intelligence (AI) in Forensic Sciences
Katrin Franke and Zeno Geradts (Editors)

An Illustrated Guide to Forensic Skeletal Trauma Analysis
Donna C. Boyd

Disaster Victim Identification in the 21st Century

A US Perspective

EDITED BY

John A Williams

Western Carolina University
Cullowhee, US

Victor W Weedn

George Washington University
Washington, US

WILEY

This edition first published 2022

Registered Offices
John Wiley & Sons, Inc., 111 River Street, Hoboken, NJ 07030, USA
John Wiley & Sons Ltd, The Atrium, Southern Gate, Chichester, West Sussex, PO19 8SQ, UK

Editorial Office
The Atrium, Southern Gate, Chichester, West Sussex, PO19 8SQ, UK

For details of our global editorial offices, customer services, and more information about Wiley products visit us at www.wiley.com.

Wiley also publishes its books in a variety of electronic formats and by print-on-demand. Some content that appears in standard print versions of this book may not be available in other formats.

Library of Congress Cataloging-in-Publication Data
Names: Williams, John A. (Physical anthropologist), editor. | Weedn, VictorWalter, editor. | John Wiley & Sons, publisher.
Title: Disaster victim identification in the 21st century : a US perspective / edited by John A Williams, Victor W Weedn.
Description: Hoboken, NJ : John Wiley & Sons, 2022. | Series: Forensic science in focus | Includes bibliographical references and index.
Identifiers: LCCN 2021061393 (print) | LCCN 2021061394 (ebook) | ISBN 9781119652786 (hardback) | ISBN 9781119652809 (pdf) | ISBN 9781119652793 (epub) | ISBN 9781119652823 (ebook)
Subjects: LCSH: Disaster victims--Identification. | Dead--Identification.
Classification: LCC RA1055 .D53 2022 (print) | LCC RA1055 (ebook) | DDC 363.34/8--dc23/eng/20220301
LC record available at https://lccn.loc.gov/2021061393
LC ebook record available at https://lccn.loc.gov/2021061394

Cover Image: © Pgiam/Getty Images
Cover Design by Wiley

Set in 10.5/13.5pt Meridien LT Std by Integra Software Services Pvt. Ltd, Pondicherry, India

Contents

About the Editors

Victor W Weedn, MD, JD, is a forensic pathologist and attorney, and the Chief Medical Examiner for the State of Maryland. He has worked as a medical examiner, crime laboratory director, research scientist, and professor of forensic science and of law. He founded the military's DNA identification program and oversaw the Armed Forces Identification Laboratory (AFDIL), which identified the remains of Czar Nicholas II of Russia, the Branch Davidian conflagration victims in Waco, and later the Michael Blassie, the Vietnam unknown of the Tomb of the Unknowns. He pioneered STR and mtDNA analysis and CE and DNA microchip technologies. He was on the prosecution witness list for the OJ Simpson trial. He holds a patent on latent fingerprint technology. He led the establishment of the NAME inspection and accreditation program. He was the 2015–2016 AAFS President and established the AAFS Academy Standards Board. He received the Helpern Award from the Path/Bio Section of the AAFS in 2017. He was detailed to the DOJ as the Senior Forensic Advisor to Deputy Attorney General Sally Yates, 2016–2017. He testified to the US Congress in 2018. He currently serves on the NAME Board of Directors, the AAFS ASB Disaster Victim Identification Consensus Body, and the NIST OSAC Medicolegal Death Investigation Subcommittee.

John A Williams, Ph.D. D-ABFA (retired), is an Emeritus Professor of forensic anthropology at Western Carolina University. He received his doctorate in 1980 in physical anthropology from the Ohio State University. He spent nearly a quarter of a century as a Professor at the University of North Dakota. There he began his academic career working with prehistoric human skeletons. This led to his involvement with law enforcement and his current interest in forensic anthropology. He is a Fellow of the American Academy of Forensic Sciences and a now retired Diplomate of the American Board of Forensic Anthropology. Over the past four decades he has worked with medical examiners, the FBI, and law enforcement agencies across the United States. In 2003 he moved to North Carolina to create and direct the forensic anthropology program at Western Carolina

University. There in 2005 he established the world's second human decomposition research facility. He has been a member of the Federal agency, Disaster Mortuary Operational Response Team (DMORT), since 1995. In his capacity with DMORT, he has assisted in the identification of mass fatality victims including aircarrier accidents and the 911 terrorist attack. He has also served as an instructor at national DMORT trainings. Since 2016 he has chaired the Disaster Victim Identification Consensus Body of the American Standards Board.

Notes on the Contributors

Kenneth W. Aschheim, DDS, D-ABFO, began his forensic career following the World Trade Center attack in 2001 and is a Diplomate of the American Board of Forensic Odontology. He serves as the Assistant Chief Forensic Odontologist for NYC's OCME and is a member of DMORT. Dr. Aschheim chairs both the ADA SCDI Forensic Odontology Informatics, and the OSAC Forensic Odontology SAC. He is a board member of the Academy Standards Board, ADA's Standards Committees, the International Association of Coroners & Medical Examiners, and Interpol's Forensic Odontology DVI Sub Working group. Dr. Aschheim is an Adjunct Clinical Professor at NYU College of Dentistry, a full-time practitioner, and has co-authored three textbooks on esthetic dentistry.

Jason Byrd, Ph.D., D-ABFE, is a Professor and Associate Director of the William R. Maples Center for Forensic Medicine at the University of Florida's College of Medicine. He is a Board-Certified Forensic Entomologist and Diplomate of the American Board of Forensic Entomology. Dr. Byrd is the educational program administrator for UF's Veterinary Forensic Sciences, Wildlife Forensic Sciences, Shelter Medicine, and Forensic Medicine educational programs. He has served as President of the American Board of Forensic Entomology, the North American Forensic Entomology Association, and the International Veterinary Forensic Science Association. He is a Fellow of the American Academy of Forensic Sciences. Dr. Byrd serves as a Medicolegal Death Investigator within the National Disaster Medical System, Disaster Mortuary Operational Response Team, Region IV, and serves as Commander for the Florida Emergency Mortuary Operations Response System.

Taylor Dickerson III, MSFS, began his career in Forensic Science in 2004 at the NYC Office of Chief Medical Examiner's (OCME) Department of Forensic Biology, where he performed DNA testing and provided expert testimony for a wide range of criminal cases. Mr.

Dickerson also supervised the identification of the victims of the 9/11 World Trade Center incident, helped develop the OCME's Family Assistance Center procedures for mass fatality events, supervised NIJ grant funded work for missing and unidentified person cases, and served as an assistant CODIS administrator. In 2012, Mr. Dickerson joined the Armed Forces Medical Examiner System's Armed Forces DNA Identification Laboratory (AFDIL) as Technical Leader of the Current Day Operations Section and contractor through SNA International. He oversees the DNA testing of criminal casework and current military death identifications. Mr. Dickerson served on the DNA committee of the Scientific Working Group on Disaster Victim Identification and is a current member of the AAFS Standards Board Consensus Body for DVI. Mr. Dickerson is also an Adjunct Professor within Pace University's Forensic Science Program.

Cynthia Gavin, Ph.D., is a strategist, having a diverse background in healthcare, chemical/biological/radiological disaster response, and US military planning. Among her favorite positions, she has provided strategic advisement for the US Army, US Secret Service's Technical Security Division, and the City of New York Office of Emergency Management and Office of Chief Medical Examiner. Building upon her thirty years of experience, Dr. Gavin has taught for the Harvard School of Public Health and the University of Maryland Baltimore County. She has published several works within the Department of Defense and private sector, some of which include Concepts of Operation development, Return on Investment, Decision Papers and creating a future vision for Disaster Victim Identification.

Bryan Johnson, MSFS, is the Major Incident Management Program Manager for the FBI Laboratory's Latent Print Unit in Quantico, VA. He has been with the FBI since 2009 as an FBI Qualified Latent Print Examiner and has focused on mass fatality and unknown deceased issues since 2015. He oversees the FBI's Disaster Victim Identification (DVI) Response Team, who also conducts all fingerprint identifications for the Armed Forces Medical Examiner in Dover, DE, as well as at mass fatality incidents around the globe. He has published in international peer-reviewed forensic science journals on topics pertaining to postmortem fingerprinting and digital capture of postmortem fingerprints. He currently provides regional trainings to agencies across the United States on DVI, postmortem fingerprinting, and has a passion for furthering the science and technology used.

Michal L. Pierce, MS, ASQ CMQ/OE, received her Bachelor of Science in Microbiology from the University of Illinois, followed by a Master of Science in Forensic Science from Sam Houston State University. She joined the Harris County Institute of Forensic Sciences (HCIFS) Forensic Biology Laboratory in October 2007 as a DNA analyst, and she served as the QA/Compliance Manager for Forensic Genetics from 2011 to 2013. In 2013, she was appointed as the first Quality Director for the HCIFS. In this position, she oversees the Quality Management Division, which includes quality assurance, safety, training and development, and analytical statistics. Licensed through the Texas Forensic Science Commission as a forensic analyst, Ms. Pierce possesses a professional certification by the American Board of Criminalistics in molecular biology, and she is certified as a Manager of Quality/Organizational Excellence through the American Society for Quality.

Jason Wiersema, Ph.D., is a forensic anthropologist, and the Director of Forensic Anthropology and Emergency Management at the Harris County Institute of Forensic Sciences in Houston, Texas. He earned his PhD from Texas A&M University in 2006, and his certification by the American Board of Forensic Anthropology in 2012. Dr. Wiersema has extensive experience in DVI response, including large-scale human rights and disaster responses in Bosnia, Guatemala, in Thailand after the 2005 tsunami, in New Orleans following Hurricane Katrina and in New York City as part of the Investigation of the World Trade Center terrorist attack. He has leveraged this, and his experience as a laboratory-based analyst of over 2000 forensic anthropology cases, in the development and implementation of standards and best practices for medicolegal death investigation generally and for DVI specifically. He is the current Chair of the Medicine Scientific Area Committee of the Organization of Scientific Area Committees (OSAC), and a member of the Forensic Sciences Standards Board. He is past Chair of the Disaster Victim Identification Subcommittee of the OSAC. He is the author of numerous peer-reviewed publications relevant to DVI.

Preface

In 2009 the National Academy of Sciences issued a report critical of the state of forensic science in the United States. One outcome of the report was the formation of OSAC, Organization of Scientific Area Committees for Forensic Science. OSAC's 22 subcommittees are charged with creating standards for the forensic sciences. The formation of standards for Disaster Victim Identification (DVI) is one component of OSAC's mission. To make these standards reality requires an SDO or Standards Development Organization. In response to this need the American Academy of Forensic Sciences established an SDO, the Academy Standards Board or ASB. DVI is included in the ASB and has its own committee or Consensus Body. It was during the routine work of the DVI Consensus Body that impetus for this book, outlining the current state of DVI in the United States, came about.

December 2021

John A. Williams
Victor W. Weedn

Series Preface

The forensic sciences represent diverse, dynamic fields that seek to utilize the very best techniques available to address legal issues. Fueled by advances in technology, research, and methodology, as well as new case applications, the forensic sciences continue to evolve. Forensic scientists strive to improve their analyses and interpretations of evidence and to remain cognizant of the latest advancements. This series results from a collaborative effort between the American Academy of Forensic Sciences (AAFS) and Wiley to publish a select number of books that relate closely to the activities and Objectives of the AAFS. The book series reflects the goals of the AAFS to encourage quality scholarship and publication in the forensic sciences. Proposals for publication in the series are reviewed by a committee established for that purpose by the AAFS and also reviewed by Wiley. The AAFS was founded in 1948 and represents a multidisciplinary professional organization that provides leadership to advance science and its application to the legal system. The 11 sections of the AAFS consist of Criminalistics, Digital and Multimedia Sciences, Engineering Sciences, General, Pathology/Biology, Questioned Documents, Jurisprudence, Anthropology, Toxicology, Odontology, and Psychiatry and Behavioral Science. There are over 7000 members of the AAFS, originating from all 50 States of the United States and many countries beyond. This series reflects global AAFS membership interest in new research, scholarship, and publication in the forensic sciences.

Douglas H. Ubelaker
Senior Scientist
Smithsonian Institution
Washington, DC, USA
Series Editor

CHAPTER 1
Introduction

John A. Williams[1] and Victor W. Weedn[2]

[1] *Department of Anthropology and Sociology, Western Carolina University, Cullowhee, NC, USA*
[2] *Office of the Maryland Chief Medical Examiner, Baltimore, MD, USA*

1.1 Introduction

Mass fatality disasters, both natural and man-made, are increasing in frequency. Extreme environmental disruptions like hurricanes, wildfires, and flooding are on the rise and in the news almost daily. Mass casualty terrorism is sadly also becoming more commonplace. In spite of improvements in technology common carrier crashes continue to take place. The COVID-19 pandemic has shown us that twenty-first-century medicine can be outmatched by a "novel" virus that does not respect national boundaries. The deaths that result from these events place a different set of needs and obligations on those charged with disaster victim identification, or DVI. In the United States during the 1980s the National Funeral Directors Association (NFDA) noticed with concern that there was no national coordinating body with regard to mass fatality events and DVI. The NFDA was the first organization to draw up plans for the handling of mass fatality victims. From their initial efforts came the Federal agency DMORT (Disaster Mortuary Operational Response Team) and the concept of a disaster morgue, marking the beginning of DVI in the United States as it is known today.

Disaster Victim Identification in the 21st Century: A US Perspective, First Edition.
Edited by John A Williams and Victor W Weedn.

Disaster Victim Identification is the comprehensive process of human identification as applied to mass fatality events. Although by definition a mass fatality event is any situation that overwhelms local resources, we generally think of situations in which identification is hampered by the event itself and the process of recovery from the event. Human remains that have been badly traumatized, heavily decomposed, or recovered outside of their normal context are examples that would require DVI.

In 2009, after issues surfaced regarding the scientific basis for the practice of forensic science, the National Academy of Science issued a report on the state of forensic science in the United States. In response to the NAS report a movement to formulate standards within the forensic sciences began. DVI was included and the creation of standards and best practices within the field are ongoing. In 2014, responding to the 2009 NAS report, the US Department of Commerce's National Institute of Standards and Technology (NIST) established the Organization of Scientific Area Committees (OSAC) to assist with the development of these standards in the forensic sciences. In OSAC's first iteration a Disaster Victim Identification subcommittee was established to promulgate recommended standards. In 2016, the American Academy of Forensic Sciences created the American Standards Board (ASB) as a standards development organization (SDO). The ASB includes a Disaster Victim Identification Consensus Body to produce American National Standards for DVI. Using the OSAC DVI subcommittee recommendations, the ASB has to date published several standards/best practices that apply to DVI.

Although DVI may be thought of as a police function, and in most countries Interpol guidelines are used, in the United States the responsibility is left to the medical examiner and coroner (MEC), who are generally outside of law enforcement. The most current books on the subject of DVI take a European perspective, and do not directly address needs of practitioners in the United States. While DVI is carried out locally, it is by its nature under a broader governmental umbrella (i.e., based in the office of a coroner or medical examiner). At the US federal level, 15 Emergency Support Functions (ESFs) outline how the public and private sectors should respond to national emergencies. Buried in the scope of ESF#8 is the role of the Public Health Service in disaster response, specifically in mass fatality management and DVI. Here is where standards or best DVI practices would prove highly beneficial in providing guidance to the varied agencies that may be involved in a mass fatality event.

Disaster victim identification has never been a static process. With each mass fatality event (each hurricane, plane crash, terrorist attack) comes different circumstances of recovery, the state or condition of the victim's remains, and the resulting challenges to victim identification. Even though we learn from each disaster nothing fully prepares us for the next to come. The best that can be done is to plan and train personnel for multiple scenarios, and hope that the planning and training never needs to be implemented.

1.2 This Book

This book approaches DVI from three organizational perspectives. The beginning chapters cover the background of mass fatalities and disaster victim identification, its history and the evolving scope of governmental response. The bulk of the book – the middle chapters – focuses on the nuts and bolts of DVI, the DVI morgue and VIC (Victim Information Center), and the methods used to ensure correct and proper identifications. The concluding chapters examine two less concrete elements of DVI in an MFI (Mass Fatality Incident): ethical considerations and the changing landscape of twenty-first-century MFIs.

To anyone who is a student of the past, mass fatality incidents have a long and varied history not only in the United States but the world at large. From a global perspective, we see that fortunately Americans have been spared from many of the worst recorded losses of life. This is partly due to the relative youth of our nation, its relatively small population density, and a favorable geography that has not been conducive to extreme natural events. Still, the United States has experienced its share of MFIs, as well as other disasters. Until recently, as a nation, the response of the federal government, and state governments, has been at least mainly mitigative. Responses to disasters have been direct and fiscal in nature. It was only in the aftermath of the September 11th terrorist attack that a more proactive approach to disasters and MFIs began to take shape. The 2004 National Response Plan (NRP) and its Emergency Support Functions (ESF) highlighted the need for preparation and coordinated response to all forms of disasters, including MFIs.

Our approach to DVI was further impacted by the 2009 National Academy of Science report on the scientific basis of forensic science. Few MECs have had, or will ever have, the need to respond to an MFI. While DVI is a death investigation process it is not simply an extension of the routine operations of the MEC jurisdiction. Besides differences in the circumstances of death (e.g., the likelihood of extreme fragmentation), the MEC must contend with external inputs from the media, family and loved ones of the victims, and political figures. Conducting a DVI without a guiding framework can easily result in inconsistency, inefficiency, and the possibility of a less than adequate result. It is precisely for these reasons that the NAS report targeted the forensic sciences, of which DVI is one multidisciplinary component. This report, through various stages, led to the creation of the Organization of Scientific Area Committees (OSAC) and that in turn to the Academy Standards Board (ASB), leading to the formation of standards in the forensic sciences, including DVI. These standards, which are still being formed and undergoing review, will provide some degree of consistency and accountability in the practice in how MECs and other agencies approach DVI. However, for these standards (best practices) to be effective there must be some overriding effort to bring all of the various partners in DVI into compliance

During the early 1980s the National Funeral Directors Association recognized the need for a coordinated effort in responding to mass fatality events. This private response to a growing concern, in part due to several airline accidents with significant loss of life, led to the formation of DMORT. With DMORT came a team approach to DVI. Following a presidential disaster declaration, it is possible for an MEC to utilize DMORT, alleviating the problems that can arise when a jurisdiction is unprepared for or incapable of responding to the MFI. In addition to a fully operational disaster morgue team, a DMORT deployment comes with a fully outfitted disaster morgue. Since the mid-1990s when DMORT was first commissioned many states have developed their own mass fatality teams (i.e., FEMORS in Florida).

Whether the mass fatality morgue is free-standing, as in DMORT, or incorporated into the MEC jurisdictional morgue, it is here that the work of DVI takes place. The mass fatality morgue is designed to be flexible, as are mass fatality teams. Together with logistical and support team members, the forensic science team members go about the process of identifying victims. Although all members of the DVI morgue contribute to victim identification, the majority of positive identification derives from odontology, fingerprints, and DNA. In the decades since the advent of DMORT, DVI has become increasingly technology driven. Where forensic odontologists once examined actual dental radiographs, the work is now accomplished digitally using software applications. Fingerprints can be scanned and uploaded to a regional or national database directly from the DVI morgue using technology no more complex than a personal cellphone. Advancements in rapid DNA processing may soon result in identifications made while the remains are still being processed through the DVI morgue stations. Together these advancements have increased the speed, efficiency, accuracy, and accountability in the identification process.

Prior to the mid-1990s the US approach to the DVI was a relatively uncentralized mix of federal and local deployed assets. On the heels of highly visible airline crashes and the terrorist attack of 2001 came DMORT, FEMA, and an ever-changing bureaucracy of the NRP and NRF (National Response Framework). The question to consider is whether our plan for the disasters of the late twentieth century is still valid for the first quarter of the twenty-first century. Currently, the MEC jurisdictions that must handle DVI vary from large urban ones with self-sufficient morgue capabilities for even the largest MFIs to small rural ones with few assets and little training to handle mass fatalities. Federal assets, like DMORT, were designed for the MFIs of the mid-1990s, i.e., transportation accidents. This model of morgue deployment has far less utility in handling other disasters, like that occurring on our southern border with the undocumented deaths of immigrants crossing illegally into the United States. Can the MEC system meet the challenges of a changing role for DVI? Add to this the contrast upgrading of technology, like rapid DNA testing, and the disparity between MEC jurisdictions becomes even more pronounced.

DVI, whether we retain the DMORT model, or some form of it, or move to a novel approach, it must be adaptable for it be relevant to the needs of the twenty-first century and the ever-changing theater of mass fatality disasters.

Interlaced throughout the chapters of this book are references to law, domestic and occasionally international. The complexity of an MFI response would be far more difficult to approach if it were not for various legislative actions like the Stafford Act, FEMA, and the National Response Framework. These mandate and make possible our ability to respond to mass fatalities and carry out DVI. State responses are more varied but also contribute to the framework of DVI. In the end, though, it is the MEC jurisdiction and its legal requirement to establish cause of death, and, in so doing, identify the deceased, upon which DVI rests.

How the dead should be treated falls under the umbrella of ethical conduct. Every person should have the right to be identified and be treated with dignity after death. A statement attributed to William Gladstone makes this point: "Show me the manner in which a nation cares for its dead and I will measure with mathematical exactness, the tender mercy of its people, their respect for the law of the land and their loyalty to high ideals." If the recent work treating the victims of COVID-19 in New York City by DMORT are an indication, despite our country's differences, on this we as Americans still agree.

CHAPTER 2
Historical Background

Victor W. Weedn
Office of the Maryland Chief Medical Examiner, Baltimore, MD, USA

2.1 History of Mass Disasters

There have always been natural cataclysms, such as hurricanes, floods, droughts, wildfires, mudslides, avalanches, earthquakes, and volcanic eruptions. Undoubtedly, the great disasters have been recorded, because there was simply insufficient population amassed in prehistoric times. The flood myths, of which there are hundreds from around the world and the Noah and Gilgamesh stories are most famed, probably are just myths based upon the common human experience of flooding. The story of Atlantis was likely based upon a parable in Plato's writings, although it is possible that he had known of the volcanic eruption at Thera (present-day Santorini island) in 1646 BCE, which destroyed the Greek city of Akrotiri and may have resulted in as many as 20,000 fatalities, although there is some evidence that many of the inhabitants fled [1].

Perhaps the most famous disaster recorded in ancient history was that of the eruption of Mount Vesuvius in 79 AD, which destroyed the Roman villages of Pompeii, Herculaneum, Oplontis, and Stabiae and is thought to have resulted in approximately 1,000 deaths [2].

The Bible refers to earthquakes, floods, wildfires, plagues, and famines. Notable ancient earthquakes include the 115 AD earthquake

Disaster Victim Identification in the 21st Century: A US Perspective, First Edition.
Edited by John A Williams and Victor W Weedn.

(magnitude 7.5) that killed 260,000 in the Byzantine city of Antioch (now Turkey), the 526 AD earthquake (magnitude 7.0) that killed 250,000 also in Antioch, and the 1138 AD earthquake (magnitude 7.1) that devastated the Syrian city of Aleppo that killed 230,000 [3].

With the exception of the Black Death of the bubonic plague that was responsible for the death of approximately 50 million or one-half of the fourteenth-century European population, the deadliest disasters are relatively recent phenomena due to population growth (Figure 2.1) [4].

Table 2.1 lists the deadliest natural disasters (prior to the COVID pandemic). Deaths from natural disasters have seen a large decline over the past century. Annual deaths from natural disasters have decreased by 75 percent over the past 100 years, to an average of 60,000 over the past decade, approximately 0.1% of global deaths [7]. Death tolls are highest in low- to middle-income countries without the infrastructure to prepare, respond, and protect their citizens.

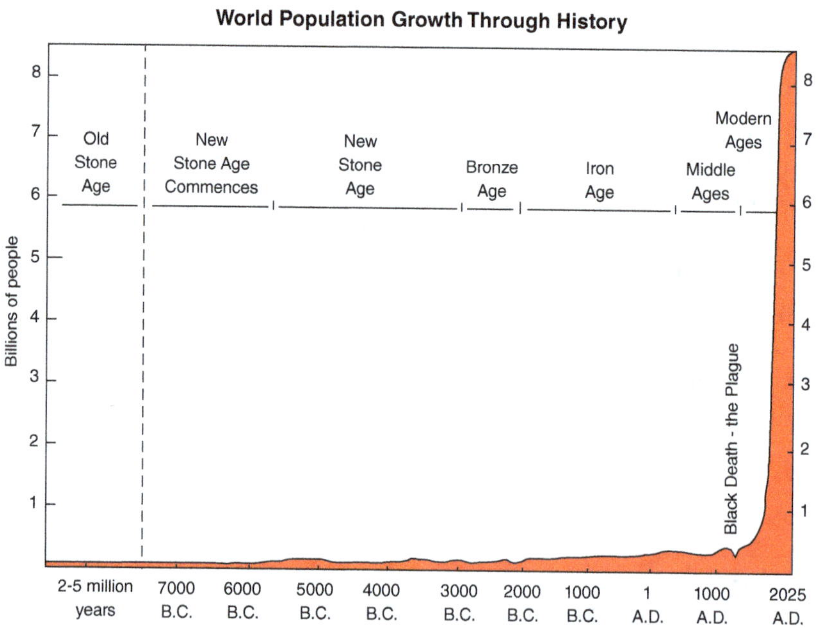

Figure 2.1 World population growth (billions)[5].

Table 2.1 World's deadliest natural disasters [6].

Table	Year	Disaster	Location	Deaths
1	1931	China floods	China	1–4 million
2	1887	Yellow River flood	China	0.9–2 million
3	1556	Shaanxi earthquake	China	830,000
4	1970	Bhola cyclone	Bangladesh	500,000
5	1881	Haiphong typhoon	Vietnam	300,000
6	1920	Haiyuan earthquake	China	273,400
7	526	Antioch earthquake	Turkey	250–300,000
8	1976	Tangshan earthquake	China	243–655,000
9	2010	Haiti earthquake	Haiti	230–316,000
10	1975	Typhoon Nina	China	229,000

The deadliest natural disasters are dwarfed by military wars (Table 2.2). Between 90,000 and 146,000 died acutely from the bombing of Hiroshima, and between 39,000 and 80,000 died from the bombing of Nagasaki [9,10]. Far fewer Americans have died in wars (Table 2.3).

Most early mass fatality incidents were of natural disasters, but there were a few noncombat manmade disasters, particularly the collapse of the wooden amphitheater at Fidenae (8 miles north of Rome) in 27 AD that killed 20,000 spectators and the collapse of the upper tier of the Circus Maximus in Rome in 143 AD that killed 1112 spectators (Table 2.4) [13]. In general, manmade disasters are a feature of modern times and generally track technologic progress [14–26].

It is sometimes difficult to categorize a mass fatality incident as natural or manmade; e.g. is the 2005 flooding of New Orleans due to inadequate levees or due to Hurricane Katrina?

If we confine our attention to the United States, Table 2.5 lists the deadliest non-military disasters in US history according to one online source (prior to the COVID pandemic). However, a FEMA (Federal Emergency Management Agency) listing of the deadliest US disasters (prior to the COVID pandemic) is quite different (Table 2.6). Listings of disasters are problematic due to differences in how far back they go,

Table 2.2 World's deadliest wars [8].

Rank	Years	War	Location	Deaths
1	1939–1945	World War II	Worldwide	56–85 million
2	1850–1864	Taiping rebellion	China	20–100 million
3	184–280	Three Kingdoms War	China	36–40 million
4	1206–1368	Mongol conquests	Eurasia	30–40 million
5	1616–1683	Ming-Qing transition	China	25 + million
6	1519–1632	Spanish conquest of Aztecs	Mexico	24.3 million
7	1914–1918	World War I	Worldwide	16–30 million
8	1937–1945	Second Sino–Japanese war	China	20–25 million
9	755–763	An Lushan rebellion	China, Vietnam	13–36 million
10	1370–1405	Conquest of Timur	Eurasia	8–20 million

Table 2.3 Deadliest US wars [11,12].

Rank	Years	War	Deaths
1	1861–1865	American Civil War	750,000
2	1941–1945	World War II	405,399
3	1917–1918	World War I	116,516
4	1961–1975	Vietnam War	58,220
5	1950–1953	Korean War	54,246
6	1775–1783	American Revolutionary war	25,000
7	1812–1815	War of 1812	15,000
8	1846–1848	Mexican-American War	13,283
9	2003–2011	Iraq War	4,497
10	1899–1902	Philippine-American War	4196

Table 2.4 World's deadliest non-combat disasters [27].

Rank	Year	Location	Deaths
Railroad			
1	2004	Sri Lanka tsunami train wreck	1700 +
2	1917	Ciurea, Romania rail disaster	600–1000
3	1917	Saint-Michel-de-Maurienne, France derailment	675–800
Air carrier			
1	1977	Tenerife runway collision	83
2	1985	Japan Airlines Flight 123	520
3	1996	Charkhi Dadri mid-air collision	349
Maritime			
1	1987	MV *Doña Paz*, Philippines	1562–4386
2	1948	SS *Kiangya*, Shanghai	2750–3920
3	2002	MV *Le Joola*, Senegal	1863
Smog			
1	1952	London	4000–6000
2	1880	London	2200
3	1956	London	1000
Structural collapse			
1	1975	Banqiao Dam, China	171,000
2	27	Amphitheater, Italy	20,000 +
3	1979	Machchhu Dam, India	5000–10,000
Industrial			
1	1984	Bhopal India chemical disaster	3787–19,000
2	1942	Benxihu, China colliery disaster	1549
3	2013	Rana Plaza, Bangladesh collapse	1134

(*Continued*)

Table 2.4 (Continued)

Nuclear			
1	1957	Mayak nuclear waste explosion	200–6000
2	1986	Chernobyl disaster	95–4000 +
3	1957	Windscale fire	33
Explosions			
1	1629	Wanggongchang, China	20,000
2	1769	Bresda, Italy	3000
3	1948	Hsuan Huai, China	3000
Building fires			
1	1863	Church of the Company, Chile	2000 +
2	1893	Theater fire, China	1995
3	1845	Theater fire, China	1670

Table 2.5 Deadliest US disasters [28].

Rank	Year	Disaster	Location	Deaths
1	1900	Galveston hurricane	Galveston, TX	6000–12,000
2	1899	San Ciriaco hurricane	Puerto Rico	3389
3	1906	San Francisco earthquake	San Francisco, CA	3000 +
4	2001	September 11 terrorist attacks	NYC, Pentagon, Shanksville, PA	2996
5	2017	Hurricane Maria	Puerto Rico, Virgin Islands, East Coast	2982
6	1928	Okeechobee hurricane	Puerto Rico, Florida	2823
7	1941	Pearl Harbor attack	Honolulu, HI	2467
8	1889	Johnstown Flood	Johnstown, PA	2209
9	1893	Cheniere Caminada hurricane	Louisiana	2000
10	1865	Sultana steamboat explosion	Arkansas	1700

Table 2.6 Deadliest US disasters (FEMA) [29].

Rank	Year	Disaster	Location	Deaths
1	1918–1919	Influenza pandemic	US	500,000
2	1775–1782	Smallpox	US	130,000
3	1957	Influenza epidemic	US	69,800
4	1968	Influenza epidemic	US	38,800
5	1878	Yellow Fever	Mississippi valley	13,000
6	1900	Galveston hurricane	Galveston, TX	8000
7	1849–1851	Cholera epidemic	Midwest	11,000
8	1980	Heatwave/drought	Central/East	10,000
9	1988	Heatwave/drought	Central/East	10,000
10	1853	Yellow Fever	New Orleans, LA	7790

Table 2.7 Categorization of US mass fatality incidents of 200 fatalities or greater [31].

Man-made	No.	Natural	No.
Military strikes	10	Tornados	8
Terrorism	4	Hurricanes	13
Building fires	5	Floods	5
Aircraft crashes	5	Blizzards	6
Ship sinkings	6	Heat waves	3
Explosions	9	Wildfires	5
Other	7	Earthquakes	1
Total	46	Total	41

what constitutes a disaster, and the uncertainty in the number of fatalities for many of the disasters. Listings of costliest disasters also is different than listings of deadliest disasters [30].

If we categorize the US disasters that have resulted in greater than 200 deaths, according to one online source, then we find that there are a similar number of natural (41) and manmade disasters (46) (Table 2.7).

Table 2.8 Categorization of US mass fatality incidents of 10 or greater from 2000–2016 [33].

Man-made	No.	Natural	No.
Transportation	47	Tornados	25
Mass shooting	12	Hurricanes	13
Fires	10	Floods	8
Collapse	10	Blizzards	4
Asphyxiation	1	Mudslides	3
Stampede	1	Wildfires	3
Total	81	Total	56

A study by the New York City Office of the Chief Medical Examiner of mass fatality incidents in the US from 2000 to 2016, where a mass fatality was defined as more than ten deaths, similarly found that the number of natural disasters (56) was roughly equal to the number of manmade disasters (81) (Table 2.8) [32]. Tornados, hurricanes, and floods were the most common natural disasters; transportation, mass shootings, fires, and structural collapses were the most common man-made disasters. The average number of deaths per incident was 62, but this was skewed by the WTC terrorist attack and Hurricane Katrina – when these were excluded the average number of deaths per incident dropped to only 29; 89% of the disasters involved less than 50 fatalities.

2.2 Early History of Mass Disaster Response

Communities have always had to cope with catastrophes as best they could, but planned and coordinated response and actions taken to mitigate future catastrophes are a development of modernity.

Commentators have called the 1755 Great Lisbon Earthquake "The First Modern Disaster" [34,35]. When the quake struck in 1755, Lisbon was a great and wealthy city with a population of 275,000. It struck on All Saints day during the morning when thousands were attending Catholic mass ceremonies. This earthquake, calculated to have had a magnitude of at least 8.5, was associated with a tsunami sea wave and numerous fires that combined to destroy 85% of the city and cause an estimated 50,000 fatalities. The quake lasted for about five minutes, collapsing buildings and creating massive fissures in the earth, but then was followed by a tsunami that flooded the city. Hundreds who had fled to the docks to escape the carnage in the city were washed away. All churches were destroyed, but the red-light district was spared. The catastrophe had a strong impact on European culture and influenced philosophers such as Voltaire, Rousseau, and Immanuel Kant.

King Joseph I, who suffered a nervous breakdown after the catastrophe, placed his prime minister, Sebastião de Melo, later the Marquis de Pombal, in charge of responding to the disaster. Allegedly, the Marquis, when asked what was to be done, he replied, "bury the dead and heal the living." This was the first organized disaster response in history. Firefighters were sent to extinguish the fires, the military was sent to prevent looting, and citizens were ordered to remove the bodies. Over the objections of the church, many of the bodies were loaded onto barges and buried at sea. Pombal sent a query to all parishes in the country about the earthquake which provided the earliest known seismologic data. In less than a year, the city was cleared of debris. With funding from the king, the city was rebuilt based upon the plan of their Chief Engineer, Manuel da Maia. "Pombaline" buildings were built to withstand future earthquakes, based upon tests of wooden scale models and simulations of earthquakes by marching troops around them.

Prior to the formation of the United States the English colonies could not expect relief from the English king or Parliament, who often had little knowledge or interest of calamities across the Atlantic in America, and most relief was from voluntary private donations of labor, goods, and money – notwithstanding the £20,000 sterling issued for the 1740 Great Fire of Charleston [36,37]. This was the experience of the American society and expectation for governmental disaster relief at the founding of the country.

2.2.1 The Portsmouth Christmas Fires and 1803 Portsmouth Federal Disaster Relief

Hours after Christmas Day of 1802, a fire broke out behind the New Hampshire Bank building in Portsmouth, New Hampshire [38,39]. A large portion of the town burned, with 120 buildings lost and damages estimated at $300,000 ($6.8 M 2019 USD). There were no fatalities. A committee of five men was appointed to receive and distribute donations for relief. They raised over $45,000 from all over the country. Most property owners had no insurance, and private charity provided the only relief. Afterward, the New Hampshire Fire and Marine Insurance Company was founded. The city sought to widen streets and use brick and "fireproof" materials for all future buildings.

In 1803, four years after ratification of the Constitution, the 7th US Congress enacted the first federal disaster relief legislation when it extended the time the Portsmouth proprietors had for remitting tariffs on imported goods (Box 2.1).

After the Christmas fire of 1802, there were two more fires in Portsmouth. In 1806, on the day before Christmas, four stores caught fire, then row of buildings and a church. Future buildings were to be built of brick, but this was not enforced. Then in 1813, three days before Christmas, "the Great Portsmouth Fire" raged. After starting in a barn from suspected arson, 15 city acres were destroyed, including 108 residential homes, 64 public buildings and stores, and 100 barns. Afterward, the Brick Act of 1814 was passed, but it lasted only ten years. The insurance company went bankrupt.

2.2.2 The 1835 Great Fire of New York City

In the evening of December 16, 1835, a fire began in a five-story warehouse but quickly spread from gale-force winds, destroying much of the commercial district of lower Manhattan [41]. New York City had become the preeminent city in the US after the opening of the Erie Canal. The fire burned 13 acres, 17 city blocks, destroyed 530 to 800 buildings, resulted in $20 M in economic loss ($584 M 2019 USD), and caused 2 to 200 fatalities. The fire department's growth had not kept up with that of the booming city; nor had its water supply. Due to the intense cold (–17° F), the East River and Hudson River had

Box 2.1 A Bill for the Relief of Sufferers by Fire, in the town of Portsmouth [40]

Be it enacted by the Senate and House of Representatives of the United States of America in Congress assembled, That all persons who, being indebted to the United States, for duties on merchandise, have given bond therefor, with one or more sureties, payable to the collector for the district of Portsmouth, and who have suffered a loss of property by the late conflagration at that place, shall be, and they hereby are allowed to take up, or have cancelled, all bonds heretofore given for duties as aforesaid, upon giving to the said collector new bonds, with one or more sureties, to the satisfaction of said collector, for the sums of their former bonds respectively, payable in twelve months from and after the day of payment specified in the bonds to be taken up or cancelled as aforesaid; and the said collector is hereby authorized and directed, to give up or cancel, all such bonds upon the receipt of others as described in this act; which last mentioned bonds shall be proceeded with, in all respects, like other bonds which are taken by collectors for duties due to the United States: Provided however, that nothing in this act contained shall extend to bonds which had fallen due before the twenty-sixth day of December last.

APPROVED, February 19, 1803

frozen over, forcing firefighters to drill holes in the ice for water. Water froze in their hand-pumped fire engines. Buildings were blown up in an attempt to stop the fire's spread. Reconstruction with stone and brick buildings followed based upon insurance payments and accessible loans. The disaster prompted construction of a new water supply, and expansion of the fire service. Most New York insurance companies went out of business and Hartford, Connecticut, came to dominate the NYC fire insurance market.

2.2.3 1865 Sultana Explosion

On April 27, 1865, three of four boilers of the side-wheel steamboat *Sultana* exploded causing her to catch fire and sink into the Mississippi River near Memphis, Tennessee [42,43]. Although she had a listed capacity of only 376 passengers, 2137 passengers were aboard that day. The official death toll was 1547, but the exact number is disputed; of the nearly 800 who initially survived and were taken to Memphis hospitals, 31 died there. This was the worst maritime disaster in US history, in fact the worst transportation disaster in US history, but it was overshadowed by the end of the Civil War and particularly the death of John Wilkes Booth on the preceding day.

2.2.4 The 1871 Fires

Due to the hot dry weather, the US Midwest was a tinderbox in the fall of 1871 [44]. The Great Chicago Fire began on October 8, 1871, and burned until the 10th [45–47]. The fire burned 2000 acres, 17,500 buildings, and a total of $222 M ($4.6B 2019 USD) in property losses. The fatalities were thought to be 300 dead, but the county coroner speculated that an accurate count was impossible, as some victims may have drowned or had been incinerated, leaving no remains. Lieutenant General Philip Sheridan was placed in charge of a de facto martial law of dubious legitimacy to preserve the peace of the city. The Chicago Relief and Aid Society was in charge of the city's relief efforts. The city began to rewrite its fire standards at the urging of insurance executives and fire-prevention reformers. Chicago developed one of the country's leading fire-fighting forces and remains so today.

That same day, October 8, 1871, the Great Peshtigo Fire raged [48,49]. The firestorm destroyed the towns of Peshtigo, Wisconsin, and a dozen other villages in the area. The fire burned approximately 1.5 million acres. It is the deadliest US fire to date, with a mortality of 1200–2500 fatalities. The fire in Chicago overshadowed the Peshtigo fire, which was given little notice due to the remoteness of the region and to the destruction of the telegraph lines to Green Bay soon after the fire began.

On the same day as the Chicago and Peshtigo fires began, fires began in the Door Peninsula of Wisconsin, in the Upper Peninsula of Michigan (the Great Michigan Fire), and in Urbana, Illinois; fires

began Windsor, Ontario, Canada, four days later. There has been speculation that fragments of Biela's comet impacting the region caused the various fires, but this theory has generally been discounted.

2.2.5 American Red Cross (ARC)

In 1881, the American National Red Cross (ANRC), also known as the American Red Cross (ARC), became the major source of relief for US disaster victims after it was founded by Clara Barton in Washington, DC, for the humanitarian aid of war victims [50–52]. She had learned of the Swiss Red Cross network while visiting Europe after the US Civil War. Barton would lead the Red Cross for 23 years. In 1900, the ARC was granted a Congressional Charter. Barton sought to expand the role of the ARC to include peacetime disaster relief and in 1905, the year after Barton resigned, the Charter was revised to include, "mitigating the sufferings caused by pestilence, famine, fire, floods, and other great national calamities, and to devise and carry on measures for preventing the same." She also campaigned for peacetime relief work as part of the global Red Cross network. The so-called American Amendment initially met with some resistance in Europe, but was eventually adopted. The current charter includes providing national and international disaster relief and mitigation. The ARC operated with relatively little direct contributions from the federal government for many years. Today, the ARC becomes a federal agency during times of declared disasters and is an integral part of the federal response.

2.2.6 1889 Johnstown Flood

On May 31, 1889, after an exceptionally heavy rainfall, the South Fork Dam on the Little Conemaugh River failed, releasing 14.5 tons of water from Lake Conemaugh with a Mississippi River–like flow onto South Fork, then Conemaugh, and finally Johnstown, which with its 50,000 inhabitants was 14 miles downstream [53,54]. The flood killed 2208 citizens and produced damages of $17 M ($475 M 2019 USD). Industrialist Henry Frick had bought the dam from the Commonwealth of Pennsylvania to establish the South Fork Fishing and Hunting Club. Development involved changes that increased the threat of failure of the dam. It was the worst disaster in US history to that date. Clara

Barton with 50 volunteers led the first ARC major disaster relief effort. To help the families $3.8 M in donations was collected. Survivors sued Frick's Club unsuccessfully, the defense claiming it was an act of God. Public outrage over the lawsuit resulted in later courts holding those unnaturally using land strictly liable for damages. Floods of Johnstown occurred later in 1907, 1924, 1936, and 1977.

2.2.7 1899 San Ciriaco Hurricane

On August 8, 1899, the San Ciriaco hurricane hit Puerto Rico, killing 3369, causing $38 M ($1.2B 2019 USD) in damages, and leaving 250,000 homeless [55]. The hurricane hit also in the Antilles, the Bahamas, and North Carolina, resulting in a total of 3,855 fatalities. Although only a Category 4 hurricane, it is the longest-lived (28 days) and most powerful Atlantic hurricane in history. The entire island of Hatteras, NC, was submerged by 4 to 10 feet of water. Hurricanes were not named then, but the nickname is Spanish for Roman Catholic feast day devoted to Saint Cyriacus. Donations largely consisted of clothing and some food.

2.2.8 1900 Galveston Storm

On September 9, 1900, a hurricane and tidal wave hit Galveston, Texas [56–60]. It is the deadliest natural disaster in US history, other than the 1918 Spanish Influenza pandemic and the current COVID-19 Pandemic (the deadliest Atlantic hurricane is the 1780 San Calixto II hurricane that killed well over 20,000 of the Antilles and other Caribbean islands [61]; and even deadlier cyclones and typhoons have been recorded in India and Southeast Asia). Galveston had a population of approximately 38,000 at the time and was a busy port, second only to the port of New York City. Galveston is a barrier island on the coast of Texas with an elevation of one foot above sea level. The island was hit by an 8–12′ storm surge that destroyed about 7000 buildings and $4.5 M ($138 M 2019 USD) in damages [62,63]. Every dwelling on the island was destroyed or damaged. Fatality estimates range from 6000 to 12,000 deaths; the most common official estimate is 8000. The dead were initially buried at sea, but then they began washing ashore; afterward they were burned. In the aftermath, a sea-wall was erected, 17 feet high and ten miles long. Nonetheless, the

Houston ship channel replaced Galveston as the major port in the area. A relief committee was organized. Donations of more than $1.2 M were received, primarily for the building of residences. Clara Barton arrived one week later with a group of ARC volunteers.

2.2.9 1906 San Francisco Earthquake

On April 18, 5:12 a.m., 1906, an earthquake, magnitude 7.9, struck San Francisco and leveled 80% of the city [64,65]. The rupture of the San Andreas Fault was over 300 miles long. The quake resulted in 25,000 buildings destroyed, $400 M in economic loss ($11.4B 2019 USD), and in 3000 fatalities. More than 30 fires caused up to 90% of the total destruction. Since insurers indemnified properties from fire, but not earthquakes, most damage was blamed on the fires. Additionally, fires were deliberately set to recover insurance money. Soldiers were deployed to keep peace and prevent looting. President Theodore Roosevelt appealed to the public to give to the ARC:

"In the face of so horrible and appalling a national calamity as that which has befallen San Francisco, the outpouring of the nation's aid should, as far as possible, be entrusted to the American Red Cross, the national organization best fitted to undertake such relief work." Private donations came to over $9 M. The US Congress appropriated $2.5 million to the War Department for "subsistence and quartermaster's supplies ... to such destitute persons as have been rendered homeless or are in needy circumstances as a result of the earthquake and commissary stores to such injured and destitute persons as may require assistance."

2.2.10 1911 Triangle Shirtwaist Fire

On March 25, 1911, the Triangle Shirtwaist Factory in New York City burned, resulting in the deaths of 145 factory workers [66,67]. The factory was a sweatshop that employed 500 workers in three floors of a high-rise building. A fire broke out in a fabric scrap bin on the eighth story and was over within 18 minutes. Forty-nine workers burned to death or died of smoke inhalation, 36 died in an elevator shaft, 58 jumped to their deaths, and two died later from their injuries. The victims were unable to exit the building because the exits were locked to prevent thefts and unauthorized breaks (a common practice at the time) and the fire escape collapsed during the rescue effort. The owners escaped to the roof; although a grand jury failed to indict them of manslaughter, they were found liable for wrongful death. This mass fatality incident is significant for the reform efforts it spawned. It resulted in access and egress laws, fireproofing requirements, mandatory fire extinguishers and automatic sprinklers, as well as labor laws that limited the hours women and children work.

2.2.11 1912 Sinking of Titanic

On April 15, 1912, four days into her maiden voyage from Southampton, England, to New York City as she was nearing Newfoundland, the RMS *Titanic* sunk approximately two and a half hours after striking an iceberg [68,69]. The luxury ocean liner, powered by two coal-burning steam engines, was operated by the White Star Line and was the largest ship afloat at the time, displacing 52,310 tons. More than approximately 1500 of the more than 2200 passengers died, some dying shortly after being rescued, and only 710 survived. Only 20 life boats were aboard which could accommodate approximately half of the passengers on board. The ship was insured for £1,000,000 ($34 M 2019 USD) by Lloyds of London, who paid the full sum within 30 days. A small fleet with clergy, morticians, and embalming supplies was dispatched to retrieve the bodies from the water. The bodies of 333 victims were recovered. Since health regulations permitted only embalmed bodies returned to port and they did not have sufficient embalming supplies for the number recovered, they decided to embalm only first-class passengers because of the need to identify them to settle their large estates and bury the rest at sea. Those buried at sea were identified by their clothing. Preserved bodies were taken to Halifax, where the Halifax coroner set up a temporary morgue in a curling ring for visual identification by relatives. Approximately two thirds of the bodies were identified. Many charities, including the ARC, were set up to help the survivors. In addition, a class action lawsuit settled for $664,000 ($17.5 M 2019 USD), after the US Supreme Court limited White Star's liability.

2.2.12 1918 Spanish Flu Pandemic

During World War I, from the spring of 1918 to the summer of 1919, the H1N1 avian influenza (Spanish flu) pandemic infected 500 million people, approximately one third of the world's population, and was responsible for 50 million deaths worldwide and 675,000 US deaths [70,71]. Mortality was high in children, young adults, and the elderly; the high mortality in healthy adults was a unique feature of this pandemic. Populations harbored little natural immunity, and no vaccine was available. The first outbreak in the US was detected in March of 1918 at Fort Riley, Kansas. More than 100 soldiers became ill and the number multiplied within days. The flu spread sporadically through the United States, Europe, and possibly Asia over the next six months. This second and most deadly wave of the fall of 1918 began at Camp Devens in Massachusetts, which reported 147,000 cases and 757 deaths. The third wave occurred as soldiers returned home after the war during the winter and spring of 1919 and subsided during the summer of 1919. The ARC issued an urgent call for volunteers to help nurse the ill. Corpses were placed in cold storage awaiting burial.

2.2.13 1921-22 Russian (Povolzhye) Famine

The drought of 1921 exacerbated food shortages caused by the Russian Civil War resulted in the deaths of an estimated 5 million people of the Volga and Ural River regions. Herbert Hoover had run a relief operation in Belgium, was asked to head the US Food Administration in 1917 to administer food supplies for the Allies during World War I and then to head its successor, the American Relief Administration (ARA), in 1919 to distribute food to starving Europe in the aftermath of World War I. Hoover offered to help those in Russia on the conditions that the ARA control the railways and hand out food impartially, but Vladimir Lenin refused. When Russia's condition worsened, Lenin finally requested help from Europe and America. Hoover was the first to respond and eventually fed more than 10 million Russians per day [72,73]. Cooking fuel, warm clothes, and medicines were also distributed. He obtained $78 M ($1.2 T 2019 USD) to fund the operation: $18 M from the Russian leadership, $20 M from the US Congress, $8 M from the US military, and $32 M from US charities. The US relief was more than twice the combined effort of other nations. This incident directly led to Hoover's role in the 1927 Mississippi River Flood and his eventual presidency.

2.2.14 1927 Mississippi River Flood

The "Great flood" occurred in April of 1927 [74]. It was the most destructive flood in US history. The Mississippi River became engorged and swollen and 145 levees broke in and Missouri, Arkansas, Louisiana, and Mississippi. The flood covered 26,000 square miles in seven states and 41,500 buildings and 162,000 homes flooded. The economic loss was over $100 M in damages ($1.5B 2019 USD). The flooding also resulted in about 250 fatalities.

President Calvin Coolidge created a quasi-governmental Hoover Flood Commission that included members of his Cabinet and the ARC. President Coolidge was also president of the ARC [75,76]. He gave Secretary of Commerce Herbert Hoover near-absolute authority ("Czar") of the relief effort. Over $21 M was received from public donations. The Flood Control Act of 1928 gave the federal government authority over the containment of the lower Mississippi River, and the Army Corps of Engineers built the world's longest system of levees.

2.3 1930s and 1940s Federal Disaster Relief Legislation

Between 1803 and 1947, Congress passed at least 128 ad hoc laws, responding to large disasters (i.e., New York City, Chicago, Galveston, San Francisco) on an incident-by-incident basis after the fact, generally without direct monetary contributions [77]. The dominant thought was that disaster relief was the province of state and local governments and that it was improper to provide money collected for the common good on specific places or for individual assistance. The federal government often deferred to the ARC and expected voluntary donations to be the primary and sufficient source of disaster relief assistance [78,79]. Yet, especially after the 1927 Mississippi River flood, the federal government began to increasingly participate in disaster relief.

After the 1929 stock market crash and the ensuing Great Depression attitudes toward the role of the federal government began to change. During the 1930s, FDR's New Deal incorporated disaster relief as part of its efforts to rebuild the economy and provided federal funds for reconstruction of public facilities, highways, and bridges. The Reconstruction Corporation was established in 1932 and given authority to make loans for repair and reconstruction of certain public facilities after earthquakes and, later, other disasters. In 1934, the Bureau of Public Roads was given authority to provide funding for highways and bridges damaged by natural disasters [80]. Thus, the federal government began to establish standing structures to respond to natural disasters.

2.3.1 World War II Civilian Preparedness and Emergency Assets

In 1941, during World War II, President Franklin D. Roosevelt by Executive Order established the Office of Civil Defense (OCD), patterned after England's Civil Defence Service that had been formed in 1924 from their WWI-era Air Raids Precautions (ARP) Committee and their National Fire Service [81,82]. In the 1940s, air raid warning and emergency shelter systems were established to protect the civilian population. The Civil Air Patrol (CAP) was created in 1941 as a civilian aircraft auxiliary to the army (later the air force) with some wartime bombing missions, but primarily for search and rescue. Similarly, the Coast Guard Auxiliary, established in 1939, was created as a maritime civilian force with some wartime missions, but also a role in search and rescue. The OCD was terminated at the war's end, but the CAP and CG Auxiliary continued their search and rescue efforts after the war. These wartime developments would become useful in peacetime disaster efforts.

2.3.2 Post-WWII Federal Disaster Relief Legislation

After World War II, in 1947, Congress charged the War Assets Administration and the Federal Works Agency with delivering surplus federal supplies to areas in need [83,84]. An amendment to the Surplus Property Act of 1944 (P.L. 80-233) was enacted "To make surplus property available for the alleviation of damage caused by flood or other catastrophe." However, it was soon realized that disaster relief required more than just WWII military surplus. In the following year, 1948, with a specific flood in mind, Congress passed the Second Deficiency Appropriation Act (P.L. 80-785), which established the first disaster relief fund for future contingencies [85]. Specifically, it gave the president $500,000 ($5.3 M 2019 USD) for disaster relief in the event of any major disaster, provided that: (a) the president determines that a disaster has occurred, (b) the State has defined a need and committed resources, and c) any federal funds supplement rather than supplant State funds. It enabled the president to use the federal apparatus in the disaster relief effort and specified that the relief was to supplement the state response. In 1949, two more appropriations followed for a total of $1 M ($10.7 M 2019 USD) to add to the federal disaster relief effort. After making some resourced available for disaster relief, the Truman administration then turned its attention to policy and preparedness for natural disasters and nuclear war.

2.3.3 Civil Defense Act of 1950 (P.L. 81-920)

In response to the Soviet Union's first successful nuclear weapons test in August of 1949 and the invasion of South Korea by North Korea in June of 1950, President Harry S. Truman established the Federal Civil Defense Administration (FCDA) [86–90]. The FCDA was then authorized by Congress in the Federal Civil Defense Act of 1950, passed in January of 1951. This 13-page Cold War legislation was established "to provide a plan of civil defense for the protection of life and property in the United States from attack" and declares "that this responsibility for civil defense shall be vested primarily in the several States and their political subdivisions," but the "Federal government shall provide necessary coordination and guidance." The act institutionalized the Civil Defense programs established by executive orders during the war and created the Federal Civil Defense Agency (FCDA), the peacetime equivalent of the wartime OCD. The FCDA was an agency designed to respond to emergencies caused by attacks, but it began the emergency–disaster dichotomy that would later follow. The FCDA attempted to prepare the civilian population for nuclear attack – "duck and cover" defense drills became routine. The FCDA spurred the development of civil defense offices in states, the forerunner of state offices of emergency management agencies. The FCDA would eventually become FEMA in 1979.

2.3.4 Federal Disaster Relief Act of 1950 (P.L. 81-875)

On September 30, 1950, President Harry S. Truman signed into law the three-page "act to authorize Federal assistance to States and local governments in major disasters, and for other purposes," also known as the Federal Disaster Relief Act of 1950 [91–95]. This marked a turning point as Congress had passed 128 disaster relief bills since 1803, but this was the first proactive disaster relief legislation:

> it is the intent of Congress to provide an orderly and continuing means of assistance by the Federal Government to States and local governments in carrying out their responsibilities to alleviate suffering and damage resulting from major disasters, to repair essential public facilities in major disasters, and to foster the development of such State and local organizations and plans to cope with major disasters as may be necessary.

This act institutionalized the framework of the 1948 appropriation. It defined a major disaster as beyond mere contingency funding:

> any flood, drought, fire, hurricane, earthquake, storm, or other catastrophe in any part of the United States which, in the determination of the President, is or threatens to be of sufficient severity and magnitude to warrant disaster assistance by the Federal Government to supplement the efforts and available resources of State and local governments.

The act authorized the President to provide supplementary federal assistance when a governor requests help and the president would approve the request by declaring a major disaster; consent of Congress was not required for action. The act and its amendments established, for the first time, a permanent source of federal disaster relief funds, although relief was limited to $5 M ($53 M 2019 USD) in total. These funds were initially designated for the repair of local government properties, but a 1951 amendment provided support for emergency housing, and a 1953 amendment authorized the donation of federal surplus supplies to individuals.

President Truman implemented the act on January 16, 1953, through Executive Order 10427. In this two-page order, the President delegated his authority under the 1950 Federal Disaster Relief Act to the Federal Civil Defense Administrator. He also declared that federal disaster relief is to be "supplementary to relief afforded by State, local, or private agencies and not in substitution therefor" and that "Federal financial contributions for disaster relief shall be conditioned upon reasonable State and local expenditures for such relief."

Although the basic apparatus for federal government disaster assistance was in place in the mid-twentieth century, the federal government envisioned itself in a decidedly back seat position to the states and was, in fact, fearful that it would be seen as the primary funder of relief. Yet, the federal government was also taking on a leadership role, providing guidance and coordination – centralizing previously decentralized and uncoordinated responses. Federal disaster relief continued primarily as reconstruction of public facilities, and low-interest loans through the Small Business Administration to homeowners and businesses to rebuild; state, local and private agencies, particularly the ARC, were still the front line of response and recovery. Nonetheless, the process had begun in which the federal government would become dominant.

2.4 1950s Federal Disaster Relief

During the Cold War, the national security concerns of civil defense and continuity of government took precedence over natural disasters. The 1950s were a relatively quiescent period for natural disasters, except for Hurricane Hazel in 1954 that resulted in $382 M ($3.7B 2019 USD) in damages and 591–1191 fatalities; Hurricane Diane in 1955 that resulted in $832 M ($8B 2019 USD) in damages and 189 fatalities; and Hurricane Audrey in 1957 that resulted in $147 M ($1.4B 2019 USD) in damages and 431 fatalities. There was little new substantive legislation, but congress continued reactive ad hoc legislative responses, although the FCDA was renamed the Office of Civil and Defense Mobilization (OCDM) in 1958 [96].

2.5 1960s Beginnings

In the 1960s and early 1970s, under the Kennedy, Johnson, and Nixon administrations, the federal government's role grew [97]. President John F. Kennedy abolished the OCDM and established an Office of Emergency Planning (OEP, later the Office of Emergency Preparedness) within the White House Executive for civil defense and disaster-related emergency response efforts and moving other components to the Department of Defense as the Defense Civil Preparedness Agency (DCPA). Legislation promulgated in 1962 expanded disaster relief funding coverage to territories and grants for repair of state facilities.

2.5.1 1960 Hurricane Donna

On September 4, 1960, Hurricane Donna began to strike islands of the Antilles and then Puerto Rico and the Florida Keys [98]. Donna re-emerged in the Atlantic and struck North Carolina and again re-emerging in the Atlantic and continuing north to strike Long Island, New York. At its peak, it was a Category 4 hurricane. It resulted in $980 M ($8.6B 2019 USD) in damages and 439 fatalities

2.5.2 1961 Hurricane Carla

On September 11, 1961, Hurricane Carla struck the southern coast of Texas as a Category 4 hurricane [99]. It was the most severe hurricane landfall in US history, at the time based on size and intensity as measured on the Hurricane Severity Index. Wind gusts of 175 mph were recorded and it spawned 26 tornados, including an F4 tornado. A half million people evacuated the Texas and Louisiana coast, the largest evacuation to that time. It was the first hurricane seen on live television broadcast news. The hurricane caused $326 M ($2.8B 2019 USD) in damages and resulted in 43 direct fatalities. Nearly 2,000 homes and more than 1,000 buildings were destroyed. Congress authorized $55 M in aid, but President Kennedy requested an additional $65 M.

2.5.3 1962 Ash Wednesday Storm

On March 5-9, 1962, an extreme (Level 5) Nor'easter, known as the Ash Wednesday Storm or the Great March Storm of 1962, struck the mid-Atlantic coast [100]. It was one of the costliest non-tropical cyclones to strike the coastline. It devastated 620 miles of coastline and produced $300 M ($2.6B 2019 USD) in damages. The storm resulted in 40 fatalities and 1,252 injuries.

As the decade progressed, massive disasters demanded the attention of the federal government, particularly the Federal Disaster Assistance Administration (FDAA) that had been established within the Department of Housing and Urban Development (HUD).

2.5.4 1964 Great Alaskan Earthquake

On March 27, 1964, Good Friday, a megathrust earthquake struck Prince William Sound, between Anchorage and Valdez, Alaska [101,102]. The magnitude 9.2 earthquake was associated with a tsunami an underwater landslide. The magnitude was 9.2 and involved a 600-mile rupture, making it the most powerful earthquake ever recorded in North America and the second most powerful earthquake in world history. It was also the first major disaster in the state of Alaska. It caused $311 M ($2.6B 2019 USD) in damages and resulted in 131 fatalities.

2.5.5 1960s Federal Activism in the Wake of the Alaskan Earthquake

Alaska had been a state for only five years and was only sparsely populated. Four days after the quake, the Alaskan Budget Director called President Lyndon Johnson and described the inability of the state to respond. President Johnson converted a planned federal-state development commission and converted it into a Federal Reconstruction and Development Planning Commission for Alaska [103]. Congress passed four acts authorizing hundreds of millions of dollars for Alaska's recovery – far more than for any prior federal relief effort – justified by the enormity of the disaster and the inadequacy of the state during its infancy to respond. The funding kept Alaska financially solvent until the discovery of massive oil deposits in Prudhoe Bay 1964.

2.5.6 1965 Palm Sunday Tornado Outbreak

The 1965 tornado outbreak on April 11–12, 1965, in the Midwest US [104]. It was the second Palm Sunday tornado outbreak and the worst; the first had occurred in 1920 and a third would occur in 1994. It involved 47 tornadoes and the second biggest outbreak to that time. It was responsible for 271 fatalities and 1500 injured. Indiana was hardest hit.

Indiana senator Birch E. Bayh, Jr. (D-IA) sought "Quake-Type Aid in Tornado Repairs" and pursuit of a national policy of extensive federal disaster assistance, opening "the great purse strings of Uncle Sam" to states, localities, and individuals, but the time was not yet ripe [105].

2.5.7 1965 Hurricane Betsy

On September 7, 1965, Hurricane Betsy, a Category 5 hurricane, struck the Florida Keys and then on September 9th struck New Orleans, Louisiana [106–108]. It was second only to Hurricane Carla as the most severe hurricane on record. The storm surge drove into Lake Pontchartrain and the Mississippi River Gulf Outlet causing several levees to fail. It caused $1.4 B ($11.4B 2019 USD) economic damage, primarily Louisiana, but also in Florida and Mississippi, and resulted in 81 fatalities. Since it was the first storm to result in over $1B in damages, it garnered the moniker, Billion Dollar Betsy.

Louisiana senator Russell B. Long (D-LA), then the Senate Majority Whip, lobbied for relief for the victims of the hurricane. The US Army Corps of Engineers' Hurricane Protection Program was established and new levees for New Orleans built, which later failed during Katrina [109].

2.5.8 Disaster Relief Act of 1966

The advocacy of Senators Birch Bayh and Russell Long resulted in the Disaster Relief Act of 1966 (P.L. 89-769), which updated existing legislation and expanded the scope of federal disaster relief beyond mere reconstitution to the reestablishment and recovery of the community [110,111]. The act improved handling of non-routine large-scale, catastrophic disasters. It specifically authorized loans below market rates and extended aid to rural and unincorporated areas. It authorized assistance to repair local public facilities.

2.5.9 1968 National Flood Insurance

Flooding, particularly from hurricanes such as Betsy, had always been a cause of disaster. The first significant federal legislation to address flooding was the 1850 Swamp Control Act. Dozens of flood acts were passed in Congress [112–118]. In response to the flooding of Hurricane Betsey, the Flood Control Act of 1965 (P.L. 89-298) gave the US Army Corps of Engineers greater authority to implement flood control, and the National Flood Insurance Act of 1968 (P.L. 90-448), created the National Flood Insurance Program (NFIP), the Federal Insurance Administration, and made flood insurance available to homeowners. After Hurricane Agnes in 1972, the Flood Disaster Protection Act of 1973 (P.L. 93-234) was enacted to require commercial lenders to offer flood insurance on loans secured by properties located within high-risk flood areas. After the Midwest Floods of 1993, the Flood Insurance Reform Act of 1994 (P.L. 103-325) strengthened the NFIP, increasing lender compliance and including mitigation assistance. Later, with debt in the NFIP increasing, the Biggert-Waters reform of 2012 attempted to allow premiums to reflect the true risk of living in areas of high risk of flooding, but premiums immediately rose tenfold and the legislation was quickly repealed.

2.5.10 1969 Hurricane Camille

On August 18, 1969, Hurricane Camille struck Bay St. Louis, Mississippi, as a Category 5 hurricane [119,120]. It was the third most severe hurricane to hit the US to that date, after Carla in 1961 and Betsy in 1965 and tying with Opal in 1995 and Katrina in 2005. Camille is in a tie as the second strongest US landfall, behind the Labor Day hurricane of 1935. The storm surge was over 24 feet high, only later surpassed by Hurricane Katrina. Camille caused $1.4B ($9.8B 2019 USD) economic damage and resulted in 259 fatalities. Camille was smaller but more intense than Katrina; it barely missed New Orleans – causing little damage there.

2.6 Disaster Relief Acts of 1969 and 1970

Senators Bayh and Long continued to push disaster relief and used Hurricane Camille as another opportunity. The Disaster Relief Act of 1969 (P.L. 91-79), enacted and signed into law by President Nixon in response to Hurricane Camille, expanded public and individual assistance, including temporary housing, food, and unemployment assistance [121–124]. The act created a federal coordinating officer to represent the president in the relief effort. However, these provisions were temporary, lasting only through calendar 1970 [125]. The Disaster Relief Act of 1970 (P.L. 91-606) consolidated previous disaster relief legislation from the Alaska earthquake and Hurricanes Betsy and Camille. Important 1969 Camille provisions were made permanent.

2.6.1 1971 San Fernando (Sylmar) Earthquake

In the early morning of February 9, 1971, a 6.5 magnitude earthquake unexpectedly struck the foothills of the San Gabriel Mountains of Southern California and affected Los Angeles [126]. It triggered over 1000 landslides in the mountains and produced prominent surface faulting, resulting in transportation failures. The shaking exceeded building code requirements. The economic damage was $500 to $550 M ($3.2B 2019 USD) and resulted in 58–65 fatalities. Most deaths occurred from collapses of hospital buildings. Large dams were damaged, but they did not fail; 80,000 inhabitants were evacuated for four days while authorities responded to this threat.

2.6.2 1972 Hurricane Agnes

On June 19, 1972, Hurricane Agnes was a Category 1 hurricane struck Panama City, Florida [127,128]. It moved through Georgia, South Carolina, and North Carolina, before reentry into the Atlantic Ocean and then striking New York City. The effects of Agnes were felt in 15 states; the most significant damage occurred in Pennsylvania due to flooding there. It caused $2.1B ($12.8B 2019 USD) in economic damage, the costliest natural disaster to that time in US history, and resulted in 128 fatalities.

2.6.3 1974 Super Outbreak

On April 3–4, 1974, an outbreak of 148 tornados, including 30 F4/F5 tornados, occurred across 10 states of the Midwest and South [129]. It was the largest tornado outbreak to that time in US history. It resulted in $880 M ($4.6B 2019 USD) damages, 5484 injuries, and 315 fatalities. It led to six federal disaster declarations.

2.6.4 Disaster Relief Act Amendments of 1974

The Disaster Relief Act Amendments of 1974 (DRA, the Disaster Relief Act of 1974; P.L. 93-288), amending the Disaster Relief Act of 1970, introduced by Senator Quentin Burdick (D-ND), was unanimously passed by Congress, and signed into law by President Nixon on May 22, 1974 [130–132]. In his statement upon signing the bill, the president stated:

> This bill amends the Disaster Relief Act of 1970 by further extending the assistance available from the Federal Government for individuals and States and local communities suffering from the effects of disasters such as the tornadoes that ravaged a wide area of the Nation early last

> month. It also strengthens disaster planning and preparedness and requires as a condition to receiving Federal assistance that insurance coverage be provided to protect property against future disaster losses. Since taking office, I have had to declare over 180 major disasters in 42 States. The amount of Federal assistance given to disaster victims has been greatly expanded, and this Administration has made every effort to provide this aid more equitably and expeditiously.

The Disaster Relief Act of 1974 consolidated changes following Hurricane Agnes. It defined the process of presidential disaster declaration. It introduced the concept of emergency relief when a disaster is not declared. It also provided for more individual assistance than had previously been available. It provided for a more robust preparedness program. For the first time, it incorporated a component to address mental health [133]. This legislation represented a significant broadening of federal government involvement and has been said to inaugurate the current era of federally coordinated emergency management.

2.7 National Emergencies Act of 1976

The National Emergencies Act of 1976 (NEA; P.L. 94-412) was passed to formally end all previously declared national emergencies and to formalize the emergency powers of the President [134]. Since President Franklin D. Roosevelt in 1933, presidents had asserted emergencies without clear limitations or congressional oversight. Furthermore, laws granting special powers to the president had proliferated. This act limits declarations of national emergencies to 136 emergency powers and grants Congress the ability to terminate declared emergencies. At this time, there are over 60 declared emergencies, with more than half remaining in effect.

2.8 National Earthquake Hazards Reduction Program (NEHRP) of 1977

Congressman Al Gore (D-TN) criticized FEMA for its leadership and inadequately preparing for natural disasters. An investigation led to the resignation of Director Giuffrida and his top aides for charges of misuse of funds. As senator, Gore pressed the need for preparing for natural disasters, particularly the possibility of 200,000 victims from a New Madrid earthquake. In 1977, he pushed through the Earthquake Hazards Reduction Act of 1977 (P.L. 95–124) that created the National Earthquake Hazards Reduction Program (NEHRP) that provides for seismic research for early earthquake detection and warning systems, as well as the development of mitigating technologies and practices [135,136]. The NEHRP later became the model for responding to other natural disasters, eventuating in the Federal Response Plan (FRP).

2.9 1979 Executive Orders 12127 & 12148 – Federal Emergency Management Agency (FEMA)

In 1978, State Civil Defense Directors Lacy Suiter of Tennessee and Erie Jones of Illinois pressed the National Governor's Association to advocate for a single centralized federal emergency agency to replace the more than 100 myriad agencies across the federal system that state and local governments must work. After reviewing its disaster-related programs, President Jimmy Carter issued Executive Orders 12127 and 12148 in 1979 to implement Reorganization Plan #3, which consolidated disparate disaster-related responsibilities into one agency, the Federal Emergency Management Agency (FEMA) [137–140]. FEMA absorbed, among other programs:

- the HUD Federal Disaster Assistance Administration (FDAA)
- the GSA Federal Preparedness Agency (FPA)
- the DoD Defense Civil Preparedness Agency (DCPA)
- the Federal Insurance Administration
- the National Fire Prevention and Control Administration
- the National Weather Service Community Preparedness Program

The Presidential order gave FEMA a three-part role:

1. mobilizing federal resources
2. coordinating federal efforts with state and local governments
3. managing the efforts of the public and private sectors in disaster responses

It replaced the term "civil defense" with comprehensive emergency management. FEMA was first appropriated disaster funds in FY1980.

From the outset, FEMA was challenged to integrate the various entities into a single agency and it lacked a vision to develop a set of core values. The most significant division was the federal response to domestic and national security emergencies. Tension existed between the secretive National Preparedness Directorate and the more public State and Local Programs and Support Directorate. The apparent redundancy of the plans and personnel was pointed out by the Office of the Inspector General.

At least initially, FEMA also had issues with clout. The consolidation of the numerous agencies within FEMA offered the promise of garnering significant attention and authority. However, the relatively small agency found it difficult to command and coordinate much larger agencies without the Cold War connection. Furthermore, access to the president, as a non-Cabinet-level agency, was limited.

Moreover, early FEMA directors lacked substantial emergency management background and tended to focus on national security and terrorism and neglect natural disasters. Director Louis O. Giuffrida famously overreached his authority when he advanced an emergency czar role for FEMA and developed a secret contingency plan calling for a declaration of martial law, suspension of the Constitution, and turning control of the US federal government over to FEMA during a national crisis [141].

Initially, FEMA was confronted, not by a natural disaster, but by the toxic chemical contamination of Love Canal in upstate New York discovered in 1978, in fact this was the first time in American history that emergency funds were used for a situation other than a natural disaster. FEMA also responded to the Three Mile Island nuclear accident of 1979, the Cuban refugee crisis (Mariel boatlift) of 1980, the Mount St. Helen volcanic eruption in 1980, and the toxic contamination of Times Beach, Missouri, revealed in 1982. FEMA had yet to face truly catastrophic incidents that shattered state resources and required a well-honed federal system.

2.9.1 1979 Three Mile Island (TMI) Nuclear Accident

On March 28, 1979, a partial meltdown of a nuclear reactor occurred at a power plant near Harrisburg, Pennsylvania [142,143]. The accident involved multiple mechanical failures, as well as a failure to recognize the situation by staff. The accident resulted in the release of radioactive gases and radioactive iodine into the environment. The event alarmed the public and galvanized anti-nuclear activists. New regulations for the nuclear industry were promulgated. It contributed to the marked slowdown in the construction of new nuclear plants. The cleanup started in August 1979 and ended in December 1993, with a total cleanup cost of about $1 billion, although the total cost of property damage has been estimated to as high as $2.4 billion. A number of agencies at the local, state, and federal levels responded, resulting in some level of confusion and chaos and provided further impetus for consolidation of the federal responders.

2.9.2 1980 Mount St. Helens Volcanic Eruption

On May 18, 1980, the Mount St. Helens volcano erupted [144]. It is the greatest volcanic eruption in the continental US It was preceded by a 5.1 magnitude earthquake. It caused the largest landslide in history; the massive landslide traveled at 110–155 mph. It was also associated with lateral blasts and pyroclastic flows. The thermal energy released is estimated to be 24 megatons or 1600 times that of the Hiroshima atom bomb. Ash was deposited in 11 states and 5 Canadian provinces. The eruption caused $1.1B ($3.4B 2019 USD) and resulted in 57 fatalities. This was the first disaster to be funded on a cost-sharing basis with 75% federal and 25% non-federal.

2.10 Disaster Relief and Emergency Assistance Act of 1988 (The Stafford Act)

In 1988, Congress enacted the Disaster Relief and Emergency Assistance Amendments (DREAA, P.L. 100-707) that amended and renamed the Disaster Relief Act of 1974 as the Robert T. Stafford Disaster Relief and Emergency Assistance Act (the Stafford Act) [145–147]. It is named for Senator Robert T. Stafford (R-VT), who helped pass the bill; Representative Tom Ridge (R-PA) introduced it into the House of Representatives and President Reagan signed it into law on November 23, 1988. It remains the primary legislation for federal disaster response today. Congress became concerned over the use of disaster authority for non-major disasters and the existing statutory scheme needed updating since the creation of FEMA in 1979. Congress comprehensively reviewed the existing legislation before drafting legislation that amends and renames the Disaster Relief Act of 1974.

The Stafford Act is a massive congressional delegation of power to the president to commit federal resources in times of disaster. In addition, to declarations of major disasters, the act authorizes the president to declare an emergency in "any occasion or instance" in which federal aid is needed – allowing for assistance without a major disaster declaration, but is more limited in aid to states, localities, and individuals. The Stafford Act gives FEMA responsibility for coordinating government-wide relief efforts and providing disaster relief, and the president is to appoint a federal coordinating officer (FCO).

2.10.1 FEMA under President George H. W. Bush (1989–1993)

Although FEMA had handled the minor disasters that it had faced until then, the Bush administration inherited an agency with serious organizational problems. During the first decade of its existence, FEMA had suffered from neglect and poor leadership. It had become a dumping ground for political appointees. The early FEMA directors had little experience in emergency management. The agency was fragmented and overly committed to national security preparedness at the expense of natural disaster preparedness. A focus on terrorism and weapons of mass destruction also minimized its partnership with the states. Criticism to FEMA's structure and operations from the media, Congress, and others mounted. President H. W. Bush was not interested in FEMA's organizational weaknesses and did not appoint a permanent agency director for more than a year and a half into his term. FEMA proved entirely unprepared for the catastrophic disasters it would next face, Hurricanes Hugo and Andrew and the Loma Prieta earthquake. The Bush administration did not place its full confidence in FEMA and often bypassed FEMA and directed the response from the White House. FEMA's future was placed in doubt when there were calls for its elimination.

2.10.2 1989 *Exxon Valdez* Oil Spill

On March 24, 1989, the oil supertanker *Exxon Valdez*, carrying oil extracted from the Prudhoe Bay Oil Field, struck a reef in Prince William Sound, Alaska, releasing 10.8 million gallons of crude oil over the next few days and affecting over 200 miles of coastline [148,149]. It is considered to be among the worst man-made environmental disasters of all time, although surpassed in 2010 by British Petroleum's *Deepwater Horizon* oil spill. FEMA was chided in 1989 congressional hearings for failing to respond aggressively, but FEMA maintained that the Environmental Protection Agency (EPA) and the US Coast Guard had specific legislated responsibilities for cleaning up oil or hazardous materials spills with assistance through the EPA-administered National Contingency Plan (NCP).

2.10.3 1989 Hurricane Hugo

On September 17 and 18, 1989, after briefly attaining Category 5 hurricane status, it passed over Guadaloupe, St. Croix, and St. Thomas as a Category 4 hurricane, and then Puerto Rico as a Category 3 hurricane, but then it re-strengthened to a Category 4 hurricane and struck just north of Charleston, South Carolina, on September 22, 1981 [150]. Hugo was the most intense storm to strike the East Coast north of Florida since the 1898 Georgia hurricane. The most severe damage was of St. Croix of the US Virgin Islands, but $5.9B in economic damages occurred in South Carolina. The first deployment of an NDMS DMAT team was to St. Croix. Hugo caused $10.3B ($21B 2019 USD) in damages overall and $7B in damages to the Puerto Rico and the US mainland – the costliest storm up to that time. It left 100,000 homeless. It resulted in 60 fatalities, including 3 deaths in Puerto Rico and 21 deaths on the US mainland. The ARC, Salvation Army, and various churches provided extensive relief. FEMA was heavily criticized for its role. FEMA opened its first disaster center in South Carolina a week after the hurricane struck the state. On the Senate floor, South Carolina senator Fritz Hollings called FEMA officials "a bunch of bureaucratic jackasses."

2.10.4 1989 Loma Prieta Earthquake

In the evening of October 18, 1989, a 6.9 magnitude earthquake struck the Forest of Nisene Marks State Park in California's Central Coast, 10 miles north of Santa Cruz [151,152]. Since the quake occurred during the third game of the 1989 World Series in San Francisco's Candlestick Park between the two Bay area teams, the San Francisco Giants and the Oakland Athletics, it is also known as the

World Series earthquake. The Loma Prieta segment of the San Andreas Fault had been quiescent since the Great San Francisco Earthquake of 1906. No surface faulting occurred, but liquefaction was a significant issue in the San Francisco Marina District and the Monterey Bay shore. A section of the Bay Bridge collapsed and one death occurred from a car driving over the edge. More than a mile of the upper deck of the Cypress Freeway Bridge collapsed and 42 people were crushed in their cars. 1.4 M people lost power. The earthquake resulted in $5.6–6B ($12B 2019 USD) in damage, 57 direct and 6 indirect fatalities, and 3757 injured. The federal government paid $1.1B in relief. President Bush lost confidence in FEMA to respond and turned instead to Sam Skinner, then Secretary of Transportation, to coordinate the early federal response.

2.11 1992 Federal Response Plan (FRP)

As directed by the Stafford Act, FEMA established the Federal Response Plan (FRP) [153]. An initial version circulated in early 1991, but it was not finalized and published until 1992. The FRP was modeled after the NEHRP. The FRP clarified the agency's role as the clearinghouse for disaster assistance. Although touted as an all-hazards plan, it emphasized natural disasters. In 1992, it was agreed to and signed by 27 federal departments and agencies, including the American Red Cross.

2.11.1 1992 Hurricane Andrew

On August 24, 1992, Hurricane Andrew, a Category 5 hurricane, struck Southern Florida, after hitting the Bahamas, and then crossed the Gulf of Mexico to strike Louisiana [154]. It was the most intense to hit the US mainland since Camille in 1969. It caused approximately $27–36B ($55B 2019 USD) in damages and 49 to 56 fatalities. It toppled 33 offshore oil rigs that cost $12 M per day in lost oil revenues for days after the storm. It caused the closure of the Homestead Air Force Base. A facility housing Burmese pythons was destroyed allowing sufficient numbers to escape and establish a breeding population within the everglades. Andrew surpassed Hugo as the costliest hurricane to that point in US history. Congress appropriated $11.1B in aid for relief for Andrew and cyclones that hit Hawaii and Guam, the largest amount to that time. FEMA was slow to respond to Florida and Louisiana, but fared somewhat better than after Hugo. President Bush directed Andrew Card, the Secretary of Transportation, using the military, to take over the response efforts in the wake of Hurricane Andrew.

2.11.2 1992 Hurricane Iniki

On September 11, 1992, Hurricane Iniki struck Hawaii as a Category 4 Pacific hurricane. Iniki is the most powerful storm to hit Hawaii in recorded history [155]. Hawaii had not been struck by any hurricane for a decade. Iniki resulted in $3.1B ($5.7B 2019 USD) in damages and resulted in six fatalities. It is second only to Hurricane Manuel in 2013 as the costliest hurricane in Hawaiian history. The movie *Jurassic Park* was being filmed at the time and shots of the storm were incorporated into the movie.

2.12 FEMA under President William J. Clinton (1993–2001)

President Bill Clinton tackled the FEMA legacy as a problem to be solved [156–159]. Clinton's vice president, Al Gore, had been in part responsible for the resignation of FEMA Director Giuffrida and was the architect of the NEHRP. Clinton appointed James Lee Witt, Arkansas's emergency services director, as the head of FEMA in 1993 [160]. Witt was the first emergency manager to head FEMA. Other Clinton FEMA appointments were also officials with experience in emergency management. Clinton also elevated Witt to a Cabinet-level position, providing access to the President.

Director Witt restored the integrity of FEMA and reinvigorated its staff. He redefined FEMA's mission and reorganized the agency around basic emergency management functions. Director Witt articulated an all-hazards mission as a single, clear unifying vision for the agency. He emphasized emergency response over civil defense and pressed an all-hazards approach that included natural, man-made, and national security emergencies specifically to overcome a nuclear focus that had prevailed. Witt also redirected the focus of disaster assistance toward mitigation and community resilience. Media and political criticism of the agency diminished.

2.12.1 1993 Midwest Floods

Continued heavy rain and snow resulted in flooding from April to October, 1993, along the Mississippi and Missouri rivers and their tributaries [161]. The flooded area totaled around 30,000 square miles and lasted between 100 and 200 days. The Mississippi River at St. Louis crested at 49.6 feet on August 1, nearly 20 feet above flood stage, but the St. Louis Floodwall held preventing the city from inundation. The flooding surpassed the 1927 flood, at the time the largest flood ever recorded on the Mississippi. Approximately 100,000 homes were destroyed as a result of the flooding, 15 million acres of farmland inundated, and whole towns were relocated to higher ground. Damages were estimated to be $15B ($27B 2019 USD). Officially, the death toll was only 32 fatalities, although the true number is thought to be closer to 50.

2.12.2 1994 Northridge Earthquake

In the early morning of January 17, 1994, a 6.7 magnitude earthquake occurred in the San Fernando Valley, 20 miles northwest of downtown Los Angeles, California [162]. The earthquake was in the same place and otherwise similar to the 1971 San Fernando (Sylmar) earthquake. Property damage was estimated to be $13–44B ($50B 2019 USD). The earthquake resulted in 57–72 fatalities and more than 8700 were injured. An outbreak of 203 cases coccidiomycosis was caused by dust clouds produced from the landslides triggered by the earthquake. As a result of the Northridge earthquake, California changed its building codes and created a state-run earthquake insurance program.

2.12.3 1995 Oklahoma City Bombing

On April 19, 1995, an explosion destroyed one third of the Alfred P. Murrah Federal Building in Oklahoma City killing 168 people, including 19 children in a daycare, and injuring 800 others [163]. A rental truck with 7000 pounds of ammonium nitrate fertilizer, nitromethane, and diesel fuel was parked it in front of the building and detonated. US Army veteran McVeigh was convicted of the terrorist attack, sentenced to death, and was executed in 2001; his assistant Terry Nichols is serving multiple life sentences in prison. McVeigh declared that the attack against the federal government was retaliation for the 1993 Waco Branch Davidian siege and the 1992 siege of Ruby Ridge. The building was demolished a month after the bombing and a memorial museum was built in its place.

2.13 1996 EMAC

Congress passed several pieces of legislation in 1950 after the Russian nuclear testing and North Korea's invasion of South Korea and ratified the Civil Defense Compact of 1950, in which states would help each other – at a time that federal assistance was paltry. After Hurricane Andrew in 1992, at the instigation of Florida Governor Lawton Chiles, the Southern Governor's Association in 1993 formed the Southern Regional Emergency Management Assistance Compact (SREMAC). In 1995, SREMAC opened its membership to any state or territory that wanted to join. In 1996, Congress ratified the expanded agreement as the Emergency Management Assistance Compact (EMAC) (P.L. 104-321). All 50 states, the District of Columbia, Guam, Puerto Rico, and the US Virgin Islands have now passed legislation to become members [164]. The National Emergency Management Association (NEMA) [165] drafted Model Intrastate Mutual Aid Legislation [166] that addresses the legal issues of legal liability, reimbursement, and professional licensure. EMAC assistance has been of great assistance in many since, although sometimes offers of assistance are turned down to cost reimbursement issues [167].

2.14 FEMA under President George W. Bush (2001–2009)

When President George W. Bush was elected, he named Joe Allbaugh as the director of FEMA [168–171]. Allbaugh had been Chief of Staff to then Texas governor Bush and then his presidential campaign manager. His close and trusting personal relationship with the president was an asset, but his lack of an emergency management background was a glaring weakness.

Allbaugh wanted to refocus FEMA on civil defense and counterterrorism. The Nunn-Lugar legislation of the early 1990s, which spoke to counterterrorism, had left federal agency leadership for terrorism undefined. Allbaugh re-established the Office of National Preparedness (ONP), which had been created by Director Giuffrida in 1981 to plan for World War III, but then eliminated by Director Witt in 1992. Allbaugh recreated ONP to focus on terrorism, which raised concerns inside emergency management circles and within FEMA itself.

In a September 10, 2001 speech at a meeting Montana of the National Emergency Management Association (NEMA), Allbaugh stated that FEMA's priorities were being firefighters, disaster mitigation, and catastrophic preparedness. The next day al Qaeda struck the World Trade Center and the Pentagon killing nearly 3000 and beginning a week later a series of letters containing anthrax were mailed to news media offices and to Democratic senators Tom Daschle and Patrick Leahy killing 5 people and infecting 17 others. President Bush declared a war on terrorism that led not only to military action but also to massive expenditures on preparedness for national security threats.

2.14.1 2001 Al Qaeda 9/11 Terrorist Attacks

On September 11, 2001, nineteen al Qaeda terrorists hijacked four commercial jet airliners as weapons in suicide attacks against the United States [172–174]. Nearly 3,000 died on that day now known as "9/11." United Airlines Flight #175 and American Airlines Flight #11 crashed into the Twin Towers of the World Trade Center in New York City, resulting in 2763 fatalities; American Airlines Flight #77 crashed into the Pentagon in northern Virginia, resulting in 189 fatalities; and United Airlines Flight #93, heading for the White House of US Capitol, crashed in Shanksville, Pennsylvania, after passengers stormed the terrorists, resulting in 44 fatalities. The principal focus of these after action reports was on the protection of first responders – fire, police, and emergency medical technicians.

2.15 Department of Homeland Security (DHS)

Nine days after the 9/11 terrorist attacks, President Bush by Executive Order created the Office of Homeland Security with Tom Ridge as Director, in response to criticism that interagency intelligence cooperation could have prevented the 9/11 terrorist attacks. However, the small office was widely viewed as ineffective. Both the White House and Congress recognized that a Homeland Security czar require a large staff and budget in order to succeed. Deliberations began to create a new Cabinet-level Department.

The Homeland Security Act of 2002 (HAS; P.L. 107-296) was signed by President Bush on November 25, 2002 [175–179]. It created the Department of Homeland Security (DHS) in response to the 9/11 terrorist attacks with the intent to create a coordinated approach to both natural and man-made emergencies and disaster, but the primary mission of DHS appears to target terrorism – with the first three responsibilities to "prevent terrorist attacks within the United States," to "reduce the vulnerability of the United States to Terrorism," and to "minimize the damage, and assist in recovery, from terrorist attacks that do occur within the United States."

The massive reorganization was implemented in March 2003 as DHS absorbed FEMA and 22 other agencies, programs and offices. Tom Ridge was named the first DHS Secretary. FEMA was left largely intact, but the FEMA Director was placed under the DHS Under Secretary Emergency Preparedness and Response and no longer reported directly to the president. Michael Chertoff succeeded Ridge as Secretary, who transferred many FEMA functions to other DHS components and culminating in the 2005 transfer of most emergency preparedness and response to a newly created Preparedness Directorate.

Today, the new department is responsible for public security, including anti-terrorism, border security, immigration and customs, cyber security, and disaster prevention and management. It is roughly comparable to the interior or home ministries of other countries. It is currently the third largest Cabinet department and has a budget of approximately $50B and a staff of over 240,000 employees. Homeland security policy is coordinated at the White House by the Homeland

Security Council. Other agencies with significant homeland security responsibilities include the Departments of Health and Human Services, Justice, and Energy.

The 2002 act mandated, among other things (1) the establishment of "a comprehensive national incident management system with Federal, State, and local government personnel, agencies, and authorities, to respond to such [terrorist] attacks and disasters," and (2) the consolidation of "existing Federal Government emergency response plans into a single, coordinated national response plan."

In 2003, President Bush implemented these congressional mandates through Homeland Security Presidential Directive 5 Management of Domestic Incidents (HSPD-5). The directive called for a "national approach to domestic incident management" in which state and local authorities have the primary role for domestic incident response and the DHS Secretary assists their efforts.

HSPD-5 called for the establishment of a National Response Plan (NRP) to replace the FRP and delineate the responsibilities of emergency management for homeland security. The original FRP, written during the 1980s and promulgated in 1992, was written for the federal agency response and did not include the state and local governmental agencies nor nongovernmental actors. Furthermore, it focused on natural disasters; there were separate plans for radiologic and other hazards. The president desired a single plan to be employed upon the request of the president or other agencies in which FEMA would assume a coordination role. The new plan was a true all hazards plan. The president wanted an entirely new plan with fresh ideas and distinctive language. However, there was considerable resistance to the wholesale replacement of existing terms, because there had already been a considerable investment in existing definitions, plans, and procedures that had evolved over time and was performing better than in the past. Ultimately, the planners incorporated terrorism into the procedures and giving FEMA formal authority over responses to terrorist incidents. An initial plan was approved by the Homeland Security Council in late 2003 and the NRP replaced the FRP in 2004. The NRP introduces emergency support functions (ESFs) in an annex that details the responsibility of various departments for various functional support. The NRP called for a Principal Federal Official

(PFO) who would represent the DHS Secretary at major disaster scenes, which might be from FEMA, but gave the president the flexibility to name an official who best represents him.

The National Incident Management System (NIMS) provides the template for the management of incidents. NIMS defines preparedness as a continuous cycle of planning, organizing, training, equipping, exercising, evaluating, and taking corrective active. It institutes the Incident Command System (ICS), which grew from the firefighting community that needed a strategy to organize participants from various jurisdictions to work together [180,181]. NIMS includes the concept of a Unified Command, as an alternative to an Incident Commander, which allows shared command, control, and coordination responsibility among multiple agencies, analogous to the military's Joint Chiefs of Staff.

Together, NIMS and the NRP provided the doctrine for the post-9/11 framework for federal emergency response.

2.15.1 2005 Hurricane Katrina

On Aug 25, 2005, Hurricane Katrina, a Category 5 hurricane, hit Florida and on August 29 hit Louisiana and Mississippi as the strongest hurricane in the Gulf of Mexico at the time. Disaster declarations covered 90,000 square miles in several states [182,183]. The storm surge swelled Lake Ponchartrain and resulted in over 50 breeches in the 350-mile levee system surrounding New Orleans. Over a period of roughly 18 hours, approximately 80% of the city of New Orleans was submerged with 6 to 20 feet of water. In the nation's largest search and rescue operation, the Coast guard rescued 33,500 of the estimated 60,000 people stranded in New Orleans. An estimated 215 bodies were found in nursing homes and hospitals. Katrina caused approximately \$125B (\$164B 2019 USD) in damages and 1,245 to 1,836 fatalities – the deadliest since the 1928 Okeechobee hurricane and the costliest hurricane to that point in US history. Looting and violence was a problem in the aftermath of the storm, requiring deployment of the National Guard. Furthermore, it caused massive tree loss and other environmental impact. Congress authorized \$62.3B in aid to victims. Donations were received from all over the world, including \$500 M from Kuwait. FEMA supplied housing for

700,000 far less than needed. The ARC supplied nearly 1,500 shelters. Approximately one million people were displaced and migrated from the Gulf coast elsewhere in the country, the largest diaspora in US history. Secretary of Homeland Security Michael Chertoff declared Hurricane Katrina and the ensuing flooding of New Orleans as "probably the worst catastrophe or set of catastrophes" in the country's history.

FEMA was severely criticized for poor leadership, delays, and mismanagement – so-called Katrinagate, and FEMA director Michael D. Brown was forced to resign [184–186]. There were many lessons that were learned from this catastrophe. Many who had warned that the refocus on terrorism would leave FEMA unprepared for natural disasters felt vindicated.

The 2005 hurricane season was the most active hurricane season in history. There were 28 storms, 15 hurricanes, seven major hurricanes, including four Category 5 hurricanes, and five major hurricanes that made landfall. Three of the six most intense Atlantic hurricanes ever recorded occurred in 2005: Wilma, Rita, and Katrina. Only the 1933 season had a higher recorded accumulated cyclone energy. Katrina was the costliest, but Wilma was the most intense. Rita re-damaged the same areas as Katrina. Together, the storm damage for the season accounted for over $180B in economic damage and 2000 to 4000 fatalities.

2.16 Post-Katrina Emergency Management Reform Act of 2006 (PKEMRA)

The first serious test of the NRP was Katrina and it proved a failure [187–190]. What triggered the NRP was unclear and what steps to take when it was triggered were unclear; the roles of the FCO and PFO were unclear. Congress was harsh with its criticisms and responded through the Post Katrina Emergency Management Reform Act (PKEMRA) [191–193]. The act reauthorized and restructured FEMA by redefining its mission, consolidating its emergency management functions, and granting it greater autonomy. The act transferred back to FEMA most preparedness functions and elevated its status as a "distinct entity" within DHS. The act mandated that the

FEMA administrator have significant emergency management credentials and designated the FEMA administrator to be the principal advisor on all emergency management matters to the president, DHS secretary, and the Homeland Security Council. The act allowed federal assistance even in the absence of a specific request. It expanded availability of public assistance to nongovernmental organizations.

2.17 2008 National Response Framework (NRF)

The National Response Framework (NRF) replaced the 1992 NRP in 2008 [194–196]. The NRF provides guidelines, rules of engagement, and an organizational framework for those involved in federal disaster response, rather than a specific protocol as found in Emergency Operations Plans (EOPs). The NRF gives roles and responsibilities to the private sector, nongovernmental organizations (NGOs), states, territories, and tribal governments, as well as the federal government. Adjustments were made to better accommodate the involvement and partnership of nonfederal participants. The NRF establishes a comprehensive, national, all-hazards approach to domestic incident response. It is always in effect and eliminated any triggering event required by the NRP. The NRF is more in line with an all-hazards approach than its NRP terrorism-focused predecessor. The NRF organizes actions in a prepare, respond, and recover cycle and emphasizes planning. Emergency support functions (ESFs) were better defined. It refers to the development of 15 incident scenarios by DHS for planning purposes.

In response to President Barack Obama's 2011 Presidential Policy Directive 8: National Preparedness (PPD-8), the NRF was again revised and in 2013 became one of a "series of integrated national planning frameworks covering prevention, protection, mitigation, response, and recovery" that are part of the "national preparedness system." PPD-8 deemphasized the 15 National Planning Scenarios. However, the NRF includes Incident Annexes for biologic, catastrophic, cyber, food and agricultural, mass evacuation, nuclear/radiological, and terrorist incidents. A National Response Framework Catastrophic Incident Supplement (NRF-CIS) is published independently of the NRF and its annexes designed primarily to address no-notice or short-notice incidents of catastrophic magnitude, where anticipatory planning and resource pre-positioning are precluded and where the nature of the needed resources and assets is not known.

2.18 2011 National Disaster Recovery Framework

Three years after release of the NRF, the Obama administration released a companion document, the National Disaster Recovery Framework (NDRF) [197–199]. In the months following an incident, after the ESFs demobilize, the NRF transitions into the NDRF. The nine core principles of the NDRF for achieving success are individual and family empowerment, leadership and local primacy, pre-disaster recovery process, partnership and inclusiveness, public information, unity of effort, timeliness and flexibility, resilience and sustainability, psychological and emotional recovery.

2.18.1 2012 Hurricane Sandy

On September 29, 2012, Hurricane Sandy struck New Jersey as a very large Category 2 hurricane, after hitting Cuba, Jamaica, and other Caribbean islands as a Category 3 hurricane [200]. It affected 24 states and Canada. The hurricane, dubbed Superstorm Sandy, was the most powerful, deadliest, and costliest of the 2012 season. It resulted in $70B in damages, of which $65B was in the US, and 233 fatalities. It was the second costliest US hurricane until Hurricanes Harvey and Maria in 2017. The Hurricane Sandy Rebuilding Task Force coordinated local, state, and federal recovery efforts and developed model resilience policies for vulnerable communities.

2.18.2 Sandy Recovery Improvement Act of 2013 (SRIA)

The Sandy Recovery Improvement Act (SRIA) and its companion 2013 Disaster Relief Appropriations Act substantially changed FEMA substantive authorities [201–204]. Congress enacted SRIA due to concerns over anticipated bureaucracies and delays that Hurricane Sandy victims might suffer. SRIA piloted alternative procedures for its public assistance program. Among other things, it allows disaster assistance on the basis of cost estimates rather than reimbursement of costs.

2.18.3 2017 Hurricane Harvey

On August 25, 2017, Hurricane Harvey struck the Texas coast, as a Category 4 hurricane, after striking several Caribbean islands and the Yucatan peninsula; South America and Louisiana were also affected [205,206]. The last major hurricane to hit the US was 12 years earlier. Due to picking up significant water from the warm Gulf and then its slow overland movement, it dropped unprecedented rainfall making it the wettest hurricane on record in the US. Water accumulations were over five feet in some places. Volunteers in rescue boats from Louisiana were dubbed the Cajun navy. The flooding damaged or destroyed 300,000 structures, nearly 50,000 homes, and 500,000 cars. It caused approximately $125B in damages, primarily from flooding of Houston, second only to Katrina (which resulted in $125B in 2005 dollars). Home insurance policies typically excluded flood damages, as the NFIP provides most flood insurance. Energy production in the Gulf of Mexico declined by 21%. It resulted in 107 fatalities. $15B was appropriated for relief by the federal government.

2.18.4 2017 Hurricane Maria

On September 18, 2017, as a Category 5 hurricane, Hurricane Maria slammed into Dominica, and two days later struck Puerto Rico [207–209]. The storm devastated Dominica, St. Croix, and Puerto Rico. It was regarded as the worst hurricane disaster of all the hurricanes to affect those islands and the deadliest in Puerto Rico since the 1899 San Ciriaco hurricane. Maria followed Hurricane Irma that had struck the islands only two weeks before. Irma left 80,000 without power as Maria hit. Furthermore, most of FEMA's emergency stockpiles stored in its Caribbean Distribution Center warehouse in Puerto Rico had been depleted for assistance to Irma's victims in the US Virgin Islands. Total losses from the hurricane are estimated at upwards of $91.61B, mostly in Puerto Rico, ranking it as the third-costliest hurricane on record. DHS failed to waive the waive the Jones Act for Puerto Rico, which prevented the commonwealth from receiving any aid and supplies from non-US-flagged vessels from US ports.

FEMA's response was widely criticized as slow and inadequate. Moreover, when President Donald Trump visited Puerto Rico on October 3, 2017, he was given wrong information and implied that it was not a real catastrophe, "If you looked – every death is a horror, but if you look at a real catastrophe like Katrina, and you look at the tremendous hundreds and hundreds and hundreds of people that died, and you look at what happened here with really a storm that was just totally overbearing, nobody has seen anything like this ... What is your death count as of this morning, 17?" The official fatality count after the hurricane was only 64, but it was revised a year later to 2,975. The president continued to declare his administration had done a "fantastic job," but the promised relief funding was withheld. Several studies estimated that between 1400 and 5740 deaths were attributable to the storm [210]. The stunning discrepancy in the death toll resulted in a congressionally mandated study [211].

2.19 The Disaster Recovery Reform Act of 2018 (DRRA)

The Disaster Recovery Reform Act of 2018 (DRRA), signed into law by President Donald J. Trump, was a response to wildfires in California as well as Hurricanes Harvey, Irma, and Maria [212]. The DRRA contains 56 provisions amending the Stafford Act that attempt to reduce the complexity of FEMA and build the nation's response capacity. It broadens DRF public assistance individual assistance and mitigation programs.

2.20 2020 COVID-19 Pandemic

The COVID-19 pandemic began in Wuhan, China, in December 2019, and the World Health Organization (WHO) officially declared a pandemic on March 11, 2020 [213]. In the US, community-acquired spread began in February 2020. As of September 2021, there were globally over 230 million cases and 4.7 million deaths due to COVID-19 the pandemic [214]. In the US, there have been over 42 million confirmed cases and 677 thousand deaths [215] – surpassing the Spanish flu pandemic [216]. Global lockdown occurred resulting in massive economic loss, measured in the tens of trillions of dollars [217] and caused a US recession, with job losses greater than the great depression of 1929 [218].

DHS Secretary Alex Azar declared a national emergency on January 31, 2020 [219] and President Trump declared NEA [220] and Stafford Act [221] national emergencies on March 13, 2020, triggering a federal response [222–225], but critics found the federal leadership lacking. President Trump had dismantled the Global Health Security and Biodefense unit in the White House that had been established to deal with pandemics by President Obama [226]. Within the Department of Health and Human Services (DHS) under Secretary Alex Azar, Admiral Brett Giroir was given the lead, but the CDC, Directed by Robert R. Redfield, had been assigned to be the lead agency by President Trump, although the DHS Assistant Secretary for Preparedness and Response (ASPR), Robert Kadlec, was supposed to be in charge [227,228]. The CDC did not lead and was often in conflict with the DHS ASPR. FEMA [229], as always in epidemics, was reluctant to lead [230]. The White House formed its own Coronavirus Task Force [231], headed by Vice President Mike Pence, but was dominated by the personalities of Anthony Fauci, Director of NIH's National Institute of Allergy and Infectious Diseases (NIAID), and Deborah Birx, an epidemiologist from the Department of State. President Trump invoked the Defense Production Act [232] and the legislature passed several COVID-19 stimulus packages costing trillions of dollars [233–236]. The president articulated the traditional disaster policy that states plan, locals implement, and the federal government assists [237] – but this was highly criticized, as critics demanded greater federal leadership [238]. Larry Hogan, governor of Maryland and the president of the National Governors Association, held daily teleconferences with state governors [239]. The federal response was further plagued by faulty testing [240], unprepared national stockpile [241], and infighting [242]. The COVID-19 pandemic persisted sufficiently long that more vicious variants developed [243]. The Biden administration made response to the pandemic a priority, but the pace of voluntary vaccinations slowed [244]. The epidemic is still on-going at the time of this writing

2.21 Summary of Federal Disaster Response

The role of the federal government in disaster management has continued to grow since the end of World War II (Figure 2.2) [245–247].

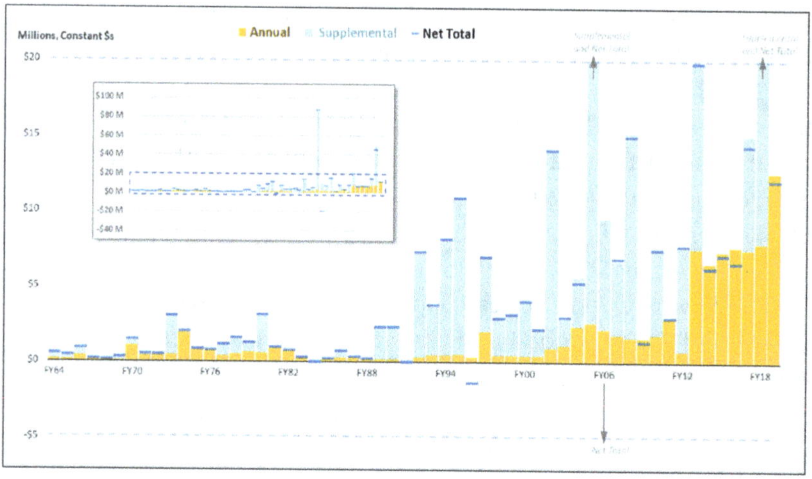

Figure 2.2 Disaster relief appropriations, FY1964–2019 (2019 USD)[248].

Nonetheless, the lead role of the states should not be overlooked [249]. Politicians, legislators, and emergency managers all want to do what they can to help in the face of tragedy, although this may result in boom and bust spending [250]. The COVID-19 pandemic has exposed a need for even greater federal involvement. The US has the economic largesse to respond to the recurrent massive disasters, but also significant mitigation efforts. This growth in federal involvement has been accompanied by fits and starts, but the current sophisticated and proactive emergency apparatus of the United States is the envy of the world. This may be necessary as hurricanes are predicted to become more frequent and stronger [251].

2.22 History of Disaster Victim Identification

Communities have always had to respond to mass fatality incidents, but it has only been in relatively recent times that ongoing contingency planning has gained significant traction and even more recently that disaster victim identification (DVI) has become a subject of study. Until the mid-twentieth century, when scientific methods of identification came into wide use, identification efforts were ad hoc and generally relied on the recognition of family members, friends, and coworkers. It is thus surprising that we know the exact number of fatalities is 1112 from the Circus Maximus collapse in Rome in 140 AD [252].

Identification was originally based upon visual recognition of the decedent. Eventually, visual identification was supplemented by photographs. As a reference, mugshots began to be used in police departments for identification in the 1850s [253].

In the US, the medical examiners and coroners take jurisdiction over the bodies of mass fatality events. The first medical examiner office was established in Suffolk County, Massachusetts (Boston), in 1877, and in 1907 the second medical examiner, George Burgess Magrath (1870–1938), was the first forensically trained pathologist to become a medical examiner [254]. The mass fatality incident that he worked was the Great Molasses Flood of 1919, when a 2.3-million-gallon tank of molasses burst and killed 21 people and injured 150 others.

Perhaps the first major forensic investigation of a mass disaster was that of the Katyn Forest Massacre during WWII [255]. The German Nazi government applied nineteenth-century German forensic medicine to prove that the Soviets, rather than the Germans, had killed 15,000 captive Polish troops in 1939. Pathologists determined the identification and causes and manners of death after the discovery of the mass grave in 1943. Moreover, the pathologists noted that skull defects matched the square bayonets of Russian soldiers and not the triangular bayonets of the Germans

2.22.1 Scientific Methods of Identification

The first systemic investigation of the identification of remains was in forensic anthropology. Physical anthropology (now biological anthropology) was spawned in mid-nineteenth-century Germany from various disciplines, including medicine, anthropometry, craniology, and paleontology [256]. The father of physical anthropology is considered to be Johann Friedrich Blumenbach (1752–1840) [257]. Samuel George Morton (1799–851) was perhaps the first American physical anthropologist; he was known for craniometry, but has been criticized for racial bias [258]. Physical anthropology came to be dominated and institutionalized by the renowned pathologist, Rudolph

Carl Virchow (1821–902) [259–261]. For two years beginning in 1985, Franz Boas (1858–1942) worked with Virchow before moving to New York and becoming the father of American anthropology [262,263]. The father of American forensic anthropology was Harvard professor Thomas Dwight (1843–1911), who published a prize winning essay, "The Identification of the Human Skeleton: A Medicolegal Study," in 1878, but Wilton Marion Krogman (1903–987) established the discipline in the US [264–266]. Another important aspect of early American forensic anthropology was the FBI use of the Smithsonian anthropologists Aleš Hrdlička (1869–1943), Thomas Dale Stewart (1901–1997), John Lawrence Angel (1915–1986) [267,268]. Physical anthropology became a section of the American Academy of Forensic Sciences in 1972, and the American Board of Forensic Anthropology was established in 1977 [269]. Forensic anthropologists have become increasingly involved in DVI operations for medical examiner offices since the 1970s [270].

The history of fingerprint identification is ancient, complex, and anecdotal [271–273]. Handprints in clay seals were used in burglary investigations during the Qin Dynasty in 200 BCE In the fourteenth century fingerprints were used for identification in the Middle East. In the seventeenth century, medical texts began to mention friction ridges. In the mid-nineteenth century, Sir William James Herschel described fingerprints as a unique permanent feature and used them to authenticate contracts in India. In 1870, Dr. Henry Faulds published an article in *Nature* discussing fingerprints as a means of personal identification and the use of ink as a method of print capture. In 1883, in the *Life on the Mississippi*, Samuel Clemens (Mark Twain) wrote about a murderer who was identified by a fingerprint. Bertillon, Vucetich, and Henry developed fingerprint classification systems, and the systematic use began at the turn of the century. Although fingerprint evidence was used in court sporadically for decades, it is generally thought that in 1911 Thomas Jennings became the first person to be convicted of a crime solely on the basis of fingerprint evidence; *People v. Jennings*, 252 Ill.534 (1911). Nonetheless, it was not until the 1935 Lindbergh baby kidnapping case that fingerprints were widely accepted as scientific evidence; *State v. Hauptmann*, 180 A. 809 (N.J. 1935).

The history of forensic odontologic identification is also ancient, complex, and anecdotal [274,275]. It is well documented that in ancient Rome, around 49 CE, that Agrippina identified the head of the slain Lollia Paulina by her teeth. In the US, Paul Revere identified Dr. Joseph Warren, who died at the Battle of Breed's Hill in 1775, by the dental bridge he had made for him. Dental identification was the critical evidence in an 1814 grave robbing case in Edinburgh, Scotland. The first dental journal was published in 1839, the first national dental association was formed in 1840, and the first graduates of an accredited dental school (Baltimore) graduated in 1842. The 1850 murder of Dr. George Parkman by Dr. John White Webster resulted in the first use of dental evidence in a US court. In 1994, the American Dental Association (ADA) passed resolution 654 in which the ADA "urges all constituents to develop dental identification teams that can be mobilized in times of need."

Forensic DNA testing, which replaced blood typing and protein serum isoenzyme technology, is dated to 1985 publications in Nature by Sir Alec Jeffreys [276–279]. Jeffreys' DNA test was first used to identify Colin Pitchfork as a suspected murderer in 1987. The 1990 to 2003 Human Genome Project was an important backdrop to the technologic evolution of forensic DNA testing [280]. Lifecodes, Cellmark, and the Serological Research Institute (SERI) offered DNA testing in 1986 and 1987; the FBI opened its doors to casework in late 1988 and the Virginia state crime lab began casework in 1989. DNA was first used in the US in a criminal case in 1986, where PCR-based DQ-alpha testing was performed to determine if the autopsied organs had been switched, *Commonwealth v. Pestinikas*, 617 A. 2d 1339 (Pa. Super. Ct. 1992). In 1987, Tommy Lee Andrews became the first person to be convicted of a crime, rape, based upon DNA evidence in *Andrews v. State*, 533 So.2d 841 (Fl. Dist. Ct. App. 1988). The first use of DNA in disaster victim identification was in the 1991 Persian Gulf War [281,282].

Specialized software to permit database searches and comparisons has become important to make use of these scientific techniques in DVI operations. In 1924, the FBI consolidated federal fingerprint files into its Identification Division [283]. In 1991, this division was housed in a new facility in Clarksburg, WV, and then broadened and renamed the Criminal Justice Information Services Division (CJIS) in 1992 [284]. Digitization had been in development for decades, when CJIS launched its first automated fingerprint identification system (AFIS) in 1974 [285], its integrated automated fingerprint system (IAFIS) in 1999 [286,287], and its next generation identification (NGI) system in 2011 [288–290]. INTERPOL launched its first automated fingerprint system in 1992 [291].

The FBI piloted its Combined DNA Index System (CODIS) software in 1990 [292,293] and then launched the National DNA Index System (NDIS) as authorized in the DNA Identification Act of 1994[294].

The development of dental identification software is less straightforward and intertwined with the development of DVI software [295–297]. Dr. Lou Lorton, at the Army Institute of Dental Research, created the first dental matching program, the DOS-based computer assisted postmortem identification program (CAPMI) in 1985 and successfully used it in the crash of a military transport plane in Gander, Newfoundland [298].

The FBI's National Criminal Information Center (NCIC) was initially created in 1967 at the Direction of Director J. Edgar Hoover [299]. The NCIC is now a part of CJIS and is used by federal, state, and local law enforcement officers for various crime data and investigatory information – including information for missing persons searches. A mid-1990s upgrade, NCIC2000, allows for simplified dental information and dental imagery; however, it is accessible only by LEOs.

CAPMI was superseded by Windows-based WinID, created by Dr. Jim McGivney in 2001, and was successfully used in the 9/11 WTC DVI effort. WinID is now in its third version and has been translated into many languages [300].

In 1994, Don Bloom developed the victim identification profile (VIP) program for DMORT with to assist its DVI operations and based upon its own DMORT forms [301]; WinID is used for dental matching.

In 2005, INTERPOL contracted Plass Data to create disaster victim identification software based upon INTERPOL forms [302]. The current DVI System International includes dental, fingerprint, and DNA matching capabilities. In December 2019, Plass Data was purchased by KMD, a Denmark-based NEC subsidiary company [303].

In 2009, the New York City Office of the Chief Medical Examiner created the Unified Victim Identification System (UVIS), during continued 9/11 WTC DVI efforts [304]. This software was developed by Nihilent (formerly Sapphire) and contains the following components: antemortem section (call center, missing persons, family assistance, records modules), postmortem section (field operations, disaster mortuary management, disaster victim identification, dental identification, pandemic influenza modules), and an administrative section.

In 2005, the National Institute of Justice (NIJ) funded Dr. Randy Hanzlick, a medical examiner, and Steve Clark, of ORA, Inc., to create NamUs, a program for both missing and unidentified persons accessible to the medicolegal community. The unidentified component was launched in 2007, the missing persons component in 2008, the combined version in 2009, and the daily operations were contracted to the University of North Texas in 2011 [305]. A dental matching capability was included. An upgrade (NamUs 2.0) was announced in 2020, NamUs, Critical Incident (NamUS-CI), which was designed specifically for mass fatality incidents and disaster victim identification [306].

2.22.2 Military Identification Efforts

Mass fatality management and human remains identification evolved first in militaries [307], not just from the war dead, but also as a source of manpower to be put to use in natural disasters as well, such as in the 1755 Lisbon disaster.

The US military has always buried its war dead in individual graves – a reflection of the value the American society places on individuals (Table 2.9) [308–313]. The Vietnam Memorial Wall lists names of the war dead. We ritualistically remember those who gave their lives, but remain unnamed in tombs of the unknown, the most famous of which is in Arlington Cemetery.

The first organized efforts to identify American war dead began in the mid-nineteenth century, and an Office of Identification was created by the end of the century. The handling of the bodies of fallen soldiers was transferred from logistics to personnel in recognition that bodies are not mere property and agencies were established specifically for the task. At the turn of the twentieth century, service

Table 2.9 Significant dates in US military victim identification efforts [314].

Year	Event
1861–1865	American Civil War: first concerted efforts to identify dead soldiers
1899–1902	Spanish-American War: initiated policy of returning soldiers killed on foreign soil back to next-of-kin in the US
1906	"Dog-tag" program established
1914–1918	WWI: Graves Registration Service established
1939–1945	WWII: Graves Registration Service re-established
1950–1953	Korea: Graves Registration Service re-established
1950	Remains to be repatriated rather than to be temporarily buried
1955–1975	Vietnam War: 96% of KIAs were recovered, compared to 78% for WWII and Korea. Only 28 bodies remained unidentified by the war's end, all but one identified by 1984
1998	Vietnam unknown in the Tomb of the Unknowns was identified as Michael Blassie using DNA
1973	Central Identification Laboratory in Thailand (CIL-THAI) established
1976	Central Identification Laboratory in Hawaii (CIL-HI) established
1986	Duplicate Panographs stored in central depository (after 1985 Gander crash)
1991	Graves Registration Service is renamed Mortuary Affairs
1991	Armed Forces Medical Examiner System established
1992	DNA registry established
2001	Geneva Conventions ID card issued with identifying information and index fingerprint [GCIII, Art. 17(3)]
2006	DOD joint publication 4 (JP4) published

members began wearing metal "dog tags" specifically to facilitate identification. Scientific means of identification began in the mid-twentieth century. Fingerprints were obtained of recruits sometime before the 1960s, perhaps long before. The index fingerprint was placed on the Geneva Convention identification card in the 1960s. Thus, fingerprint identifications were made in Vietnam. After Vietnam, anthropologists became involved to identify the decomposed remains of those remains that were dug up from the theater or returned. They often turned to dental identification. A duplicate panograph repository was established after the December 1985 Gander, Newfoundland, crash, in which the medical records files were carried onboard with the soldiers were lost. Assistance in identification became a secondary mission of the Dental Corps. The Armed Forces DNA Identification Laboratory (AFDIL) was established in 1992 and the repository of DNA samples from recruits in 1994 [315,316]. There have been no service members buried in a tomb of unknowns, since the DNA identification program began, and the Vietnam unknown from the Tomb of Unknowns in the Arlington Cemetery were identified by DNA as Lieutenant Michael Blassie in 1998 [317].

2.22.3 FBI DVI Squad

The first scientific method of individual identification used systematically in DVI was fingerprint identification. In 1940, the FBI deployed to a plane crash in Virginia that killed all 25 on board, including two Bureau employees [318,319]. The FBI positively identified eight bodies (one of which had initially been visually misidentified) through fingerprints. This mass fatality incident resulted in a fingerprint team known as the Disaster Squad. They deploy worldwide and have the capability to search their database remotely. It has recently been renamed the Disaster Victim Identification Squad within the Major Incident Program.

2.22.4 INTERPOL

The International Criminal Police Organization (ICPO-INTERPOL; Organisation internationale de police criminelle) is more commonly known as INTERPOL (Table 2.10) [320]. It is an international

Table 2.10 Significant dates in history of INTERPOL [321].

Year	Event
1914	First International Criminal Police Congress held in Monaco, attended by LEOs from 24 countries
1923	International Criminal Police Commission (ICPC) was founded in Vienna by 16 member states
WWII	Nazis gained control of the ICPC and members ceased participating
1946	ICPC was revived and relocated to Paris
1947	Issued its first Red Notice
1956	Renamed International Criminal Police Organization (ICPO)
1972	Relocated to Lyon, France
1982	Legal framework established for processing personal data, such as names and fingerprints
1990	Launched X400 electronic communication system
1992	Automated search capability introduced
2000	AFIS System for fingerprints
2001	Became 24/7 operational
2002	Launched I-24/7 electronic communication system
2002	DNA database established

organization with 190 member states. It has an annual budget of €113 M ($127 M) and a staff of 756 (from 100 countries).

INTERPOL has been instrumental to the development of DVI outside of the United States [322], where DVI is generally considered to be police function – this is not illogical because the police are in charge of missing persons investigations, they have fingerprint and DNA capabilities, and they are a cadre of government workers that can be assigned to the task. In fact, INTERPOL is probably responsible for the widespread use of the term "disaster victim identification."

In 1984, INTERPOL issued its first Guide to Disaster Victim Identification, which updates every five years. At least INTERPOL-sponsored 32 DVI Teams have deployed since 2004. The INTERPOL antemortem and postmortem forms, as well as their guide are publicly posted on the internet. INTERPOL makes Plass-Data DVI software, which automates the matching of the data, available to members for free.

INTERPOL has generally not been looked to for disasters within the United States, since DVI is generally not a police function within the US, but is instead a function of medical examiner and coroner offices. US representatives to INTERPOL are FBI fingerprint examiners.

2.22.5 Other International Guidance

A document entitled "Management of Dead Bodies after Disasters: A Field Manual for First Responders," sponsored by the Pan-American Health Organization, the World Health Organization, the International Red Cross, and the International Federation of Red Cross and Red Crescent Societies was published in 2006 [323]. The manual was updated in 2016 [324].

As a result of the genocidal violence from 1991 to 1995 following the collapse of the former Yugoslavia, US president Bill Clinton, at the G-7 Summit in Lyon, France, in 1996, initiated an International Commission on Missing Persons (ICMP) to account for the approximately 40,000 persons who were then missing [325]. The governments of the region lacked the capacity or the will to address the issue. In 2001, the ICMP developed a high-throughput DNA human identification facility that is has used to identify more than 20,000 missing persons from around the world. As a consequence of the ICMP's success in the former Yugoslavia, in 2003 ICMP's operations were extended to missing persons globally, including cases arising from natural disasters. The ICMP has helped identify the remains of victims of Saddam Hussein's regime in Iraq of 2003, the Asian tsunami of 2004, Hurricane Katrina of 2005, internal conflicts in Colombia from the 1970s through the early 2000s, Pinochet's regime in Chile during the 1980s, and violence following the fall of Gaddafi Libyan regime in 2011. Since 2014, the ICMP has become a treaty-based international organization recognized by the United Nations to assist remains identification around the world, and in 2017 its headquarters was moved to The Hague in the Netherlands.

2.22.6 Disaster Mortuary Operations Response Team (DMORT)

In 1984, the National Disaster Medical System (NDMS) was established to provide medical assistance for overseas casualties [326]. The NDMS has never been used for its primary purpose and its focus has shifted to victims of domestic disasters [327]. NDMS is under the Department of Health and Human Services (HHS) Office of the Assistant Secretary for Preparedness and Response (ASPR), in support of Emergency Support Function (ESF) #8 Public Health and Medical Services. It provides medical rescue, emergency medical services, patient movement, and definitive care, as well as veterinary services, and fatality management support when requested by authorities from States, localities, tribes and territories, or other federal departments. NDMS maintains the following response units:

- Disaster Medical Assistance Teams (DMAT)
- Trauma and Critical Care Teams (TCCT)
- Disaster Mortuary Operational Response Team (DMORT)
- Victim Information Center Team (VICT)
- National Veterinary Response Team (NVRT)
- Disaster Mortuary Operations Response Teams (DMORT)

Thomas J. Shepardson, a mortician and a member of the National Funeral Directors Association (NFDA), volunteered in what was then known as the HHS Office of Emergency Preparedness in the late 1980s [328–332]. He led a NFDA committee to create the first disaster portable morgue unit (DPMU) and then successfully proposed the creation of a DMORT program in 1993.

The National Guard has been given a significant role in national defense and homeland security [333]. To this end, the ARNG maintains Weapons of Mass Destruction Civil Support Teams (WMD-CSTs) [334]. Pertinent to DVI operations, the Air National Guard (ANG) maintains Fatality Search and Recovery Teams (FSRTs) to assist recovery of bodies when requested [335]. FSRTs maintain the capability of recovery in the event of chemical or biologic contamination.

After several major commercial airline crashes, families complained to Congress about the failure to provide an effective coordinated effort to meet the needs of family members and survivors. This resulted in the Aviation Disaster Family Assistance Act of 1996 [336–339]. The legislation assigned National Transportation Safety Board (NTSB), which investigates transportation incidents, to the role of managing the federal response to aviation disaster victims and their families. The legislation has been amended in 2000 and 2003; a separate act enacted in 2008 made NTSB responsible for family assistance to major railway accidents in addition to aviation accidents. The NTSB Office of Transportation Disaster Assistance uses DMORTs to accomplish this mission and SOPs were published in 2006 [340].

2.22.7 National Association of Medical Examiners

The National Association of Medical Examiners (NAME) has had a disaster-related committee since 2002. NAME promulgated a Mass Fatality Plan in 2002, updates entitled "Standard Operating Procedures for Mass Fatality Management" in 2010 and 2021 [341]. NAME created a position statement in 2020 and is in the process of creating a position paper. NAME has required a mass fatality plan in its current Inspection and Accreditation Program since its inception in 2005 [342].

2.22.8 Federal Direction

In response to the WTC 9/11 mass fatality incident, the National Institute of Justice (NIJ) assisted the New York City Office of the Chief Medical Examiner's Office by funding the formation of a Kinship and Data Analysis Panel (KADAP) [343,344] and later a review of disaster victim identification efforts in mass fatality incidents [345]. NIJ also began to look at the unidentified more broadly [346].

Unfortunately, the original NRF and NIMS documents did not refer to mass fatality management – ironically so given that it was a response to 9/11. The 2008 NSF and NIMS documents merely mentions mass fatality management. The National Response Framework (NRF) specifically includes Fatality Management Services as one of the 14 core capabilities. Nonetheless, mass fatality management has received very little attention or assistance by the federal government.

Under ESF #8, HHS is responsible for providing shelter for the displaced, medical rescue, patient movement, medical care of the injured, and disposition of human remains. Attention and resources for the living will always be prioritized above those of dead and accordingly DVI planning and resourcing have not been well supported.

Within the ICS, the DVI/fatality management operations are typically a "branch" under the Operations Section. The NIMS ICS structure has traditionally placed mass fatality management as a branch of the Operations Section, but a 2017 NIMS update introduces an Intelligence/Investigations Function that would place mass fatality management under a forensic section in certain cases such as criminal, terrorist, or epidemic incidents [347,348].

2.22.9 US Standards Setting Efforts

The Department of Justice (DOJ) established a Technical Working Group on DNA Analysis Methods (TWGDAM, later SWGDAM) in 1988 to facilitate adoption of the then new DNA technology. DOJ subsequently established 22 other scientific working groups (SWGs) in various forensic disciplines to establish standards, one of which was the SWGDVI [349]. Other than SWGDAM, the SWGs had no authority to produce enforceable standards, but they could create voluntary consensus standards.

From 2010 to 2013, SWG DVI was chaired by Elias Kontanis of the NTSB and composed of 30 members representing a broad spectrum of DVI expertise including federal, state, and local US jurisdictions; federal agencies; international organizations; and academia. SWG DVI recognized early that they should generate guidelines rather than standards. SWG DVI identified nearly a dozen subjects for guidance and began to produce guidelines for medical examiner and coroner offices.

After criticism of the SWGs by the 2009 National Academy of Sciences' report "Strengthening Forensic Science in the United States: A Path Forward," a decision was made in 2012 to transfer the SWGs to the National Institute of Standards and Technology (NIST) [350]. After two years of planning, the first working meeting of the new NIST Organization of Scientific Area Committees (OSAC) took place in Leesburg, Virginia in January 2016. The OSAC was created as a structured organization rather than the disparate set of SWGs that characterized the previous DOJ effort. The various previous SWGs were replaced by subcommittees under five scientific area committees that report to the Forensic Science Standards Board. NIST also recognized that voluntary consensus standards must comply with the ANSI essential requirements and the new OSAC could not meet the consensus body balance requirement. Thus, the OSAC would not itself create standards, but would forward documents produced to Standards Development Organizations. However, after standards have been produced by the SDOs, then the OSAC will reconsider them for inclusion in the OSAC Registry of Approved Standards.

The NIST OSAC DVI committee membership was determined in late 2015 and its first meeting was held in early 2016 and was chaired by Jason Wiersema [351]. The subcommittee began with nearly a dozen members with various identification disciplines represented; many of the members had previously been members of SWGDVI. The committee decided to begin with the documents that had previously been produced by SWGDVI.

In the meantime, in 2016, with a recognition of a void for appropriate then existing standards development organizations for several forensic science disciplines, the American Academy of Forensic Sciences (AAFS) created the Academy Standards Board (ASB) as an ANSI-accredited standards development organization. An ASB DVI Consensus body was established in 2016 [352]. Several products of the ASB have been created and are now American National Standards and placed on the OSAC Registry of Approved Standards (Table 2.11).

Table 2.11 DVI guidelines produced by the OSAC DVI committee [353–355].

Category	OSAC	ASB	OSAC Registry
Identification	+		
DNA Testing	+	+	
Fingerprint Searches	+	+	+
Fingerprint Recovery	+	+	
Forensic Pathology	+	+	+
Forensic Anthropology	+	+	+
Forensic Odontology	+		
Data Management	+		
Scene Processing	+	+	
Media Communications	+	+	pending
Victim Accounting	+	+	pending

2.23 Conclusion

As the population of earth grows, the potential for more and larger mass disasters grow. Technology shifts and global warming are cause for more disasters. We are currently in an historic pandemic. Systems have developed and evolved for coping with and preventing mass fatalities. In the United States, localities were left to fend for themselves for the first century and a half after the nation's founding. The federal government became routinely involved after World War II and substantially increased since the mid-1960s. Federal funding has increased exponentially. The consequent legacy places the states in charge of the disaster efforts with assistance of the federal government, but this strategy has not performed well in the face of a truly national crisis like the current pandemic. DVI has been a component of mass fatality incident response from early days, but has not gained traction as an area of focus until recent decades, but the sophistication of DVI efforts has grown rapidly in that time.

References

1. Manning, S.W. (2010). Chapt. 34 eruption of Thera/ Santorini. In: *The Oxford Handbook of the Bronze Age Aegean (Ca. 3000 – 1000 BC)* (edited by E.H. Cline), Oxford, UK: Oxford Press. ISBN 13: 9780199873609.
2. Giacomelli, L., Perrotta, A., Scandone, R., and Scarpati, C. (2003). The eruption of Vesuvius of 79 AD and its impact on human environment in Pompei. *Episodes* 26 (3): 235–238. 10.18814/epiiugs/2003/v26i3/014.
3. Ambraseys, N. (2009). *Earthquakes in the Mediterranean and Middle East: A Multidisciplinary Study of Seismicity up to 1900*. Cambridge, UK: Cambridge Univ Press. ISBN-13: 978-0521872928.
4. Benedictow, O.J. and Benedictow, O.L. (2006). *The Black Death, 1346-1353: The Complete History*. Woodbridge, UK: Boydell Press. ISBN-13: 978-1843832140.
5. SUSPS Website, Population Numbers, Projections, Graphs and Data, https://www.susps.org/overview/numbers.html (accessed, 12/19/2021).
6. List of natural disasters by death toll, Wikipedia, https://en.wikipedia.org/wiki/List_of_natural_disasters_by_death_toll#Ten_deadliest_natural_disasters (accessed, 12/19/2021).
7. Our World in Data website H. Ritchie and M. Roser (2014). Natural disasters. revised (November, 2019). https://ourworldindata.org/natural-disasters (accessed, 12/19/2021).

8. List of wars by death toll, Wikipedia. https://en.wikipedia.org/wiki/List_of_wars_by_death_toll (accessed, 12/19/2021).
9. Fujita, S., Kato, H., and Schull, W.J. (1989). The LD_{50} associated with exposure to the atomic bombing of Hiroshima. *J Radiat Res* 30 (4): 359–381. 10.1269/jrr.32.SUPPLEMENT_154 (accessed, 12/19/2021).
10. Douple, E.B., Mabuchi, K., Cullings, H.M. et. al. (2011). Long-term radiation-related health effects in a unique human population: Lessons learned from the atomic bomb survivors of Hiroshima and Nagasaki. *Disaster Med Pub Hlth Preparedness* 5: S122–S133. 10.1001/dmp.2011.21 (accessed, 12/19/2021).
11. United States military casualties of war, Wikipedia. https://en.wikipedia.org/wiki/United_States_military_casualties_of_war (accessed, 12/19/2021).
12. Hussain, M. (Nov 19, 2019). It's time for America to reckon with the staggering death toll of the post-9/11 wars. The Intercept, https://theintercept.com/2018/11/19/civilian-casualties-us-war-on-terror (accessed, 12/19/2021).
13. Rogers, S.A. Ancient engineering fail: 12 Historic structural disasters. Web Urbanist, undated, https://weburbanist.com/2014/04/16/ancient-engineering-fail-12-historic-structural-disasters/2 (accessed, 12/19/2021).
14. Eaton, G. (2015). *A History of Civilization in 50 Disasters*. Thomaston, ME: Tilbury House Publishers. ISBN-13: 978-0884484899.
15. Lloyd, J.T. (2015). *Lloyd's Steamboat Directory, and Disasters on the Western Waters: Containing the History of the First Application of Steam, As A Motive Power*. UK: Sagwan Press. ISBN-13: 978-1297996061.
16. Erwin, V.B. and Erwin, J. (2020). *Steamboat Disasters of the Lower Missouri River*. Charleston, SC,: The History Press. ISBN-13: 978-1467143257.
17. Fowler, S. (2013). *Railway Disasters*. Barnsley, UK: Pen & Sword Transport. ISBN-13: 978-1845631581.
18. Semmens, P.W.B. (1994). *Railway Disasters of the World: Principal Passenger Train Accidents of the 20th Century*. Sparkford, UK: Patrick Stephens Ltd. ISBN-13: 978-1852603236.
19. (1912). The Sinking of the Titanic and Great Sea Disasters (ed. by L. Marshall and L. Myers).
20. Mechem, L. (2014). *Disasters at Sea: A Visual History of Infamous Shipwrecks*. New York, NY: Skyhorse. ISBN-13: 978-1629141770.
21. Reed, R.C. (1968). *Train Wrecks: A Pictorial History of Accidents on the Main Line*. New York, NY: Bonanza Books. ISBN-13: 978-0764301360.
22. Simpson, P. (2014). *The Mammoth Book of Air Disasters and near Misses*. London, UK: Robinson. ISBN-13: 978-0762449422.
23. Frank, B. (2014). *Plane Crashes*. New York, NY: Bell Publishing Co. ISBN-13: 978-0517334256.

24. Marriott, L., Stewart, S., and Sharpe, M. (1999). *Air Disasters: Including Dialogue from the Black Box*. China: Barnes & Noble. ISBN-13: 978-0760718766.
25. Holanda, R. (2009). *A History of Aviation Safety: Featuring the U.S. Airline System*. Bloomington, IN: AuthorHouse. ISBN-13: 978-1449007973.
26. Miller, C.C.R. (2018). *The Biggest Plane Crashes (History's Biggest Disasters)*. North Mankato, MN: Capstone Press. ISBN-13: 978-1515799870.
27. List of accidents and disasters by death toll, Wikipedia, https://en.wikipedia.org/wiki/List_of_accidents_and_disasters_by_death_toll# (accessed, 12/19/2021).
28. List of disasters in the United States by death toll, Wikipedia, https://en.wikipedia.org/wiki/List_of_disasters_in_the_United_States_by_death_toll (accessed, 12/19/2021).
29. Blanchard, W. (July 5, 2006). Worst disasters – Lives lost (U.S.). https://training.fema.gov/hiedu/docs/hazdem/appendix-worst%20disasters%20lives%20lost.doc (accessed, 12/19/2021).
30. Blanchard, B.W. (October 8, 2008). Billion dollar U.S. disasters. https://training.fema.gov/hiedu/docs/billion%20dollar%20u.s.%20disasters.doc (accessed, 12/19/2021).
31. Wikipedia, List of disasters by death toll, *op. cit.*
32. Carroll, E., Johnson, A., DePaolo, F., Adams, B.J., Mazone, D., and Sampson, B. (2017). Trends in United States mass fatality incidents. *Acad For Path* 7 (3): 318–329.
33. Ibid.
34. Dynes, R.R. (2005). The Lisbon earthquake in 1755: The first modern disaster. http://udspace.udel.edu/bitstream/handle/19716/294/PP%20333.pdf?sequence=1&isAllowed=y (accessed, 12/19/2021).
35. Molesky, M. (2016). *This Gulf of Fire: The Great Lisbon Earthquake, or Apocalypse in the Age of Science and Reason*. New York, NY: Vintage. ISBN-13: 978-0307387509.
36. Mulcahy, M. (1998). The "Great Fire" of 1740 and the politics of disaster relief in colonial Charleston. *The South Carolina Historical Magazine* 99 (2): 135–157. https://www.jstor.org/stable/27570297 (accessed, 12/19/2021).
37. Kierner, C.A. (2019). *Inventing Disaster: The Culture of Calamity from the Jamestown Colony to the Johnstown Flood*. Chapel Hill, NC: Univ of North Carolina Press. ISBN-13: 978-1469652511.
38. Robinson, J.D. (2005). The three fires of christmas. http://www.seacoastnh.com/the-three-fires-of-christmas.
39. Achilles, S.E. (2009). *Portsmouth Firefighting*. Charleston, SC: Arcadia Publishing. ISBN-13: 978-0738562100.

40. Seventh Congress (1803). Session II. Ch. 6,7, https://www.loc.gov/law/help/statutes-at-large/7th-congress/session-2/c7s2ch6.pdf.

41. McNamara, R. (Feb. 11, 2020). New York's Great Fire of 1835, ThoughtCo., https://www.thoughtco.com/new-yorks-great-fire-of-1835-1773780.

42. Salecker, G.E. (1996). *Disaster on the Mississippi: The Sultana Explosion.* April 27, 1865, Annapolis, MD: Naval Institute Press. ISBN-13: 978-1557507396.

43. Berryman, H., Potter, J., and Oliver, S. (1988). The ill-fated passenger steamer Sultana: An inland maritime mass disaster of unparalleled magnitude. *J For Sci* 33 (3): 842–850. 10.1520/JFS12500J.

44. Haines, D.A. and Sando, R.W. (1969). *Climactic Conditions Preceding Historically Great Fires in the North Central Region.* St. Paul, MN: U.S. Dept of Agriculture. updated 2006; available at. https://www.nrs.fs.fed.us/pubs/555.

45. Murphy, J. (2006). *The Great Fire.* New York, NY: Scholastic Paperbacks. ISBN-13: 978-0439203074.

46. Skarbek, E.C. (2014). The Chicago Fire of 1871: A bottom-up approach to disaster relief. *Public Choice* 160: 155–180. https://doi.org/10.1007/s11127-014-0175-1.

47. Holden, C.P. (2011). Rescue and relief. The Great Chicago Fire & The Web of Memory. https://www.greatchicagofire.org/rescue-and-relief.

48. Gess, D. (2003). *Firestorm at Peshtigo: A Town, Its People, and the Deadliest Fire in American History.* New York, NY: Holt Paperbacks. ISBN-13: 978-0805072938.

49. Holbrook, S. (1944). The Peshtigo Fire. *The American Scholar* 13 (2): 201–209.

50. Irwin, J.F. (2013). *Making the World Safe: The American Red Cross and a Nation's Humanitarian Awakening.* Oxford, UK: Oxford Univ Press. ISBN-13: 978-0199766406.

51. Jones, M.M. (2013). *The American Red Cross from Clara Barton to the New Deal.* Baltimore, MD: Johns Hopkins University Press. ISBN-13: 978-1421407388.

52. Hutchinson, J.F. (1992). The nagler case: A revealing moment in red cross history. *Canadian Bull Med Hist* 9 (2): 177–190. 10.3138/cbmh.9.2.177.

53. McCullough, D. (1987). *Johnstown Flood.* New York, NY: Simon & Schuster. ISBN-13: 978-0671207144.

54. Kaktins, U., Todd, C.D., Wojno, S., and Coleman, N. (2013). Revisiting the timing and events leading to and causing the Johnstown flood of 1889. *Pennsylvania History: A Journal of Mid-Atlantic Studies* 80 (3): 335–363. 10.3138/cbmh.9.2.177.

55. Schwartz, S.B. (1992). The hurricane of San Ciriaco: Disaster, politics, and society in Puerto Rico, 1899–1901. *Hispan Amer Hist Rev* 72 (3): 303–334. 10.1215/00182168-72.3.303.
56. Bixel, P.B. and Turner, E.H. (2000). *Galveston and the 1900 Storm*. Austin, TX: Univ of Texas Press. ISBN-13: 978-0292708846.
57. Weems, J.E. (1958). The Galveston storm of 1900. *Southwestern Hist Quart* 61 (4): 494–506. jstor.org/stable/30240830.
58. Horowitz, A. (2015). The complete story of the Galveston Horror: Trauma, history, and the great storm of 1900. *Historical Reflections* 41 (3): 95–108. 10.3167/hrrh.2015.410307.
59. Larson, E. (2000). *Isaac's Storm: A Man, A Time, and the Deadliest Hurricane in History*. Vancouver, WA: Vintage. ISBN-13: 978-0375708275.
60. Little, B. (Aug 29, 2017). How the Galveston hurricane of 1900 became the deadliest U.S. Natural disaster. updated Apr 12, 2019; https://www.history.com/news/how-the-galveston-hurricane-of-1900-became-the-deadliest-u-s-natural-disaster.
61. Rappaport, E.N. and Fernandez-Partagas, J. (1995). The deadliest Atlantic tropical cyclones, 1492-1994. National Hurricane Center, NOAA Technical Memorandum. NWS NHC-47, https://www.aoml.noaa.gov/general/lib/lib1/nhclib/nwstechmemos/techmemo47.pdf.
62. Needham, H. and Keim, B.D. (2012). A storm surge database for the US Gulf Coast. *Int. J. Climatol* 32: 2108–2123. 10.1002/joc.2425.
63. Pielke, R.A., Gratz, J., Landsea, C.W., Collins, D., and Musulin, R. (2008). Normalized hurricane damage in the United States: 1900–2005. *Nat Hazards Rev* 9 (1): 29–42. 10.1061/(ASCE)1527-6988(2008)9:1(29).
64. Fradkin, P.L. (2005). *The Great Earthquake and Firestorms of 1906: How San Francisco Nearly Destroyed Itself*. Berkeley, CA: Univ of California Press. ISBN-13: 978-0520230606.
65. O'Dell, K.A., Weidenmier, M.D., and Shock, R. (2004). Monetary aftershock: The 1906 San Francisco earthquake and the panic of 1907. *J Econ Hist* 64 (4): 1002–1027. 10.1017/S0022050704043062.
66. McEvoy, A.F. (1995). The triangle shirtwaist factory fire of 1911: Social change, industrial accidents, and the evolution of common-sense causality. *Law Social Inquiry* 20 (2): 621–651. 10.1111/j.1747-4469.1995.tb01072.x.
67. Lange, B. (2008). *The Triangle Shirtwaist Factory Fire*. Broomall, PA: Chelsea House Publications. ISBN-13: 978-0791096413.
68. Fitch, T., Layton, J.K., and Wormstedt, B. (2015). *On a Sea of Glass: The Life & Loss of the RMS Titanic*. Gloucestershire, UK: Amberley Publishing. ISBN-13: 978-1445647012.
69. Hall, W. (1986). Social class and survival on the S.S. TITANIC. *Soc Sci Med* 22 (6): 687–690. 10.1016/0277-9536(86)90041-9.

70. Barry, J.M. (2005). *The Great Influenza: The Story of the Deadliest Pandemic in History*. New York, NY: Penguin Books. ISBN-13: 978-0143036494.

71. Taubenberger, J.K. and Morens, D.M. 1918. (2006). Influenza: The mother of all pandemics. *Rev Biomed* 17: 69–79.https://www.medigraphic.com/cgi-bin/new/resumenI.cgi?IDARTICULO=13827.

72. Weissman, B.M. (1974). *Herbert Hoover and Famine Relief to Soviet Russia: 1921-1923*. Washington, DC: Hoover Institution Press. ISBN-13: 978-0817913410.

73. Smith, D. (2019). *The Russian Job: The Forgotten Story of How America Saved the Soviet Union from Ruin*. New York, NY: Farrar, Straus and Giroux. ISBN-13: 978-0374252960.

74. Barry, J.M. (1998). *Rising Tide: The Great Mississippi Flood of 1927 and How It Changed America*. New York, NY: Simon & Schuster. ISBN-13: 978-0641763625.

75. Kosar, K.R. (2011). *Disaster Response and Appointment of a Recovery Czar: The Executive Branch's Response to the Flood of 1927*. Darby, PA: Diane Publishing. ISBN-13: 9781437938388.

76. Lohof, B.A. and Hoover, H. (1927). Spokesman of humane efficiency: The Mississippi flood of. *American Quarterly* 22 (3): 690–700. 1970. 10.2307/2711620.

77. Moss, D.A. (1999). Chapt. 8 courting disaster?: The transformation of federal disaster policy since 1803. In: *The Financing of Catastrophe Risk* (ed by K.A. Froot), Chicago, IL: Univ of Chicago. ISBN-13: 978-0226266237. https://www.nber.org/chapters/c7954.

78. Butler, D. (2020). Chapt. 3 The expanding role of the federal government: 1927–1950. In: *Emergency Management: The American Experience*, 3rd edition. (edited by C.B. Rubin), New York, NY: Routledge. ISBN-13: 978-1138354067.

79. Painter, W.L. (Nov. 22, 2019). The disaster relief fund: Overview and issues. R45484, Congressional Research Service, Updated https://www.hsdl.org/?view&did=831926.

80. Kirk, R.S. (2015). Emergency relief for disaster-damaged roads and transit systems: In brief. Congressional Research Service. R43384, https://fas.org/sgp/crs/misc/R43384.pdf.

81. Winkler, A.M. (1984). A 40-year history of civil defense. *Bull Atomic Scientists* 40 (6): 16–22. 10.1080/00963402.1984.11459239.

82. Jordan, N. (1966). U.S. civil defense before 1950: The roots of public law 920, S-212. https://apps.dtic.mil/dtic/tr/fulltext/u2/637900.pdf.

83. Moss, *op. cit.*, pp. 314-317.

84. Painter (2019), *op. cit.*, pp. 7–8.

85. Bourgin, F. (1983). A legislative history of fed disaster relief, 1950-1974. FEMA training website, 1–227. available at https://training.fema.gov/hiedu/highref.aspx.

86. Blanchard, B.W. (1985). American Civil Defense 1945-1984: The Evolution of Programs and Policies. Federal Emergency Management Agency. 33 pages, available at https://training.fema.gov/hiedu/highref.aspx.

87. Davis, T.C. (2007). *Stages of Emergency: Cold War Nuclear Civil Defense*. Durham, NC: Duke Univ Press. ISBN-13: 978-0822339700.

88. Knowles, S.G. (2007). Defending Philadelphia: A historical case study of civil defense in the early cold war. *Public Works Management Policy* 11 (3): 217–232. 10.1177/1087724X06297346.

89. Knowles, S.G. (2011). *The Disaster Experts: Mastering Risk in Modern America*. Philadelphia, PA: Univ of Pennsylvania Press. ISBN-13: 978-0812243505.

90. Garrison, D. (2006). *Bracing for Armageddon: Why Civil Defense Never Worked*. Oxford, UK: Oxford Univ Press. ISBN-13: 978-0195183191.

91. Bourgin, *op. cit.*, pp. 3-31.

92. Moss, *op. cit.*, p. 315.

93. Painter (2019), *op. cit.*, p. 8.

94. Bourgin, F.P. (1983). A history of federal disaster relief legislation, 1950-1974, FEMA. https://training.fema.gov/hiedu/docs/bourgin,%20frank%20-%20a%20legislative%20history%20of%20fed%20disaster%20relief,%201950%20-%201974.pdf.

95. Bea, K. (2020). Chapt. 4 The formative years: 1950–1978. In: *Emergency Management: The American Experience*, 3rd edition. (edited by C.B. Rubin), New York, NY: Routledge. ISBN-13: 978-1138354067.

96. *ibid.*

97. *ibid.*

98. Dunn, G.E. (1961). The hurricane season of 1960. *Monthly Weather Review* 89 (99): 104–107. http://citeseerx.ist.psu.edu/viewdoc/download?doi=10.1.1.395.3364&rep=rep1&type=pdf.

99. Huff, M. and Carroll, H.B. (1962). Hurricane Carla at Galveston, 1961. *Southwestern Historical Quarterly* 65 (3): 293–309. https://www.jstor.org/stable/30236203?casa_token=d-ribR88q94AAAAA:C8pvBpqevw0lTLCdfp2rJQdFa6uFLOZ4OovqJUpmZ2Yx6Syjd1IeZZEHCkqKrJke5D5eEhUVzzx5VvZxkhCsw8YXKO3nVpI7pkRu5JtipJSsYrbCGx8X&seq=1#metadata_info_tab_contents.

100. Dolan, R. (1987). The Ash Wednesday storm of 1962: 25 years later. *J Coastal Research* 3 (2): ii–v. https://journals.flvc.org/jcr/article/view/79509.

101. Wyss, M. and Brune, J.N. (1967). The Alaska earthquake of 28 March 1964: A complex multiple rupture. *Bull Seismological Soc Amer* 57 (5): 1017–1023. https://pubs.geoscienceworld.org/ssa/bssa/article-abstract/

57/5/1017/116520/The-Alaska-earthquake-of-28-March-1964-A-complex?redirectedFrom=fulltext.

102. Adams, D.S. (1969). Emergency actions and disaster reactions: An analysis of the Anchorage public works department in the 1964 Alaskan earthquake. https://apps.dtic.mil/dtic/tr/fulltext/u2/699832.pdf.

103. Morris, A. (Dec. 4, 2018). How the federal government became responsible for disaster relief. Washington Post. https://www.washingtonpost.com/outlook/2018/12/04/how-federal-government-became-responsible-disaster-relief.

104. Fujita, T.T., Bradbury, D.L., and Van Thullenar, C.F. (1965, 1970). Palm Sunday Tornadoes of April 11. *The Monthly Weather Review* 98 (1): 29–69. http://citeseerx.ist.psu.edu/viewdoc/download?doi=10.1.1.395.3192&rep=rep1&type=pdf.

105. Morris, *op. cit.*

106. Sugg, A.L. (1966). The hurricane season of 1965. *The Monthly Weather Review* 94 (3): 183–191. http://citeseerx.ist.psu.edu/viewdoc/download?doi=10.1.1.395.3050&rep=rep1&type=pdf.

107. Horowitz, A. (2014). Hurricane Betsy and the politics of disaster in the New Orleans's lower ninth ward, 1965-1967. *J Southern Hist* 80 (4): 893–934. https://search.proquest.com/docview/1623470406?pq-origsite=gscholar.

108. Forrest, T.R. (1979). *Hurricane Betsy, 1965: A Selective Analysis of Organizational Response in the New Orleans Area.* Newark, DE: Univ of Delaware. http://udspace.udel.edu/handle/19716/1321 (accessed, 12/19/2021).

109. Morris, *op. cit.*

110. Painter (2019). *op. cit.*, p. 9.

111. Bourgin, *op. cit.*, pp. 32-50.

112. Moss, *op. cit.*

113. Knowles, S.G. and Kunreuther, H.C. (2014). Troubled waters: The national flood insurance program in historical perspective. *Am Disaster Politics* 26 (3): 327–353.

114. Anderson, D.R. (1974). The national flood insurance program – Problems and pitfalls. *J Risk Insur* 41 (4): 579–599. 10.2307/251956.

115. Michel-Kerjan, E.O. (2010). Catastrophe economics: The national flood insurance program. *J Econom Perspectiv* 24 (4): 165–186. 10.1257/jep.24.4.165.

116. King, R. (2013). The National flood insurance program: Status and remaining issues for congress. RF42850, Congressional Research Service. http://www.fas.org/sgp/crs/misc/R42850.pdf.

117. Horn, D.P. and Webel, B. (2019) Introduction to the national flood insurance program. R44593, Congressional Research Service. https://

www.everycrsreport.com/files/20191008_R44593_b10f905bd8f9bc2bde6967358ade3a73cdf0294d.pdf.

118. National Flood Insurance Program website FEMA. https://www.fema.gov/national-flood-insurance-program.

119. Schwarz, F.K. (1970). Unprecedented rains in Virginia associated with the remnants of Hurricane Camille. *The Monthly Weather Review* 98 (11): 851–859. http://citeseerx.ist.psu.edu/viewdoc/download?doi=10.1.1.395.3218&rep=rep1&type=pdf.

120. Hearn, P.D. (2004). *Hurricane Camille: Monster Storm of the Gulf Coast.* Jackson, MS: Univ Press of Mississippi. ISBN-13: 978-1578066551.

121. Morris, *op. cit.*

122. Painter (2019). *op. cit.*, p. 9.

123. Moss, *op. cit.*, p. 317.

124. Bourgin, *op. cit.*, pp. 52-70.

125. Bourgin, *op. cit.*, pp. 71-103.

126. Russell, L.A., Goltz, J.D., and Bourque, L.B. (1995). Preparedness and hazard mitigation actions before and after two earthquakes. *Environ Behav* 27 (6): 744–770. 10.1177/0013916595276002.

127. Bailey, J.F., Patterson, J.L., and Paulhus, J.L.H. (1972). *Hurricane Agnes Rainfall and Floods.* June-July, Professional Paper 924. Washington, DC: Govt Printing Off. 10.3133/pp924.

128. Bourgin, *op. cit.*, pp. 104-122.

129. Corfidi, S.F., Weiss, S.J., Kain, J.S., Corfidi, S.J., Rabin, R.M., and Levit, J.J. (2010). Revisiting the 3–4 April 1974 super outbreak of tornadoes. *Weather and Forecasting* 25: 465–510. 10.1175/2009WAF2222297.1.

130. Bourgin, *op. cit.*, pp. 123-227.

131. Painter (2019). *op. cit.*, p. 9.

132. Zimmerman, R. (1985). The relationship of emergency management to governmental policies on man-made technological disasters. *Publ Admin Rev* 45: 29–39. 10.2307/3134995.

133. Morris, A.J.F. (2011). Psychic aftershocks: Crisis counseling and disaster relief policy. *History of Psychology* 14 (3): 264–286. 10.1037/a0024169.

134. Kleiman, A.S. (1979). Preparing for the hour of need: The national emergencies act. *Presidential Studies Quarterly* 9 (1): 47–65. https://www.jstor.org/stable/27547441?seq=1#metadata_info_tab_contents.

135. Leith, W. (2017). NEHRP Turns 40. *Seismological Research Letters* 88 (4): 943–947. 10.1785/0220170088.

136. Maggs, W.W. (1989). Money for Quakes. *Eos, Trans Amer Geophys Union* 70 (45): 1466. 10.1029/89EO00350.

137. Bea, K. (1998). FEMA and disaster relief, 97-159 GOV. https://www.everycrsreport.com/reports/97-159GOV.html.

138. Sharples, T. (2008). A brief history of FEMA. *Time Mag* 172 (10): 20.

139. Sylves, R.T. (2020). Chapt. 5 federal emergency management comes of age: 1979–2001. In: *Emergency Management: The American Experience*, 3rd edition. (edited by C.B. Rubin), New York, NY: Routledge. ISBN-13: 978-1138354067.

140. About the Agency, FEMA website, History tab; https://www.fema.gov/about-agency.

141. Roberts, P.S. (2004). Reputation and federal emergency preparedness agencies, 1948-2003. https://training.fema.gov/emiweb/downloads/robertspfema%208%2020%2004%20apsa.pdf.

142. Kereney, J.G., et al. (1979). *Report of the President's Commission on the Accident at Three Mile Island: The Need for Change: The Legacy of TMI.* Washington, DC: Govt Printing Off. ISBN-13: 978-0935758009.

143. Walker, J.S. (2004). *Three Mile Island: A Nuclear Crisis in Historical Perspective.* Berkeley, CA: Univ California Press. ISBN-13: 978-0520246836.

144. Perry, R.W. (1983). *Citizen Response to Volcanic Eruptions: The Case of Mt.* St. Helens: Irvington Pub. ISBN-13: 978-0829010503.

145. Bea, K. (2010). Federal Stafford act disaster assistance: Presidential declarations, eligible activities, and funding. RL33053, Congressional Research Service. https://www.hsdl.org/?view&did=27383.

146. McCarthy, F.X. (2011). Federal Stafford act disaster assistance: Presidential declarations, eligible activities, and funding. RL33053, Congressional Research Service. https://fas.org/sgp/crs/homesec/RL33053.pdf.

147. Moss, M., Schellhamer, C., and Berman, D.A. (2009). The Stafford act and priorities for reform. *J Homeland Sec Emerg Mgmt* 6 (1): 1–21. 10.2202/1547-7355.1538.

148. Maki, A.W. (1991). The Exxon Valdez oil spill: Initial environmental impact assessment, Part 2. *Environmental Science & Technology* 25 (1): 24–29. 10.1021/es00013a001.

149. Peterson, C.H., Rice, S.D., Short, J.W., Esler, D., Bodkin, J.L. et. al. (2003). Long-term ecosystem response to the Exxon Valdez oil spill. *Science* 302 (5653): 2082–2086. 10.1126/science.1084282.

150. Philen, R.M., Combs, D.L., Miller, L., Sanderson, L.M., Parrish, R.G., and Ing, R. (1992). Hurricane Hugo-related deaths: South Carolina and Puerto Rico. *Disasters* 16 (1): 53–59. 10.1111/j.1467-7717.1992.tb00375.x.

151. Steidl, J.H., Archuleta, R.J., and Hartzell, S.H. (1991). Rupture history of the 1989 Loma Prieta, California, Earthquake. *Bull Seisomological Soc Amer* 81 (5): 1573–1602. https://pubs.geoscienceworld.org/ssa/bssa/article-abstract/81/5/1573/119516.

152. Schneider, S.K. (1992). Governmental response to disasters: The conflict between bureaucratic procedures and emergent norms. *Public Administration Review* 52 (2): 135–145. 10.2307/976467.

153. Federal Response Plan (Interim), FEMA, 9230.1-PL, Homeland Security Digital Library; https://www.hsdl.org/?abstract&did=781058.

154. Willoughby, H.E. and Black, P.G. (1996). Hurricane Andrew in Florida: Dynamics of a disaster. *Bull Am Meteorolog Soc* 77 (3): 543–549. 10.1175/1520-0477(1996)<0543:HAIFDO>2.0.CO;2.

155. Coffman, M. and Noy, I., Hurricane Iniki: Measuring the long-term economic impact of a natural disaster using synthetic control, 17(2):187–205, 2012; DOI:10.1017/S1355770X11000350.

156. A Short History of FEMA, Frontline; https://www.pbs.org/wgbh/pages/frontline/storm/etc/femahist.html.

157. Roberts, *op. cit.*

158. Bea, K. (1998). FEMA and disaster relief, 97-159 Gov. Congressional Research Service. https://www.everycrsreport.com/reports/97-159.html.

159. Schneider, S.K. (1998). Reinventing public administration: A case study of the federal emergency management agency. *Pub Admin Quart* 22 (1): 35–57. https://www.jstor.org/stable/40861734.

160. Daniels, R.S. and Clark-Daniels, C.L. (2000). *Transforming Government: The Renewal and Revitalization of the Federal Emergency Management Agency.* Arlington, VA: PricewaterhouseCoopers Endowment. https://www.fema.gov/pdf/library/danielsreport.pdf.

161. Larson, L.W. (1997). The great USA flood of 1993. In: *Destructive Water: Water-Caused Natural Disasters, Their Abatement and Control* (edited by G.H. Leavesley, H.F. Lins, F. Nobilis, R.S. Parker, V.R. Schneider and F.H.M. van de Ven), International Assoc of Hydrological Sci Proceedings & Reports, Paris, France:;IAHS Press. ISBN-13: 978-1901502008. https://www.nws.noaa.gov/oh/hrl/papers/area/great.htm.

162. Tierney, K.J. (1994). Northridge earthquake. January 17, 1994, Social Impacts and Emergency Response, art. #279, http://www.desastres.hn/docum/crid/Septiembre-Octubre2005/CD-1/pdf/eng/doc6099/doc6099-contenido.pdf.

163. Linder, D.O. (2007). The Oklahoma city bombing and the trial of Timothy McVeigh. SSRN. DOI: 10.2139/ssrn.1030565.

164. Lindsay, B.R. (2008). The Emergency Management Assistance Compact (EMAC): An overview. RL34585, Congressional Research Service.

165. National Emergency Management Association (NEMA) website; https://www.nemaweb.org.

166. Intrastate Mutual Aid EMAC website; https://www.emacweb.org/index.php/resources/best-practices/intrastate-mutual-aid.

167. Waugh, W.L. (2007). EMAC, Katrina, and the Governors of Louisiana and Mississippi. *Pub Admin Rev* 67 (s1): 107–113. 10.1111/j.1540-6210.2007.00819.

168. Frontline, *op. cit.*

169. Roberts, *op. cit.*

170. Carafano, J.J. and Mayer, M.A. (2007). FEMA and federalism: Washington is moving in the wrong direction. *Heritage Foundation Backgrounder* 2032.

171. Sylves, R. and Cumming, W.R. (2004). FEMA's path to homeland security: 1979-2003. *J Homeland Sec Emerg Mgmt* 1 (2): 10.2202/1547-7355.1023.

172. National Commission on Terrorist Attacks (2004). *The 9/11 Commission Report.* New York, NY: W. W. Norton & Company. ISBN-13: 978-0393060416. https://www.9-11commission.gov/report.

173. Aronson, J.D. (2016). *Who Owns the Dead?: The Science and Politics at Ground Zero.* Cambridge, MA: Harvard Univ Press. ISBN-13: 978-0674971493.

174. Cutler, N. (September 6, 2018). Deaths from 9/11 diseases will soon outnumber those lost on that fateful day, USA today. https://www.msn.com/en-us/news/us/deaths-from-9-11-diseases-will-soon-outnumber-those-lost-on-that-fateful-day/ar-BBMX459?ocid=spartandhp.

175. Harrald, J.R. (2020). Chapt. 6 emergency management restructured: Intended and unintended outcomes of actions taken since 9/11. In: *Emergency Management: The American Experience,* 3rd edition. (edited by C.B. Rubin), New York, NY: Routledge. ISBN-13: 978-1138354067.

176. Thessin, J. (2003). Department of Homeland Security. *Harvard J Legisl* 40: 513–535. https://heinonline.org/HOL/Page?handle=hein.journals/hjl40&id=519&collection=journals&index=.

177. Bea, K., Krouse, W., Morgan, D., Morrissey, W., and Redhead, C.S. (2003). Emergency preparedness and response directorate of the department of homeland security. RS21367, Congressional Research Service. https://fas.org/sgp/crs/RS21367.pdf.

178. Perrow, C. (2006). The disaster after 9/11: The department of homeland security and the intelligence reorganization. *Homeland Security Affairs* 2 (1): (art.3). 1–29. https://core.ac.uk/download/pdf/36718212.pdf.

179. Carafano, J. and Heyman, D. (2004). DHS 2.0: Rethinking the department of homeland security. The Heritage Foundation. https://www.heritage.org/homeland-security/report/dhs-20-rethinking-the-department-homeland-security.

180. NIMS and Incident Command System FEMA. website; https://www.fema.gov/txt/nims/nims_ics_position_paper.txt.

181. History of ICS, EMSI website, (2018). http://www.emsics.com/history-of-ics.

182. Brunkard, J., Namulanda, G., and Ratard, R. (2008). Hurricane katrina deaths, Louisiana, 2005. *Disaster Med Public Health Preparedness* 2 (4): 215–223. 10.1097/DMP.0b013e31818aaf55.

183. Cataldie, L. (2006). *Coroner's Journal: Forensics and the Art of Stalking Death*. New York, NY: Berkeley Books. ISBN 13: 9780399152825.

184. Kellner, D. (2007). The Katrina spectacle and crisis of the Bush presidency. *Critical Methodologies* 7 (2): 222–234. 10.1177/1532708606295642.

185. Moynihan, D.P. (2008). A heckuva job: How management failures doomed the Bush Administration. La Follette Sch Pub. Affairs working paper No. -018; DOI:10.2139/ssrn.1311566.

186. Brown blames Homeland for Katrina response *Associated Press* 2/10/2006; http://www.nbcnews.com/id/11255379#.XtarCS-ZN-U.

187. Weitz, R. (2005). FEMA, DHS, and Katrina: Managing domestic catastrophes better. Hudson Institute Report. https://www.hudson.org/content/researchattachments/attachment/439/fema_weitz_15feb06.pdf.

188. (2006). The federal response to Hurricane Katrina: Lessons learned. U.S. Executive Office of the President. ISBN-13: 978-0160756009; https://fas.org/irp/agency/dhs/fema/katrina.pdf.

189. Select Bipartisan Committee (2006). *A Failure of Initiative: Final Report of the Select Bipartisan Committee to Investigate the Preparation for and Response to Hurricane Katrina*. Report 109-377, Washington, DC: Gov Printing Off. ISBN-10: 0160754259.

190. Colten, C.E. (2009). *Perilous Place, Powerful Storms: Hurricane Protection in Louisiana*. Jackson, MS: Univ Press of Mississippi. ISBN-13: 978-1604732382.

191. Springer, C.G. (2009). Evaluating the new FEMA post PKEMRA. https://digitalscholarship.unlv.edu/sea_presentations/2.

192. Gall, M. and Cutter, S.L. (2020). Chapt. 7 2005 events and outcomes: Hurricane katrina and beyond. In: *Emergency Management: The American Experience*, 3rd edition. (edited by C.B. Rubin), New York, NY: Routledge. ISBN-13: 978-1138354067.

193. Schneider, S.K. (2011). *Dealing with Disaster: Public Management in Crisis Situations*, 2nd ed. New York, NY: Routledge. ISBN-13: 978-0765622433.

194. National Response Framework (2008). https://www.fema.gov/pdf/emergency/nrf/nrf-core.pdf.

195. National Response Framework Information Sheet, FEMA https://www.fema.gov/media-library-data/20130726-1914-25045-6465/final_informationsheet_response_framework_20130501.pdf.

196. (2011). The national response framework: Overview and possible issues for Congress. RL34758, Congressional Research Service. https://www.everycrsreport.com/files/20110121_RL34758_9fb3078c550dcccc74f7ff80252f94d472f0f3a9.pdf.

197. (2010). FEMA's Preparedness for the Next Catastrophic Disaster – An Update, DHS OIG, OIG 10-123. https://www.oig.dhs.gov/sites/default/files/assets/Mgmt/OIG_10-123_Sep10.pdf.

198. National Disaster Recovery Framework, FEMA website; https://www.fema.gov/pdf/recoveryframework/ndrf.pdf.

199. Zimmerman, E. Obama administration announces new approach to strengthen disaster recovery across the nation, FEMA. website; https://www.fema.gov/blog/2011-09-23/obama-administration-announces-new-approach-strengthen-disaster-recovery-across.

200. Miles, K. (2014). Superstorm: Nine days inside Hurricane Sandy. Dutton: ISBN-13: 978-0525954408.

201. Pirani, R. and Tolkoff, L. (2014). Lessons from sandy: Federal policies to build climate-resilient coastal regions. Lincoln Institute of Land Policy and Regional Plan Association. https://staging.community-wealth.org/sites/clone.community-wealth.org/files/downloads/report-pirani-tolkoff.pdf.

202. One Year Later: Examining the Ongoing Recovery from Hurricane Sandy, Statement of Craig Fugate before the Senate Committee on Homeland Security and Governmental Affairs, Subcommittee on Emergency Management, Intergovernmental Affairs and the District of Columbia (Nov 6, 2013). https://www.fema.gov/media-library-data/1387208691195-dda79568fbb827633b3e095d61fa9f7a/11-6-2013_ONE%20YEAR%20LATER_EXAMINING%20THE%20ONGOING%20RECOVERY%20FROM%20HURRICANE%20SANDY.pdf.

203. Progress Report: Hurricane Sandy Recovery – One Year Later, Statement of Elizabeth Zimmerman before the House Committee on Transportation and Infrastructure (Nov 14, 2013). https://republicans-transportation.house.gov/uploadedfiles/2013-11-14-zimmerman.pdf.

204. McCarthy, F.X. (2014). FEMA's disaster declaration process: A primer. R43784, Congressional Research Service. https://fas.org/sgp/crs/homesec/R43784.pdf.

205. Amadeo, K. (Jan 20, 2019). Hurricane Harvey facts, damage and costs: What made Harvey so devastating. updated https://www.lamar.edu/_files/documents/resilience-recovery/grant/recovery-and-resiliency/hurric2.pdf.

206. Jonkman, B., Godfroij, M., Sebastian, T., and Kolen, B. (2018). Loss of life due to Hurricane Harvey. *Nat Hazards Earth Syst Sci* 18: 1073–1078. 10.5194/nhess-18-1073-2018.

207. Farber, D.A. (2018). Response and recovery after Maria: Lessons for disaster law and policy. *Revista Juridica UPR* 87 (3): 743–771. https://escholarship.org/uc/item/936195d5.

208. Schroeder, S.C. (2019). Does America's new disaster relief law provide the relief America needs. *Hou L Rev* 56 (5): 1177–1212.

209. Puerto Rico disaster recovery: FEMA actions needed to strengthen project cost estimation and awareness of program guidance (Feb. 2020). GAO-20-221, https://www.hsdl.org/?view&did=833806.

210. Santos-Lozada, A.R. and Howard, J.T. (2018). Statistics to calculate excess deaths in Puerto Rico following Hurricane Maria. *JAMA* 320 (14): 1491–1493. 10.1001/jama.2018.10929.

211. (2020). Assessing mortality and morbidity after large-scale disasters. National Academies Press. DOI 10.17226/25863.

212. Disaster Recovery Reform Act of 2018 Transforms Field of Emergency Management (Oct 5, 2020). FEMA press release. https://www.fema.gov/news-release/2018/10/05/disaster-recovery-reform-act-2018-transforms-field-emergency-management.

213. 199 WHO Timeline – COVID-19 (April 27, 2020). WHO. website; https://www.who.int/news-room/detail/27-04-2020-who-timeline—covid-19.

214. COVID-19 Coronavirus pandemic, Worldometer website; https://www.worldometers.info/coronavirus/?.

215. Johns Hopkins coronavirus resource center website; https://coronavirus.jhu.edu.

216. Johnson, C.K. COVID has killed about as many Americans as the 1918-19 flu, AP Press 9/20/2021; https://apnews.com/article/science-health-pandemics-united-states-coronavirus-pandemic-c15d5c6dd7ece88d0832993f11279fbb.

217. Goldstein, S. (May 20, 2020). Pandemic could cost global economy $82 trillion in depression scenario. Market Watch, https://www.marketwatch.com/story/today-in-scary-numbers-pandemic-could-cost-global-economy-82-trillion-2020-05-19 (accessed, 12/19/2021).

218. Long, H. and Van Dam, A. (May 8, 2020). U.S. unemployment rate soars to 14.7 percent, the worst since the depression era. Washington Post.https://www.washingtonpost.com/business/2020/05/08/april-2020-jobs-report.

219. Secretary Azar Declares Public Health Emergency for United States for 2019 Novel Coronavirus, DHS website (January 31, 2020). https://www.hhs.gov/about/news/2020/01/31/secretary-azar-declares-public-health-emergency-us-2019-novel-coronavirus.html.

220. Proclamation on Declaring a National Emergency Concerning the Novel Coronavirus Disease (COVID-19) Outbreak (March 13, 2020).White house. website; https://www.whitehouse.gov/presidential-actions/proclamation-declaring-national-emergency-concerning-novel-coronavirus-disease-covid-19-outbreak.

221. Letter from President Donald J. Trump on Emergency Determination Under the Stafford Act (March 13, 2020). White house. website; https://www.whitehouse.gov/briefings-statements/letter-president-donald-j-trump-emergency-determination-stafford-act.

222. Robert, T. Stafford disaster relief and emergency assistance act: Fact sheet. https://www.astho.org/Programs/Preparedness/Public-Health-

Emergency-Law/Emergency-Authority-and-Immunity-Toolkit/Robert-T–Stafford-Disaster-Relief-and-Emergency-Assistance-Act-Fact-Sheet/?terms=stafford+act.

223. Perez, M. (March 13, 2020). The stafford act, invoked by president Trump, has rarely been used for public health emergencies. Forbes, https://www.forbes.com/sites/mattperez/2020/03/13/the-stafford-act-invoked-by-president-trump-has-rarely-been-used-for-public-health-emergencies/#43d7dde31fd3.

224. Lindsay, B.R. and Lee, E.A. (2020). Stafford act assistance for public health incidents, IN11229, Congressional Research Service. https://crsreports.congress.gov/product/pdf/IN/IN11229.

225. Lister, S.A., Sekar, K., Dabrowska, A., Gottron, F., Singer, A., and Sarata, A.K. (2020). Overview of U.S. Domestic response to coronavirus disease 2019 (COVID-19). R46219, Congressional Research Service. https://crsreports.congress.gov/product/pdf/R/R46219.

226. Partly false claim: Trump fired entire pandemic response team in 2018 (March25,2020). *Reuters*. https://www.reuters.com/article/uk-factcheck-trump-fired-pandemic-team/partly-false-claim-trump-fired-pandemic-response-team-in-2018-idUSKBN21C32M.

227. Samuels, B. (May 19, 2020). White house, CDC rift spills into the open. The Hill, https://thehill.com/homenews/administration/498416-white-house-cdc-rift-spills-into-the-open (accessed, 12/19/2021).

228. Dornauer, M. (May 15, 2020). ASPR: The federal agency designed for crises like COVID-19. FREOPP, https://freopp.org/a-federal-office-to-prepare-for-covid-19-exists-but-what-is-it-bea9ec47a0c.

229. Jha, A.K. (April 29, 2020). We need the real CDC back and we need it now. STAT, https://www.statnews.com/2020/04/29/we-need-the-real-cdc-back-and-we-need-it-now.

230. Samuels, B. (April 8, 2020). FEMA finds itself in uncharted waters with coronavirus. The Hill, https://thehill.com/homenews/coronavirus-report/491817-fema-finds-itself-in-uncharted-waters-with-coronavirus (accessed, 12/19/2021).

231. Facher, L. (March 20, 2020). 'A number of new stars': The definitive guide to the Trump administration's coronavirus response team. STAT, https://www.statnews.com/2020/03/20/guide-to-trump-administration-coronavirus-response-team (accessed, 12/19/2021).

232. Forgey, Q. (March 24, 2020). Trump triggers defense production act for the first time, politico https://www.politico.com/states/new-york/albany/story/2020/03/24/trump-triggers-defense-production-act-for-the-first-time-1268815 (accessed, 12/19/2021).

233. Iacurci, G. (June 4 2020). Good news for small businesses as Trump signs PPP reform bill into law, CNBC. updated June 5, 2020: https://www.cnbc.com/2020/06/04/senate-passes-ppp-reform-bill-addressing-concerns-of-small-businesses.html.

234. The CARES Act works for all, Treasury website; https://home.treasury.gov/policy-issues/cares.

235. Outlook of Congress' "Phase 4" COVID-19 Stimulus Package (April 3, 2020). Akin gump. website; https://www.akingump.com/en/news-insights/outlook-of-congress-phase-iv-covid-19-stimulus-package.html.

236. COVID-19 Stimulus Tracker and Analysis (June 5, 2020). https://www.taxpayer.net/budget-appropriations-tax/covid-19-stimulus-tracker-and-analysis.

237. Knotts, B. and Chakrabarti, M. (April 16, 2020). The role of governors and the federal government during the coronavirus pandemic. WBUR, https://www.wbur.org/onpoint/2020/04/16/kathleen-sebelius-coronavirus-states-government (accessed, 12/19/2021).

238. Yglesias, M. (April 3, 2020). America has no federal response to this crisis: Trump is playing president on television instead of doing the job, Vox. https://www.vox.com/2020/4/3/21204489/coronavirus-response-chris-murphy.

239. Ball, M. (April 30, 2020). Trump told America's Governors they were on their own. So Maryland's Larry Hogan Is Taking Charge, Time Magazine. https://time.com/5829777/governors-reopening-coronavirus.

240. Boburg, S., O'Harrow, R., Satija, N., and Goldstein, A. (April 3, 2020). Inside the coronavirus testing failure: Alarm and dismay among the scientists who sought to help. Washington Post, https://www.washingtonpost.com/investigations/2020/04/03/coronavirus-cdc-test-kits-public-health-labs/?arc404=true (accessed, 12/19/2021).

241. Swane, J., O'Harrow, R., and Davis, A.C. (May 4, 2020). Before pandemic, Trump's stockpile chief put focus on biodefense. An old client benefited. Washington Post, https://www.washingtonpost.com/investigations/before-pandemic-trumps-stockpile-chief-put-focus-on-biodefense-an-old-client-benefited/2020/05/04/d3c2b010-84dd-11ea-878a-86477a724bdb_story.html (accessed, 12/19/2021).

242. Dearment, A. (May 6, 2020). The eye-popping allegations in ousted BARDA director rick bright's whistleblower complaint. MedCity News, https://medcitynews.com/2020/05/the-eye-popping-allegations-in-ousted-barda-director-rick-brights-whistleblower-complaint/?rf=1.

243. Fontanet, A., Autran, B., Lina, B., Kieny, M.P., Karim, S.S.A., and Sridhar, D. (2021). SARS-CoV-2 variants and ending the COVID-19 pandemic. *Lancet* 397 (10278): 952–954. 10.1016/S0140-6736(21)00370-6.

244. Horton, J. (August 3, 2021). Covid: Where and why is the US vaccine rollout slowing down? BBC News, https://www.bbc.com/news/57889961.

245. History of Federal Disaster Policy, Evidence Matters, HUD PDR website; https://www.huduser.gov/portal/periodicals/em/winter15/highlight1_sidebar.html.

246. Unit Three: Overview of Federal Disaster Assistance, FEMA training website; https://training.fema.gov/emiweb/downloads/is7unit_3.pdf.

247. Painter, W.L. (2020). The disaster relief fund: Overview and issues. R45484, Congressional Research Service. https://crsreports.congress.gov/product/pdf/R/R45484.

248. Painter (2020). *op. cit.*, fig. 2.

249. What We Don't Know About State Spending on Natural Disasters Could Cost Us, The Pew Charitable Trusts (June 19, 2018). https://www.pewtrusts.org/en/research-and-analysis/reports/2018/06/19/what-we-dont-know-about-state-spending-on-natural-disasters-could-cost-us.

250. Abelson, J., Priest, D., Sullivan, J., and Dungca, N. (May 2, 2020). Boom-and-bust federal funding after 9/11 undercut hospital's preparedness for pandemics. Washington Post, https://www.washingtonpost.com/investigations/2020/05/02/hospital-preparedness-coronavirus-federal-funds/?arc404=true.

251. Fountain, H. (May 19, 2020). Climate change is making hurricanes stronger, researchers finds. New York Times, https://www.nytimes.com/2020/05/18/climate/climate-changes-hurricane-intensity.html.

252. Rogers, S.A. Ancient engineering fail: 12 historic structural disasters, Web Urbanist, undated, https://weburbanist.com/2014/04/16/ancient-engineering-fail-12-historic-structural-disasters/2.

253. Smith, S.M., The mug shot: A brief history, JSTOR Daily, undated; https://daily.jstor.org/the-origins-of-the-mug-shot.

254. Goldfarb, B. (2020). *18 Tiny Deaths: The Untold Story of Frances Glessner Lee and the Invention of Modern Forensics*. Naperville, IL: Sourcebooks.

255. Laqueur, T. (2002). *Chapter 5. The Dead Body and Human Rights, in the Body* (ed by S.T. Sweeney and I. Hodder), Cambridge, UK: Cambridge University Press.

256. Ellison, P.T. (2018). The evolution of physical anthropology. *Am J Phys Anthropol* 165 (4): 615–625. 10.1002/ajpa.23408.

257. Bertoletti, S.F. (1995). The anthropological theory of Johann Friedrich Blumenbach. In: *Romanticism in Science, Boston Studies in the Philosophy of Science,* vol. 152. (eds S. Poggi and M. Bossi), Dordrecht: Sprin ger.10.1007/978-94-017-2921-5_7.

258. Renschler, E.S. and Monge, J. (2008). The Samuel George Morton cranial collection. *Expedition* 50 (3): 30–38. https://www.penn.museum/sites/expedition/the-samuel-george-morton-cranial-collection.

259. Boas, F. (1902). Rudolf Virchow's anthropological work. *Science* 16 (403): 441–445. https://www.jstor.org/stable/1628050.

260. Sanders, W.E. (1953). Rudolph Ludwig Karl Virchow: Pathologist, anthropologist, champion of German liberty. *Bios* 24 (4): 177–189. https://www.jstor.org/stable/pdf/4605576.pdf.

261. Boak, E.R. (1921). Rudolf Virchow – Anthropologist and archaeologist. *The Scientific Monthly* 13 (1): 40–45. https://www.jstor.org/stable/6581.

262. Benedict, R. (1943). Franz Boas. *Science* 97 (2507): 60–62. https://www.jstor.org/stable/1670558.

263. Lewis, H.S. (2001). The passion of Franz Boas. *American Anthropologist* 103 (2): 447–467. 10.1525/aa.2001.103.2.447.

264. Tersigni-Tarrant, M.A. and Shirley, N.R. (2013). *Brief History of Forensic Anthropology in Forensic Anthropology: An Introduction*. Boca Raton: CRC Press.

265. Stewart, T.D. (1982). Background of American forensic anthropology. *Crim Justice Rev* 7 (10): 4–6. 10.1177/073401688200700104.

266. Iscan, M.Y. (1988). Rise of forensic anthropology. *Yearbook of Physical Anthropology* 31: 203–230. 10.1002/ajpa.1330310510.

267. Ubelaker, D.H. (1999). Aleš Hrdlička's role in the history of forensic anthropology. *J For Sci* 44 (4): 724–730. 10.1520/JFS14544J.

268. Ubelaker, D.H. (2018). A history of forensic anthropology. *Am J Phys Anthropol* 165: 915–923. 10.1002/ajpa.23306.

269. Bethard, J.D. (2016). Historical trends in graduate research and training of diplomates of the American Board of Forensic Anthropology. *J For Sci* 62 (1): 5–11. 10.1111/1556-4029.13262.

270. Mundorff, A. (2012). Integrating forensic anthropology into disaster victim identification. *Forensic Sci Med Pathol* 8 (2): 131–139. 10.1007/s12024-011-9275-0.

271. Berry, J. and Stoney, D.A. (2001). Chapter 1. history and development of fingerprinting. In: *Advances in Fingerprint Technology*, 2nd ed. (edited by H.C. Lee and R.E. Gaensslen), Boca Raton, FL: CRC Press. ISBN-13: 978-0849309236.

272. Barnes, J.G. (2011). Chapter 1. History. in The Fingerprint Sourcebook, NCJ 225320, NIJ, https://nij.ojp.gov/library/publications/fingerprint-sourcebook (accessed, 12/19/2021).

273. Cole, S. (2004). *Suspect Identities: A History of Fingerprinting and Criminal Identification*. Cambridge, MA: Harvard University Press. ISBN-13: 978-0674004559.

274. Svoboda, M., Bowers, S.M., Perrier, M., and Swank, S. (2010). Chapter 1. historical dental investigations. In: *Forensic Dental Evidence: An Investigators Handbook*, 2nd ed. (edited by C.M. Bowers), Burlington, MA: Academic Press. ISBN-13: 978-0123820006.

275. Lipton, B.E., Murmann, D.C., and Pavlik, E.J. (2013). Chapter 1. history of forensic odontology. In: *Manual of Forensic Odontology*, 5th ed. (edited by D.R. Senns and R.A. Weems), Boca Raton, FL: CRC Press. ISBN-13: 978-1439851333.

276. Zagorski, N. (2006). Profile of Alec J. Jeffreys. *PNAS* 103 (24): 8918–8920. 10.1073/pnas.0603953103.

277. Butler, J.M. (2009). Chapter 1. overview and history of DNA typing. In: J.M., Butler *Fundamentals of Forensic DNA Typing* Burlington, MA: Academic Press. ISBN-13: 978-0123749994.

278. Coleman, H. and Swenson, E. (1994). *DNA in the Courtroom: A Trial Watcher's Guide.* Seattle, WA: Genelex Press. ISBN-13: 978-0964450707.

279. Aronson, J. (2007). *Genetic Witness: Science, Law, and Controversy in the Making of DNA Profiling.* New Brunswick, NJ: Rutgers University Press. ISBN-13:978-0813541884.

280. Cook-Deegan, R. (1994). *The Gene Wars: Science, Politics, and the Human Genome.* New York, NY: W. W. Norton and Co. ISBN-13: 978-0393313994.

281. Kashyap, V.J., Sitalaximi, T., and Chattopadhyay, P.,.R. (2004). DNA profiling technologies in forensic analysis. *J Int Hum Genet* 4 (1): 11–30. 10.1080/09723757.2004.11885864.

282. Weedn, V.W. (2011). *DNA Identification of Mass Disaster Victims, in Death in Large Numbers: The Science, Policy, and Management of Mass Fatality Events* (ed By E. Gursky and M. Fierro), Chicago, IL: AMA. 77–110.

283. Fox, J.F. The birth of the FBI's technical laboratory – 1924 to 1935, FBI history. website; https://www.fbi.gov/history/history-publications-reports/the-birth-of-the-fbis-technical-laboratory1924-to-1935.

284. Criminal Justice Information Services (CJIS), FBI website; https://www.fbi.gov/services/cjis.

285. Komarinski, P. (2005). *Automated Fingerprint Identification Systems (AFIS).* Burlington, MA: Elsevier Academic Press. ISBN-13: 978-0124183513.

286. Brown, J.P. (2007). A latent print examiner's guide to IAFIS. *J For Ident* 57 (4): 539–549.

287. Privacy Impact Assessment for the Fingerprint Identification Records System (FIRS) Integrated Automated Fingerprint Identification System (IAFIS) Outsourcing for Noncriminal Justice Purposes – Channeling (May 5, 2008). https://www.fbi.gov/services/information-management/foipa/privacy-impact-assessments/iafis.

288. Next Generation Identification (NGI), FBI website; https://www.fbi.gov/services/cjis/fingerprints-and-other-biometrics/ngi.

289. Automated Fingerprint Identification System – a short history, Thales website. (May 14, 2020). https://www.thalesgroup.com/en/markets/digital-identity-and-security/government/biometrics/afis-history.

290. Heckman, J. (February 17, 2020). Automated fingerprint matching at FBI allows employees to shift to higher-value work. Federal News Network.https://federalnewsnetwork.com/automation/2020/02/automated-fingerprint-matching-at-fbi-allows-employees-to-shift-to-higher-value-work.

291. Our History INTERPOL. website; https://www.interpol.int/en/Who-we-are/Our-history.

292. Combined DNA Index System (CODIS), FBI. website; https://www.fbi.gov/services/laboratory/biometric-analysis/codis#CODIS-Overview.

293. Cryer, A. CODIS database: Solving crime one genome at a time. DOJ website; https://learnaboutforensics.weebly.com/history.html.

294. Shapiro, E.D. and Reifler, S. (1996). Forensic DNA analysis and the United States government. *Med Sci Law* 36 (1): 43–51. 10.1177/002580249603600109.

295. Loomis, P.W., Reid, J.S., Tabor, M.P., and Weems, R.A. (2018). Chapter 3. dental identification & radiographic pitfalls. In: *Forensic Odontology: Principles and Practice*, 1st ed. (edited by T.J. David and J.M. Lewis), Burlington, MA: Elsevier Academic Press. ISBN-13: 978-0128051986.

296. Mass Fatality Incident Data Management: Best Practice Recommendations for the Medicolegal Authority, NIST OSAC DVI subcommittee 2019; https://www.nist.gov/system/files/documents/2020/04/07/mass_fatality_incident_data_management-_best_practice_recommendations_for_the_medicolegal_authority_OSAC%20Proposed.pdf.

297. Adams, B.J. and Aschheim, K.W. (2016). Computerized dental comparison: A critical review of dental coding and ranking algorithms used in victim identification. *J For Sci* 61 (1): 76–86.

298. Lorton, L., Rethman, M., and Friedman, R. (1988). The computer-assisted postmortem identification (CAPMI) system: A computer-based identification program. *J For Sci* 33 (4): 977–984.

299. NCIC National Crime Information Center (NCIC) FBI. website; https://www.fbi.gov/services/cjis/ncic.

300. McGivney, J. and Fixott, R.H. (2001). Computer-assisted dental identification. *Dent Clin North Am* 45 (2): 309–325.

301. VIP Personal Information http://dmort4.com/DMORT4/downloads/VIP%20Personal%20Information%20Form.pdf.

302. INTERPOL Partner, Plass Data website; https://plassdata.com/interpol-partner.html.

303. KMD buys IT system for disaster assistance from Plass Data (December 4, 2019). NEC, https://www.nec.com/en/press/201912/global_20191205_01.html(accessed, 12/19/2021).

304. Unified Victim Identification System (UVIS) (2009). UVIS information guide, NYC OCME. website; http://www.nyc.gov/html/ocme/downloads/pdf/Special%20Operations/UVIS%20Information%20Guide_20090917.pdf.

305. NamUs website; https://www.namus.gov.

306. Critical Incidents – NamUs Resources and Outreach https://static1.squarespace.com/static/5d0cfe3b240ddb00016f9215/t/5d8a6fc02c7f0364af89399f/1569353666110/namusCIoverview_forweb.pdf.

307. Daniel, V. (2020). The social history of disaster victim identification in the United States, 1865 to 1950. *Acad For Pathol* 10 (1): 4–15. 10.1177/1925362120941336.

308. Sledge, M. (2007). *Soldier Dead: How We Recover, Identify, Bury, and Honor Our Military Fallen*. New York, NY: Columbia University Press. ISBN-13: 978-0231135153.

309. McCarroll, J.E. (2006). Book review: Sledge M, military fallen. *Armed Forces & Soc* 32 (4): 666–669. 10.1177/0095327X06288740.

310. Eckert, W.G. (1983). History of the U.S. Army graves registration service (1917–1950s). *Am J For Med Pathol* 4 (3): 231–243. 10.1097/00000433-198309000-00010.

311. Stewart, J.M. (2004). *Mortuary Affairs – Is USNORTHCOM and the Department of Homeland Security Positioned for Contaminated Mass Fatality Management?* Carlisle: U.S. Army War College. https://info.publicintelligence.net/FLU.pdf.

312. Mortuary Affairs (2011). Joint publication 4-06. https://fas.org/irp/doddir/dod/jp4_06.pdf.

313. Ismay, J. (August 2, 2018). How the defense department identifies the remains of our war dead. New York Times, https://www.nytimes.com/2018/08/02/magazine/korea-remains-identification.html.

314. Mortuary Affairs Wikipedia webpage; https://en.wikipedia.org/wiki/Mortuary_Affairs.

315. Armed Forces Repository of Specimen Samples for the Identification of Remains (AFRSSIR) Armed forces medical examiner. website; https://health.mil/Military-Health-Topics/Combat-Support/Armed-Forces-Medical-Examiner-System/DoD-DNA-Registry/Repository-of-Specimen-Samples-for-the-Identification-of-Remains.

316. Weedn, V.W. (2020). Origins of the armed forces medical examiner system. *Acad For Path* 10 (1): 16–34. 10.1177/1925362120937916.

317. Thomas, B. (2012). *Last Soldier Buried in Tomb of the Unknowns Wasn't Unknown*. Washington Post. November 8. https://www.washingtonpost.com/lifestyle/magazine/last-soldier-buried-in-tomb-of-the-unknowns-wasnt-unknown/2012/11/06/5da3e7d6-0bdd-11e2-a310-2363842b7057_story.html (accessd, 12/19/2021).

318. Minnich, J.T. (1967). The F.B.I.'s disaster squad. *The Medico-Legal Society* 35 (3): 103–113. 10.1177/002581726703500303.

319. The Disaster Squad FBI. website; https://archives.fbi.gov/archives/news/stories/2010/june/disaster-squad.

320. Our History INTERPOL. website; https://www.interpol.int/en/Who-we-are/Our-history.

321. Our History INTERPOL. website, *ibid.*

322. Disaster Victim Identification (DVI) INTERPOL. website; https://www.interpol.int/en/How-we-work/Forensics/Disaster-Victim-Identification-DVI.

323. Morgan, O., Tidball-Binz, M., and Van Alphen, D., editors. (2006). *Management of Dead Bodies after Disasters: A Field Manual for First Responders*, 2nd ed. (edited by M. O Morgan, D. Tidball-Binz and van Alphen), Washington DC: PAHO. https://www.icrc.org/en/doc/assets/files/other/icrc_002_0880.pdf.

324. Cordner, S., Conninx, R., Kim, H.-J., van Alphen, D., and Tidball-Binz, M., editors.(2016). *Management of Dead Bodies after Disasters: A Field Manual for First Responders*, 2nd ed. Washington, DC: PAHO. ISBN: 978-92-75-31924-6.https://www.icrc.org/en/publication/0880-management-dead-bodies-after-disasters-field-manual-first-responders.

325. History, ICMP website; https://www.icmp.int/about-us/history.

326. Suner, S. (2015). History of disaster medicine. *Turk J Emerg Med* 15 (Suppl 1): 1–4. 10.5505/1304.7361.2015.69376.

327. Franco, C., Toner, E., Waldhorn, R., Inglesby, T.V., and O'Toole, T. (2007). The national disaster medical system: Past, present, and suggestions for the future, biosecurity and bioterrorism. *Biodefense Strategy, Practice, and Science* 5 (4): 319–328. 10.1089/bsp.2007.0049.

328. Disaster Mortuary Operational Response Teams, DHS website; https://www.phe.gov/Preparedness/responders/ndms/ndms-teams/Pages/dmort.aspx.

329. Saul, F.P. (November 24, 2009). DMORT teams and their role in MFIs. domesticpreparedness.com, https://www.domesticpreparedness.com/healthcare/dmort-teams-and-their-role-in-mfis.

330. Waters, M. (February 5, 2019). The funeral directors deployed to America's deadliest disasters, Gizmodo. https://earther.gizmodo.com/the-funeral-directors-deployed-to-americas-deadliest-di-1832357395.

331. Spiro, L.N. (April 27, 2003). Dentists pitch in when disaster strikes. New York Times, https://www.nytimes.com/2003/04/27/nyregion/dentists-pitch-in-when-disaster-strikes.html (accessed, 12/19/2021).

332. Hardy, R. and McKinney, (October 8, 2008). The unaccounted deaths. Green Party Watch. website; http://www.greenpartywatch.org/2008/10/08/mckinney-the-unaccounted-deaths.

333. Spencer, J. and Wortzel, L. (April 8, 2002). The role of the National Guard in homeland defense. The Heritage Foundation. https://www.heritage.org/homeland-security/report/the-role-the-national-guard-homeland-security.

334. Williams, L. (February 4, 2020). National Guard civil support teams ready to respond. National Guard website, https://www.nationalguard.mil/News/Article/2074024/national-guard-civil-support-teams-ready-to-respond.

335. Bynum, J. (May 21, 2010). Mass fatality training integrates Air Guard recovery teams, National Guard website. https://www.nationalguard.mil/News/Article-View/Article/577250/mass-fatality-training-integrates-air-guard-recovery-teams.

336. Schroeder, K.B. (2002). Failing to prevent the tragedy, but facing the Trauma: The aviation disaster family assistance act of 1996 and the air transportation safety and system stabilization act of 2001, 67. *J Air L & Com* 189: https://scholar.smu.edu/jalc/vol67/iss1/9.

337. Hall, J. and Evans, D. (2004-2008). Family assistance in air disasters: Much progress, more to be done. *Issues in Aviat L & Policy* 19091: 33021–2006. https://heinonline.org/HOL/LandingPage?handle=hein.journals/isavialp2&div=46&id=&page=.

338. Airlines Help Traumatized Family Members After Major Disasters (March 8, 2014). NBC News, https://www.nbcnews.com/storyline/missing-jet/airlines-help-traumatized-family-members-after-major-disasters-n48041.

339. Federal Assistance Plan for Aviation Disasters, NTSB (2000). http://www.disastersrus.org/emtools/aircrash/SPC9903.pdf.

340. DMORT Standard Operating Procedures for National Transportation Safety Board Activations (2006). https://nsri.nebraska.edu/-/media/nsri/documents/ndms2020/dmort-ntsb-sop-nov-2006.pdf.

341. National Association of Medical Examiners Standard Operating Procedures for Mass Fatality Management (2010). NAME. website; https://www.thename.org/assets/docs/31434c24-8be0-4d2c-942a-8afde79ec1e7.pdf.

342. NAME Inspection and Accreditation Checklist, A7. (2018). https://www.thename.org/inspection-accreditation.

343. Ritter, N. (2007). Identifying remains: Lessons learned from 9/11, NCJ 216527. *NIJ J* 256: 20–26. https://nij.ojp.gov/topics/articles/identifying-remains-lessons-learned-911.

344. Biesecker, L., Bailey-Wilson, J.E., Ballantyne, J., Baum, H., Bieber, F.R., Brenner, C., Budowle, B., Butler, J.M., Carmody, G., Conneally, P.M., Duceman, B., Eisenberg, A., Forman, L., Kidd, K.K., Leclair, B., Niezgoda, S., Parson, T.J., Pugh, E., Shaler, R., Sherry, S.T., Sozer, W., and Walsh, A. (2005). DNA identifications after the 9/11 world trade center attack. *Science* 310 (5751): 1122–1123. 10.1126/science.1116608.

345. Technical Working Group on Mass Fatality Forensic Identification (2005). *Mass Fatality Incidents: A Guide for Human Forensic Identification*. NCJ 199758. Washington, DC: NIJ. https://nij.ojp.gov/library/publications/mass-fatality-incidents-guide-human-forensic-identification.

346. Ritter, N. (2007). Missing persons and unidentified remains: The silent mass disaster, NCJ 216527. *NIJ J* 256: 2–7. https://www.ncjrs.gov/pdffiles1/nij/jr000256.pdf.

347. National Incident Management System, FEMA website; https://www.fema.gov/national-incident-management-system.

348. National Incident Management System (2017). 3rd ed., https://www.fema.gov/media-library-data/1508151197225-ced8c60378c3936adb92c1a3ee6f6564/FINAL_NIMS_2017.pdf.

349. Scientific Working Groups, NIST website; https://www.nist.gov/oles/scientific-working-groups.

350. Butler, J.M. (2017). Recent activities in the United States involving the National commission on forensic science and the organization of scientific area committees for forensic science. *Austral J For Sci* 49 (5): 526–540. 10.1080/00450618.2016.1243153.

351. Disaster Victim Identification Subcommittee, NIST OSAC website; https://www.nist.gov/topics/organization-scientific-area-committees-forensic-science/disaster-victim-identification.

352. ASB Consensus Bodies, AAFS ASB website; http://asb.aafs.org/wp-content/uploads/2016/02/ConsensusBodyDefinitions2-2016.pdf.

353. OSAC DVI Subcommittee *op cit.*

354. ASB Published Documents, AAFS ASB website; http://www.asbstandardsboard.org/published-documents/disaster-victim-identification-published-documents.

355. OSAC Registry, NIST webpage; https://www.nist.gov/osac/osac-registry.

CHAPTER 3

Quality Assurance in Disaster Victim Identification

The Case for Standards

Jason M Wiersema and Michal L Pierce

Harris County Institute of Forensic Sciences, Houston, TX, USA

3.1 Introduction

Disaster Victim Identification (DVI) is the application of the forensic and medicolegal sciences to investigations of incidents involving multiple fatalities. Successful application of these sciences in the context of the aftermath of a chaotic scenario requires planning and preparedness to ensure that the quality of service that a local jurisdiction maintains for daily casework is also maintained in the DVI response. There is a real need for both best practice and minimum standards guidance for local jurisdictions interested in appropriately equipping themselves to respond to a scenario involving multiple fatalities. This type of planning and preparedness is often complicated, for local medicolegal jurisdictions, by the fact that they: (1) likely have little or no experience in DVI response and (2) are often under-resourced even for their daily operations. In addition, medicolegal death investigation (MDI) is managed in highly variable ways, and this degree of variability in the structure and function of local medicolegal jurisdictions presents a considerable obstacle to standardization in how these varied entities can and will respond.

Disaster Victim Identification in the 21st Century: A US Perspective, First Edition.
Edited by John A Williams and Victor W Weedn.

The terms "guideline," "best practice," and "standard" are often used interchangeably when discussing the creation of shared documents or methods. These terms are related, but not equivalent. A best practice is generally defined as a method or technique that has consistently shown results superior to those achieved with other means, and that is used as a benchmark (BusinessDictionary 2020). A guideline is meant to be a suggestion that provides direction. Meanwhile, a standard, for our purposes, is an approved model, something considered by an authority or by general consent as a basis for comparison. Standards are meant to establish "a way of doing things"; this is why the term "standardize" is commonly used in process management discussions (ISO 2020).

If many entities follow the same best practices, or guidance, they may come closer to standardizing the system, but not exactly; there will be several similarities in actions or behaviors, but not necessarily in the outcomes. Best practices and guidelines are not enforceable either. Furthermore, a lack of adherence to guidelines and best practices does not always imply a lack of quality, depending on the situation at hand. When a set of minimum standards are accepted and used within a field or discipline, however, those standards establish expectations for the practice, behavior, and outcomes. Additionally, standards allow for a means to compare one entity (or operation) to another, speaking to their quality, and, where applicable, their technical competence. Most importantly, standards can be enforced as part of a government or other authoritative mandate.

3.2 The Need for Standards in MDI

The gaps in the daily practice of the medicolegal authority, and the consequent need for standards and best practices, are well understood among medicolegal practitioners. The 2009 National Academy of Sciences (NAS) publication entitled "Strengthening Forensic Science in the United States: A Path Forward" brought political and public attention to what was no surprise to medicolegal authorities, the shortcomings of the US system of forensic and medicolegal sciences. The paper pointed out in detail that these shortcomings apply to daily casework and by extension to scenarios involving surges in caseload.

The report notes that the forensic science disciplines "[t]oo often have inadequate educational programs, and they typically lack mandatory and enforceable standards, founded on rigorous research and testing, certification requirements, and accreditation programs," and that specific to medicolegal authorities, "more rigorous efforts are needed in the areas of accreditation and adherence to standards" (NRC 2009)

The NAS report identifies the lack of consistency in the structure and function of the medicolegal system in the United States as the root of the inconsistent application of best practices in death investigation. This is not a new opinion from the NAS. The agency first publicly identified this problem in 1928. In that year, the NAS National Research Council (NRC) convened the Committee on Medical Legal Problems who issued a critical review entitled "The Coroner and the Medical Examiner," and suggested the abolishment of the coroner concept altogether, based in their view, on its demonstrable incapacity to perform the functions required of it (NRC 1928). The NRC continued to argue for standardization of the death investigation system in subsequent reports, and in 1968 created the Committee on Forensic Pathology to again issue a report (NRC 1968). The concerns identified in the report are specific to the practice, training, and availability of forensic pathologists, all of which remain today (Hanzlick 2006).

In 1954, the Uniform Law Commission generated the "Model Postmortem Examinations Act" that provided states with guidance for the development of medical examiner systems (NCCUS 1954). The publication of this report was followed by an increase in the 1960s, 1970s, and 1980s of states converting from coroner to medical examiner systems (Hanzlick 2014b). The National Commission on Forensic Sciences voted to adopt a similar recommendation in 2017 (NCFS 2017). The trend from coroner to medical examiner systems has since waned for reasons logistical and political (Hanzlick 2007). The governmental and political constraints to advancing the death investigation system were addressed in a contentious symposium held in 1985, and organized by the National Association of Counties, entitled "Death Investigation in the Community: Forging New Partnerships." The goal of the symposium was to improve the quality of death investigation in the United States, but a formal report was never released (Hanzlick 2014c).

The lack of consistent quality of practice in death investigation in the United States has been long recognized, and remains in large part unchanged. Most recently (2019) the National Institute of Justice (NIJ) authored a report to Congress entitled "Needs Assessment of Forensic Laboratories and Medical Examiner/Coroner Offices" that summarizes the progress made since the 2009 NAS report (NIJ 2019). The report authors suggest that "[t]here is still great variability in the practice of death investigation across the United States, as jurisdictions struggle to procure and retain needed resources," and that "[v]ariability in MDI capabilities and services can result in the inequitable application of death investigations, which may have deleterious effects on the fair administration of justice."

3.3 The Need for Standards in DVI

DVI scenarios result in cases that have to be managed in excess of daily caseload burden. For this reason, local MDI jurisdictions must maintain realistic plans for DVI response. These DVI plans are best structured continuity of operations guides, ensuring that a jurisdiction has in place the resources and strategies necessary to accommodate a surge in caseload while maintaining quality operations. Plans must both account for the array and combination of complexities that a scenario may present, and ensure adherence to MDI best practices and standards. However, even if MDI operations are managed well in a particular jurisdiction, the circumstances of a particular DVI incident can differ sufficiently from daily operations, that standards of practice for MDI are best considered a prerequisite rather than a template for DVI. For this reason, there is a need for DVI specific best practices and standards.

Ramped-up or otherwise enhanced MDI operations are often insufficient for the effective management of a DVI response. DVI-specific guidance is needed for the application of even the most fundamental MDI operations in a DVI response. Identification, for example, can be a wholly different process following a mass fatality incident than with daily cases. The focus of the identification of daily medical examiner cases is the expeditious identification of a body, most frequently by contextual identifiers and/or fingerprints. Body fragmentation of the type that can characterize a mass fatality incident instead requires both the identification of body parts and the reconciliation or reuniting of those parts as an individual. In addition, mass fatality incidents often distort, render unreliable, or altogether erase the contextual information that can lend support to an identification. Personal effects, body location, tattoos, etc. can be removed, displaced, or destroyed, compromising their utility as identifying characteristics. These factors have a variety of logistical implications, including the need for a case numbering system that can accommodate body parts and individuals, and can facilitate reconciliation of the two without overcomplicating the process. Experience-based guidelines for identification in the DVI context are of critical importance to local jurisdictions when faced with a response scenario that is fully distinct from daily casework.

Recovery of remains in the DVI context can be highly variable and can even change during the course of a single response, and the process is often completely distinct from the typical MDI scene that a jurisdiction may be accustomed to managing. The environment may be contaminated, unstable, or otherwise unsafe, or have characteristics that prolong recovery and/or necessitate more detailed mapping of a site than is required of a standard MDI scene. These scenes may require specialized equipment and or training that are best acquired prior to an event.

Evidence management can vary widely from the scenes of accidents or disasters for which civil litigation may follow, to scenarios that are more likely to involve future criminal proceedings. Similarly, management of personal property in the DVI context often varies considerably from daily operations, and best practice for property management, particularly unassociated items, may best exclude the medicolegal authority from involvement.

Personnel constraints are often the most difficult to contend with. Responder safety and wellbeing must be taken into account. MDI jurisdictions are frequently understaffed for daily casework, and for these jurisdictions it may be best practice to develop rapidly actionable contracts for mutual aid in transport, scene response, and/or postmortem examination. It may be that a local jurisdiction can leverage cross training of internal staff or staff from other local agencies. Whatever the solution, it must be reconciled with the need for the MDI jurisdiction to remain in its purview and avoid mission creep between agencies.

Invariably, along with all of these considerations come unrealistic expectations on the part of local political, emergency management, public health, and/or other officials as well as the public for the management of an incident. These expectations are often accompanied by external pressure to expedite processes. For this reason, best practice for DVI always necessitates clear communication of the considerations that partner agencies and the lay public should take into account as they assess local DVI operations, including likely prolonged identification and notification of families, etc.

3.4 History of Standards Development in DVI

Much like some of the other forensic science disciplines, there has not been a reputable single source of guidance for MDI and/or DVI until recently. In the past, some forensic communities have nominated groups of people to work toward standards and best practices for their disciplines, but they have operated independently from each other which led to some degree of problematic overlap between documents. These groups, known as scientific working groups (SWG), technical working groups (TWG), or steering committees, were collections of experts with variable funding that recognized the need for standards, and may even have developed them, and went so far as to seek review and input from other experts, the users of the standards, and the general public. The earliest of these groups were formed in the 1980s and 1990s, but the majority of them did not assemble until after 2000.

The DVI community first established a working group in 2010. The group, developed via partnership between the National Transportation Safety Board and the Federal Bureau of Investigation, was named the Scientific Working Group on Disaster Victim Identification (SWGDVI), and was a large collection of internationally recognized responders to multiple fatality incidents large and small, brief and prolonged, criminal and natural. The group was convened to develop best guidance for local coroner/medical examiner jurisdictions interested in preparing for mass fatality response. Unlike most of the SWGs that focus on a single science and its application to forensics, the SWGDVI was tasked with developing best practices for the application of various disciplines (pathology, anthropology, DNA, friction ridge, etc.) in the mass fatality setting. For this reason, there was considerable overlap in the content of the SWGDVI documents and those of other SWGs, and the composition of the SWGDVI was much more multidisciplinary than other SWGs.

From its inception in 2010 SWGDVI membership made the decision to develop best practice guidance rather than minimum standards. The members felt it was too difficult to create documents vague enough that would assist a wide range of local jurisdictions, and that detailed documents should be used as planning guidance for local jurisdictions rather than as minimum standards for DVI practice. The group ultimately generated a significant number of documents that provided guidance for general management of DVI incidents to specific guidance on the collection of fingerprints from heavily decomposed decedents. SWGDVI was disbanded with the development of its successor, the DVI Subcommittee of the Organization of Scientific Area Committees (OSAC), in 2014.

3.5 Organization of Scientific Area Committees (OSAC)

Even with the valuable work conducted by the various SWGs, the forensic sciences generally, and DVI specifically, were not adhering to a key tenet of the 2009 NAS report, which was the standardization of practice. The SWGs operated independently and produced overlapping guidance without a mechanism to reconcile the overlap. In 2014, the National Institute of Standards and Technology (NIST) partnered with the NIJ to construct the OSAC. The OSAC is a collaborative body of more than 500 forensic science practitioners and other experts deliberately selected to ensure representation by all levels of the government (federal, state, and local), academia, and industry. The body was divided into Scientific Area Committees that address broad areas of forensic science (crime scene and death investigation, for example) and smaller Subcommittees that address more specific subfields (including DVI). The OSAC replaced most of the SWGs, and its structure ensures consistent oversight of process that did not characterize the varied efforts of the SWGs.

Unfortunately, the OSAC is not a standards development organization (SDO), which means that it cannot publish its own standards. This requires that the subcommittees who generate standards or best practice guidance must select an external SDO to review and publish the OSAC documents. In some cases, relevant SDOs did not exist. The American Academy of Forensic Sciences (AAFS) was among the entities that developed novel SDOs (the AAFS SDO is called the Academy Standards Board [ASB]). While the SDO process prolongs the publication of standards and best practices, sometimes by years, the process does result in extensive review of all OSAC products. Once the OSAC documents make their way through the SDO process, and are published by that SDO, they are eligible for posting on the OSAC Registry. The OSAC Registry is the manifestation of all that the OSAC was developed for – a central location for jurisdictions seeking minimum standards or best practices for the forensic sciences that (1) communicates to the reader that the guidance is developed by experts in the field; (2) has had detailed review by legal, quality, and human factors experts; and (3) has been vetted by a separate panel of experts (SDO) without vested influence in the specific language of the document. A large number of standards and best practices are currently present on the registry from each of the SACs, and range in scope from baseline language documents for a particular discipline to detailed procedures for the collection of evidence.

3.6 Discussion

The need for standards and best practice is well known for the forensic sciences generally, and this certainly applies to medicolegal death investigation and disaster victim identification. Without sound guidance and standards for practice, even experienced professionals who conduct quality medicolegal death investigations on a daily basis may stumble into difficulty because of a lack of awareness of how mass fatality complicates response at all levels, granular and strategic. For example, the development of a complicated case numbering system without the prerequisite software to manage it is not valuable.

Similarly, jurisdictions who have prepared themselves for DVI operations but have not ensured that its partner agencies are similarly prepared will likely have difficulty adhering to their own best practices. If, for instance, the medical examiner/coroner has not coordinated disaster-related death reporting/tracking prior to an incident in adherence to best practice, doing so after the incident will be unnecessarily complicated, and the strategy adopted is less likely to be scientifically and strategically sound.

Without standardized guidance developed via the processes described above, local jurisdictions have only local plans from other jurisdictions, and all-hazards federal guidance to refer to. The former are often too specific to a particular jurisdiction's capabilities to be applicable elsewhere, and the latter are focused on the structure and operation of a scalable disaster response rather than best practices for the individual components of a mass fatality response. Although the federal disaster preparedness guidance is critical to successful local DVI operations, and medical examiner/coroner jurisdictions should ensure that they are aware of the federal strategy for disaster response, best practices for DVI cannot be to simply defer to the federal government for assistance.

The Department of Homeland Security (DHS) maintains the National Response Framework (NRF), which provides the overarching strategy for management of local disasters (DHS 2019). Its premise is that all disasters are local. The NRF details the scalable strategy adopted by the federal government for stepwise disaster (including mass fatality) assistance that progresses from local requests for assistance, to state, and then to federal, assistance if needed. The guidance in the framework is based on response to its National Planning Scenarios. These scenarios were first developed by the Homeland Security Council in 2003. The Council established fifteen all-hazards planning scenarios that are an integral part of the department's capabilities-based strategy for the ensuring the successful implementation of Homeland Security Presidential Directive 8 (HSPD-8). DHS used these scenarios to develop homeland security tasks, target capabilities, standards, and performance metrics that serve as a basis for assessing national preparedness. It is this assessment that informs the department's investment in assistance to state, local, and tribal governments.

The scenarios include terrorist attacks, nuclear attacks, improvised explosive attacks, radiological attacks, biological attacks, etc., scenarios that are often foreign and intimidating to smaller, particularly rural jurisdictions that might instead be seeking guidance for the management of smaller incidents for which there will not be a federal response. Understanding of and compliance with the NRF is key to the successful management of all scales of DVI incidents, but the NRF is not a source for specific DVI management best practices.

3.7 Adoption of Standards

There has been a stepwise progression in the right direction, starting with recognition of the problem by members of the death investigation community and by external entities like the NAS. Development of the SWGs resulted in a large number of guidance documents and the consolidation of these efforts under the OSAC umbrella greatly increased the consistency and longevity of the process. There is more to be done, however, to achieve OSAC's dual goal of developing sound standards and guidelines and promoting their use throughout the forensic community. The latter aspiration, to promote the use of standards, may prove to be even more challenging than developing the standard themselves. Just as the OSAC is not an SDO, neither is it a regulatory body. Therefore, it does not have the authority to enforce the use of standards (or even best practices). Yet truly, by pledging to "promote," or "encourage" the use of, we mean we want the forensic community to actually utilize or follow the standards. Standards that sit dormant in a registry, or that are adopted only by a few, are not serving to uniformly advance forensic practice.

Realistically, asking for voluntary adoption of standards developed and promoted by OSAC will not lead to the desired result. Just as in any industry, legal and regulatory factors have the potential to influence the strategic plans in forensic science. Two historic changes within the crime laboratory community serve to illustrate this point: First, in 2003, a provision was added to the Texas Code of Criminal Procedure that required state-recognized accreditation of any crime laboratory or other entity that was conducting forensic analyses of physical evidence for use in criminal proceedings (TLC 2003). Second, in the same year, the American Society of Crime Laboratory Directors/ Laboratory Accreditation Board (ASCLD/LAB), one of the main accrediting bodies of crime laboratories at the time, voted to transition their accreditation program to incorporate the ISO/IEC 17025 standard – *General requirements for the competence of testing and calibration laboratories*, in an effort to advance the quality of accredited laboratories (Pyrek 2018). Other accreditation bodies with forensic programs made the same move around that time. Consequently, every crime laboratory in the state of Texas that served to furnish government witnesses eventually became accredited under a program that adhered to an International Standard.

Some laboratories were prepared for this change and embraced the accreditation and oversight, while some laboratories did not perceive this as a positive change. Nonetheless, they adapted, and likely required a boost in funding to do it, which was easy to justify given the new regulation. The change would never have happened in Texas without the accreditation bodies adopting the standard or the government statute mandating a specific type of laboratory accreditation. The stakeholders of crime laboratory services ultimately benefitted; there is now a statewide guarantee that providers of these services adhere to the standard for which experts in most countries deem to foster quality and technical competence.

Although Texas was the first state to require crime laboratory accreditation by law, other states followed its example. That is not to say only laboratories in those states are currently accredited; plenty of crime laboratories around the world embrace voluntary accreditation to demonstrate adherence to standards. It has come to a point that the "reputable" crime laboratories are accredited, and accredited to programs incorporating International Standards. This was an evolution of concept; it did not happen overnight. For instance, studies conducted by the Bureau of Justice Statistics showed the percentage of publicly funded crime laboratories (federal, state, county, and municipal) that were accredited jumped from 70% in 2002 to almost 90% by 2014, with the state crime laboratories hitting 99% (Burch and Durose 2016). These statistics were remarkable, given that the accreditation rate of crime laboratories in the mid- to late 1990s was estimated to be around 50% (Steadman 2000). The same evolution is possible in MDI and DVI, where accreditation is neither mandatory nor a popular concept yet. It takes perseverance of the leading scientific committee members and also a united stand on the importance of implementing standards in the field.

3.8 Conclusion

Without the existence of standards and their enforcement we cannot address the concerns of the NAS. The stakeholders of MDI and DVI deserve the same quality of service, as do those of other forensic disciplines, such as the end users of crime laboratory testing. The DVI subcommittee of OSAC, and the DVI consensus body of the ASB, should continue on the path toward developing sound standards and best practice guidelines for the community, as these would equip the jurisdictions, at all levels, with adequate knowledge and plans for mass fatality management. Equally important, there should be a push from within to work with both accreditation providers and legislative bodies to ensure adoption. Compliance with a standard or requirement is best confirmed by external assessment by a qualified entity, which is where accreditation programs come into play. Federal, state, or local statutes are powerful on their own, not only setting a precedent for what is expected, but also helpful in facilitating the necessary funding and resources required to bring each jurisdiction up to par, in terms of preparedness. Regulation would assist with closing the gap between large, urban agencies and smaller, remote ones so that any stakeholder of DVI services would be granted the same quality of response and service, no matter where they reside.

References

Burch, A.M. and Durose, M.R. (2016). *Publicly Funded Forensic Crime Laboratories: Quality Assurance Practices, 2014 [Online]*. Washington DC: United States Department of Justice. Office of Justice Programs, Bureau of Justice Statistics Bulletin (2016). Available at: http://www.bjs.gov/index.cfm?ty=pbdetail&iid=5828 (accessed 2 December 2019).

BusinessDictionary (2020) *Best practice* [online]. Available at: http://www.businessdictionary.com/definition/best-practice.html (Accessed 16 September 2020).

DHS (2019). *National Response Framework,* fourth edition. Department of Homeland Security.

Hanzlick, R. (2006). Medical examiners, coroners, and public health: a review and update. *Archives of Pathology and Laboratory Medicine* 130(9): 1274–1282.

Hanzlick, R. (2007). The conversion of coroner systems to medical examiners in the us: a lull in the action. *American Journal of Forensic Medicine and Pathology* 28 (4): 279–283.

Hanzlick, R. (2014a). A synoptic review of the 1954 model postmortem examinations act. *Academic Forensic Pathology* 4 (4): 451–454.

Hanzlick, R. (2014b). A synoptic review of the 1985 wingspread symposium on death investigation. *Academic Forensic Pathology* 4 (4): 459–462.

ISO (2020). *Standards* [online]. Available at: https://www.iso.org/standards.html (accessed 16 September 2020).

NCCUS (1954). *Model Post-mortem Examinations Act.* Chicago: National Conference of Commissioners on Uniform State Laws.

NCFS (2017). *Model Legislation for Medicolegal Death Investigations Systems.* National Commission on Forensic Sciences Medicolegal Death Investigation Subcommittee, Recommendation to the Attorney General https://www.justice.gov/archives/ncfs/page/file/934406/download.

NIJ (2019). *National Institute of Justice Office of Justice Programs, Report to Congress: 2019 NIJ Report to Congress Needs Assessment: Needs Assessment of Forensic Laboratories and Medical Examiner/coroner Offices.* Washington, DC: Office of Justice Programs.

NRC (1928). The coroner and the medical examiner. In: *Bulletin of the National Research Council* (Eds. O.T. Schultz and E.M. Morgan), No. 64. Washington DC: National research Council.

NRC (1968). *A Progress Report on Forensic Pathology.* Washington DC: National Academy of Sciences, National Research Council.

NRC (2009). *Strengthening Forensic Science in the United States a Path Forward.* Washington DC: The National Academies Press.

Pyrek, K.M. (2018). *Pioneers in Forensic Science: Innovations and Issues in Practice.* Boca Raton: CRC Press.

Steadman, G.W. (2000). *Survey of DNA Crime Laboratories.* 1998. Washington DC: United States Department of Justice, Office of Justice Programs, Bureau of Justice Statistics Special Report.

TLC (2003). *Summary of Enactments: 78th Legislature, Regular Session 1st, 2nd, 3rd Called Sessions.* Austin, Texas: Texas Legislative Council. November.

CHAPTER 4

Medical Examiners, Coroners, and Public and Private Agencies

John A. Williams[1] and Jason Wiersema[2]

[1]*Department of Anthropology and Sociology, Western Carolina University, Cullowhee, NC, USA*
[2]*Harris County Institute of Forensic Science, Houston, TX, USA*

4.1 Introduction

In the United States the legal identification of human remains, whether in the context of a single individual or mass mortality, is a function of the medical examiner/coroner (ME/C) system (Hanzlick and Combs 1998). The statutory duties and capacities of the medical examiner/coroner or medicolegal jurisdiction vary widely by state and especially by population density and case load (Carroll et al. 2017; NIJ 2005). No two medicolegal jurisdictions will necessarily respond to a mass fatality incident (MFI) in the same manner. What then is an MFI? Given that any jurisdiction might have a different response from the next jurisdiction, a simple definition of a mass fatality event would be any situation where the number of deaths exceeds the local capability to handle them (Gershon et al. 2014; NAME 2010). For a small jurisdiction, this might even be as little as a single death. Whereas the medicolegal jurisdiction in a large population center might easily accommodate a hundred fatalities without straining local resources. Local capacity can also be viewed from the perspective of expertise. Even a medical examiner/coroner who performs hundreds of autopsies annually may be overwhelmed not only by the sheer magnitude and extent of a mass fatality event

Disaster Victim Identification in the 21st Century: A US Perspective, First Edition.
Edited by John A Williams and Victor W Weedn.

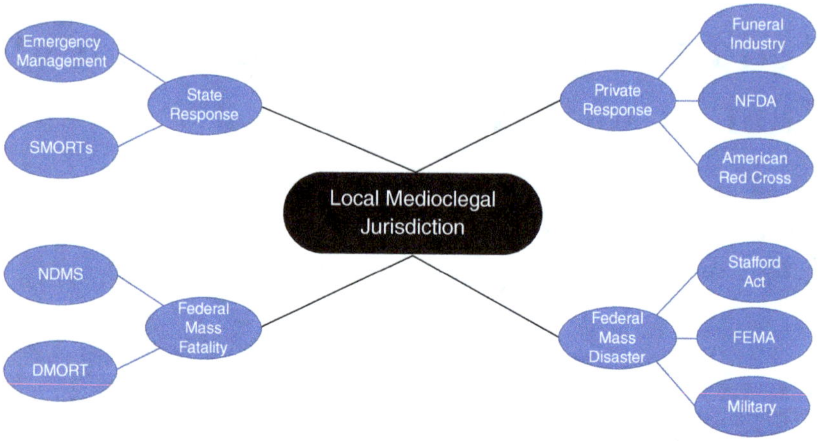

Figure 4.1 The mass fatality response framework and extra-jurisdictional responding assets. In the event of an MFI the ME/C can potentially draw from various sources. The nature of the disaster will dictate which assets are tapped into.

but also by the ancillary functions accompanying such an event. In the aftermath of a mass fatality incident the identification of victims sometimes becomes secondary to the need to store victims, process the disaster scene, and handle media relations. Disaster victim identification (DVI) complicates and often synergistically amplifies the coordination of efforts of the medicolegal jurisdiction. An additional factor is the lack of trained forensic pathologists to handle the growing case load medicolegal jurisdictions have been facing (Hanzlick 2003). At some point, either by numbers or by experience, the local medicolegal jurisdiction will be taxed beyond the abilities of the local system (Merrill et al. 2017). When this point is reached, extra-jurisdictional agencies enter (Figure 4.1). The sheer surge volume of COVID-19 deaths in the city of New York in early 2020 led to the deployment of DMORT (see Section 4.4) to assist with the processing of and care for the deceased victims of this disease. This is one example of the complex interrelationship of the ME/C and state and federal responses to mass fatality incidents.

4.2 The Medical Examiner/Coroner System

Today, within the United States approximately 2000 medical examiner/coroner jurisdictional units exist (Hanzlick 2003). Some form part of a centralized state-run system. Others are a hybrid of coroners and medical examiners (Fierro 2003). Still, medicolegal death investigation is primarily a local function. Even states that operate state-level medical examiner systems often have death investigators dispersed on the county level. Outside of this local focus, there is little else that can be considered standard practice in the American death investigation system. The system is characterized by vast differences in approach, personnel, jurisdiction, capability, and funding. Regardless of their size and capability, most medicolegal jurisdictions are either under-resourced or retain very limited capacity for surge, and are thus presented with personnel, logistical, and resource difficulties with even minor shifts and/or surges in caseload.

For these reasons, MFIs present significant obstacles to the continuity of ME/C operations. In addition to a surge in caseload, MFIs often present circumstances that vary considerably from the daily casework that an office may be accustomed to and thus prepared for. Decedents may be fragmented and/or otherwise damaged, commingled or incomplete. Contamination, biological and/or chemical, is often associated with MFIs, as are atypical logistical complications like prolonged or delayed recovery or unusual commingling of human remains and evidence/property. These circumstances often co-occur and can have significant impacts on even the most basic ME/C functions. Some impacts are readily recognized. An ME/C facility may, for example, become suddenly inadequate or inappropriate to manage cases because of either volume or contamination, among other things. Other more subtle impacts can have immediate and confounding downstream implications that permeate multiple functions. For example, the need to adopt an alternate or additional case numbering system because of fragmentation invariably has downstream effects on decedent identification and reconciliation. The choice of case numbering can additionally impact sampling and testing for laboratory tests and on communication with families, i.e., when and how often to notify families of the identification of fragmentary remains (see Chapter 9).

MFI preparedness among ME/C jurisdictions varies at least as much as the basic components of ME/C operations. Some, primarily larger jurisdictions have robust integrated preparedness programs that include detailed integrated interdepartmental standard operating procedures, jurisdiction-specific planning strategies, equipment and materials caches, training and exercise programs, and reliable and well-conceived relationships with relevant partner agencies. Others have solid internal capabilities but are inadequately integrated with external agencies, and yet others are completely ill prepared. There are many small medicolegal jurisdictions that maintain unreliable and inappropriate expectations regarding the provision of external support from either state or federal agencies or both. These expectations are not compatible with the local provenience of the ME/C function. In addition, responses to MFIs also often involve the need for resources that are not practical, and may be irresponsible, to retain outside of emergency circumstances. For example, the acquisition and retention of large caches of atypical PPE (personal protective equipment) or investment in the training needed to remain current on its use may be difficult to reconcile with workload and other resource needs. ME/C offices are regularly dependent on partnerships with other governmental and private entities (e.g., toxicology laboratories) for their daily casework, but have often not incorporated surge into their relationships with these entities. Outside of the agencies that they are bound to by virtue of their daily casework, ME/Cs are often poorly or inadequately integrated into their local governmental structure, even with agencies that have roles in emergency response.

Meaningful and reliable MFI preparedness requires significant investment of both time and resources on the local level, and is thus not pervasive among ME/Cs, and among those that have invested in preparedness there is considerable variation in approach. Most efforts toward preparedness begin internally. Thus, it is important to understand that a siloed approach to preparedness ignores the possibility that other government agencies may have capabilities to bring to bear in response to an MFI and that can mitigate the resource burden of preparedness. The use of PPE illustrates the varied preparedness capabilities of ME/C jurisdictions. Each acquires and uses PPE for their daily caseload. Specialized, unfamiliar PPE may be needed following an MFI, and those needs can vary considerably based on the circumstances of a particular MFI. The notion that MFI preparedness requires that an ME/C should not only acquire PPE appropriate for any combination of MFI circumstances, but that the acquisition of PPE should also be accompanied by training and replacement program sufficient to ensure its utility (if it's ever needed) is unreasonable. There are, however, local agencies who are qualified to use this equipment because they use them regularly, and in all likelihood will have their own role in the event anyway. Coordination of these capabilities with the needs of the ME/C has the added benefit of preventing agencies from stumbling into each other's lanes.

Some incidents will exceed a local ME/Cs capacity regardless of local preparedness efforts, and for this reason local ME/C efforts benefit from identifying specific threshold metrics and a robust extra-local component of their preparedness strategy. Extra-local coordination can take many forms depending on the structure of a particular state's death investigation system. The most successful leverage existing, non-medicolegal, mutual aid structures. Texas for example has TMORT, a mutual aid system that operates as a component of a broader state rapid deployment function, the Texas Emergency Medical Task force (EMTF).

4.3 The US Federal Government and Mass Disasters

When the United States was formed the Constitution designated specific functions to the federal government, with the remainder being under the province of the individual states. At a time when most Americans lived outside of large urban areas the Founding Fathers could not have envisioned that one day one of the roles of the government would be to assist in the mitigation of large-scale disasters. Yet barely 25 years had passed since the inception of the United States when, in December of 1802, the port-city of Portsmouth, New Hampshire, was impacted by a series of disastrous fires. These fires affected Portsmouth's and the Northeast's ability to conduct trade and commerce. The federal response to this disaster was the Congressional Relief Act of 1803. This legislation granted tariff (tax) relief until the city could rebuild. This was the first in a long series of federal responses to large-scale disasters (Merrill et al. 2016). For the next 150 years disaster mitigation was similarly individual in nature and scope, created ad hoc and anew for each disaster (FEMA 2019a). There was no overarching process of planning for and implementation of disaster response. Responses to the Great Chicago Fire and San Francisco earthquake, as destructive as these two events were to these cities, were primarily local with minimal federal contributions.

The federal response to catastrophic disasters would continue to be revisited over much of the twentieth century. The first comprehensive legislation regarding disasters was the 1950 Federal Disaster Assistance Program. This granted the president the power to determine whether a disaster warranted a federal response and the nature and degree of that response. While this legislation, for the first time, created a mechanism to initiate federal response mitigation, it remained primarily reactive in nature. The Cold War and ever-present natural disasters shifted the emphasis of the federal response more and more toward planning and not just mitigation. As the 1950s progressed into the 1970s newer versions of the Federal Disaster Relief Act were passed by Congress. During this time the Federal Disaster Assistance Administration was created as a function of the Department of Housing and Urban Development. Despite these improvements in disaster response these federal actions remained mitigative in nature, most in the form of post-disaster tax relief or other monetary assistance.

As the 1970s came to a close the federal response to disasters, natural and man-made, changed. President Carter, by Executive Order 12127, created FEMA (Federal Emergency Management Agency) (FEMA 2019a). Multiple agencies from the Department of Defense to the National Weather Service were consolidated under the umbrella of FEMA. Initially, FEMA was a stand-alone agency, but following the terrorist attack of September 11, 2001, it was housed under the Department of Homeland Security (DHS). For the first time, with the formation of FEMA, preparedness *and* planning became a component of the federal disaster response process. Although FEMA is a federal agency responsible for a coordinated response to national disasters it retains somewhat of a local/regional influence. FEMA's activities are organized into 10 geographic regions. Each region consists of a minimum of four contiguous states, with coastal regions "responsible" for adjacent US territories. Thus, when FEMA responds to a disaster those in the region affected, those with the best knowledge of regional resources are usually the first to respond.

FEMA's role in disaster response and mitigation was further defined by the Disaster Relief Act of 1974 and later by the Robert T. Stafford Disaster Relief and Emergency Assistance Act (FEMA 2019b). Passed by Congress in 1988 and most recently revised in 2018, the Stafford Act establishes funding for disaster response as it pertains to a presidential disaster declaration. The Stafford Act further places an emphasis on state and local preparedness as an element of the federal disaster response.

The events of September 11, 2001, changed the landscape of the federal response to mass disasters. This was not the first time that terrorism had resulted in a loss of life within the continental borders of the United States. The 1995 bombing of the Murrah Federal building had already made us aware of the dangers we face in a free country. The magnitude of the World Trade Center disaster, in terms of both loss of life and damage to the World Trade Center complex, led in 2003 to the formation of the Department of Homeland Security. FEMA, once a stand-alone agency, was incorporated into DHS together with the National Disaster Medical Service (NDMS). The NDMS was formed in 1984 as a component of the US Public Health Service within the Department of Health and Human Services (HHS) and responds to health-related aspects of mass disasters. Disaster preparedness and mitigation now included terrorism together with hurricanes, earthquakes, and mass transit accidents. Shortly after the formation of the DHS came the establishment of the National Response Plan (NRP) of 2004 and the National Incident Management System (NIMS) (DHS 2004). Relying on the Incident Command System (ICS), the NRP and NIMS provided for a coordination of efforts across state and federal jurisdictions and private agencies to prepare for, prevent, and react to the variety of hazards the country was now facing. In 2008 the NRP was replaced by the National Response Framework (NRF) (FEMA 2019c).

One feature of both the NRP and NRF was the formation of the Emergency Support Functions (ESF) (FEMA 2008). There are 15 Emergency Support Functions as components of the National Response Plan and its successor the National Response Framework. The ESFs work to coordinate one or more federal agencies in response to a national disaster. They can be activated for both federally declared emergencies and non–Stafford act conditions. Common aspects of the ESFs include one primary responding agency, one or more supporting agencies, and a private sector liaison. Each ESF covers a mission that may occur as a result of a large-scale national disaster. For example, ESF 1 is Transportation, and accordingly the primary responding agency is the Department of Transportation. Each ESF is expanded through an Emergency Support Function Annex, which describes the role and function of the ESF. Continuing with ESF 1, following a disaster that impacts the transportation network, one basic and perhaps obvious Annex responsibility is to restore the transportation infrastructure. While in various ways each of the 15 ESFs can connect to DVI, it is ESF #8 that is most directly involved with the identification of mass fatality victims. ESF #8 is Public Health and Medical Services (FEMA 2016). The ESF #8 Annex lists four responsibilities: public health, medical health services, mental health services, and *Mass Fatality Management* (Tables 4.1, 4.2). The primary responding agency in 2020 for ESF #8 is the Department of Health and Human Services, although there are no fewer than 19 public and private supporting agencies for this ESF, including the US Postal Service and the American Red Cross. As HHS took on the responsibility for the medical response to national disasters the office of the Assistant Secretary for Preparedness and Response (ASPR) was formed (ASPR 2020). ASPR

Table 4.1 Role of emergency support function 8 (ESF #8), Public Health and Medical Services.

Public health
Medical health
Mental health services
Mass fatality management

Table 4.2 Core capability of ESF#8 as it applies to DVI (FEMA 2016).

Fatality Management Services
Assists jurisdictional medico-legal authorities and law enforcement agencies in the tracking and documenting of human remains and associated personal effects; reducing the hazard presented by chemically, biologically, or radiologically contaminated human remains (when indicated and possible); establishing temporary morgue facilities; determining the cause and manner of death; collecting antemortem data in a compassionate and culturally competent fashion from authorized individuals; performing postmortem data collection and documentation; identifying human remains using scientific means (e.g., dental, pathology, anthropology, fingerprints, and, as indicated, DNA samples); and preparing, processing, and returning human remains and personal effects to the authorized person(s) when possible; and providing technical assistance and consultation on fatality management and mortuary affair services. May provide behavioral health support to families of victims during the victim identification mortuary process.
May provide for temporary interment when permanent disposition options are not readily available

was created in 2006 following Hurricane Katrina and provides direct leadership and responsibility for the implementation of ESF 8.

4.4 Disaster Mortuary Operational Response Team

Although the ESFs were not defined until the formation of the National Response Plan in 2004, HHS was already the home agency for mass fatality management. As the twentieth century came to a close several airline accidents with large loss of life brought into focus the need for a better coordinated response to mass fatalities, and the processing and identification of victims. This culminated in the creation of the federal unit known as DMORT (HHS 2017). The concept of Disaster Mortuary Operational Response Teams grew, not from a federal initiative, but rather from the private sector. The National Funeral Directors Association (NFDA) in the late 1980s and early

1990s recognized the need for a coordinated effort in responding to mass fatality events. Sam Shepardson, later to be named the DMORT National Commander, and others in the NFDA began lobbying the federal government to enact policies that would eventually result in the creation of DMORT. In 1991 the National Foundation for Mortuary Care (NFMC) was founded. This collection of private professionals further set the stage for the creation of DMORT. Starting with a base of funeral directors and embalmers, members included dentists, anthropologists, medical examiners, and other death investigator specialists. This voluntary group of private individuals was organized around the ten FEMA regions. Each regional group was represented by a Regional Trustee. Not only did this serve as the model for DMORT organization, still in use today, but several of the NFMC officers and trustees went on to serve in the early administration of DMORT. The NFMC also established the first portable morgue and before the formation of DMORT, self-deployed to a number of mass fatality incidents. The use of the deployable portable morgue, of which there are now three, has been a signature feature of the DMORT response to mass fatalities.

The NFMC was active for less than half a decade when it was absorbed into or perhaps more correctly morphed into DMORT. By early 1994 DMORT was actively recruiting new members to fill out the roster of regional teams. Until just following the September 11th attack, HHS was the federal home for DMORT, within the larger umbrella of the National Disaster Medical Service. For a brief time starting in late 2001, NDMS moved to the Department of Homeland Security and then back to HHS in 2007. After more than a quarter century DMORT still reflects its origins in the NFMC and the actions of the NFDA. Its members are volunteers until deployed, at which time they become intermittent federal employees. Deployment itself is voluntary and a member can decline deployment. DMORT teams are arranged by FEMA region, with each team headed by a commander (reminiscent of the NFMC Regional Trustee). In the early years of DMORT administrative and team leader positions were often staffed, and many still are, by funeral directors. Even as intermittent federal employees, DMORT team members, when on deployment, are covered by the mandate of USERRA (Uniformed Services Employment and Reemployment Rights Act). The provisions of this Act prohibit employers from dismissing a DMORT member from their job due to deployment.

Each FEMA region-based team comprises various positions, some specialty-specific and some more broadly managerial. Technically, each team should be complete to the point that a morgue with all of its varied functions, including bureaucratic ones, can be staffed and deployed for the two-week standard period of deployment. Because each team is region-based the original philosophy was that a DMORT team would be available to be the first to respond to a regional disaster. Until recently, team sizes were limited more by geography and demography than by government dictate. This meant that some regional teams were heavily staffed at all positions while others were chronically under-represented. Changes in HHS philosophy regarding staffing have led to an overall reduction in team size and a more general size equity across DMORT (FEMA) regions.

In its early iteration, when DMORT was deployed to a mass fatality incident, a Family Assistance Center (FAC) was usually deployed as well. The FAC is now called the Victim Identification Center, or, more correctly, the Victim Information Center (VIC), to avoid confusion with other family-related functions of mass fatality response. The VIC gathers antemortem data from family and respondents. These data provide one branch of the identification process, the other provided by those who labor in the mass fatality morgue. Recently, the FAC/VIC was removed from DMORT and now deploys separately (see Chapter 9). Not all mass fatality events require a DMORT team response, nor do all DMORT team responses require a VIC. Separating the VIC from DMORT permits a flexible response to each event. Although no longer considered a direct DMORT asset, the VIC draws heavily from DMORT teams to staff itself, especially in long deployments. The morgue experience of DMORT members makes them ideal in understanding the needs of the identification process.

Although no longer in existence, throughout much of the 2000s, an eleventh DMORT team existed. The WMD (Weapons of Mass Destruction) team trained and was outfitted to process victims of radiation, chemical, and biologic disasters. Thankfully never deployed, this team provided DMORT with the ability to be truly all-hazards.

The NFMC pioneered the concept of the portable morgue. The DPMU (Disaster Portable Morgue Unit), as the portable morgue is now called, was designed to take the function of mass fatality processing and identification out of the local morgue. The goal was not to replace or subvert the local morgue, but to allow the medical examiner/coroner to continue with the normal activities of that office. The routine daily functions of the ME/C do not cease simply because an MFI has taken place within its jurisdiction. In this way, the mass fatality process would stay separate from the day-to-day functions of death investigation. There are currently three DPMUs, strategically stored across the lower 48 states: Frederick, MD; Fort Worth, TX; and San Jose, CA. Each DPMU is a full cache of the tools, supplies, and equipment necessary for a functional mass fatality morgue. The DPMUs are containerized and can be quickly transported where needed and set up rapidly.

Excluding transportation disasters, deployment of a DMORT team first requires a presidential disaster declaration. In anticipation of a deployment, an advance assessment team is sent to the disaster scene. This select group of logistic and forensic specialists determines the parameters of the mass fatality event. It is not uncommon upon reaching the scene to discover that there is no need for a DMORT deployment. There might be, for example, far fewer fatalities than originally thought or predicted, so that the local ME/C is not significantly impacted. The assessment team also determines how many forensic specialists and in what combinations are needed for the particular MFI response. For example, in 1993 DMORT responded to the Hardin MO cemetery displacement (often recorded as the first DMORT deployment). Overland flooding from the Mississippi River caused coffins to come to the ground surface. Forensic anthropologists, with their knowledge of the human skeleton, were the most needed. This illustrates one of the signature features of DMORT: flexibility and the ability to adjust to fit the needs of each deployment. This also highlights a feature of all mass fatality events, that no two are ever the same, even when the base cause of the mortality is the same (i.e., a transportation accident). The flexibility of the DMORT design is further seen in the ability to supplement a deployment team with members from another region. This is a routine occurrence in most large-scale, multi-week deployments.

Each of the ten DMORT teams is staffed by a variety of specialists (Table 4.3). The team begins with a commander, deputy commander, and administrative officers. The various forensic specialties, including anthropology, odontology, and pathology, are represented. Recently, the position of a DNA technician to properly extract DNA samples has been added. Other morgue workers include photographers, radiologists, body trackers, and IT technicians. Security is an important element of all that DMORT accomplishes, and the respectful treatment of the deceased is paramount. The DMORT morgue team is rounded out with embalmers who are often the last to view the remains before they are released. The standard deployment for a DMORT team or individual is two weeks (as covered by USERRA).

An additional, and not insignificant, function of the assessment team is the choice of where to place the DPMU. This will be dictated by the nature of the disaster event and the extent to which local resources and infrastructure have been impacted. Following Hurricane Katrina in 2004 much of the Gulf Coast was in total devastation and finding a building which could house the DPMU was problematic. The requirements for a

Table 4.3 DMORT team positions and specialists.

Team Commander
Deputy Commander
Administrative Officer
Anthropologist
DNA technician
Embalmer
Fingerprint specialist
Information technology
Medicolegal investigator
Odontologist
Pathologist
Photographer
Radiologist

DPMU site and the steps involved in morgue operations have been previously outlined by the various agencies involved in DVI (FEMA 2019a; Jensen 2000; NAME 2010). In the simplest terms a body or various forms (e.g., a dismembered appendage) of human remains enter the morgue and are triaged. An examination takes place at various "stations" at which time biological parameters and other features that may aid in identification are recorded. DMORT and other DVI agencies (see Section 4.6) rely on a software application called VIP (Victim Identification Profile). VIP takes antemortem data collected by the VIC and postmortem data collected in the morgue and finds preliminary matches. These are then reconciled as either a probable match or not. Probable matches are presented to the medical examiner/coroner who makes the final determination of a positive identification.

As a federal unit, DMORT's first and primary call is to the United States and its territories. A partial list of DMORT deployments over the past 27 years bears this out (Table 4.4). This changed in 2010

Table 4.4 Selected DMORT deployments illustrating the variety of MFIs.

Event	year
Cemetery, Hardin MO	1993
Murrah Federal Building, Oklahoma City	1995
KAL Flight 801, Guam	1997
AMTRAK, Bourbonnais, IL	1999
Egypt Air, Providence, RI	1999
World Trade Center	2001
United Flight 93, Somerset, PA	2001
TriState Crematory, Noble, GA	2002
The Columbia Shuttle, Texas	2003
Hurricane Katrina, Gulf Coast	2005
Continental Flight 3407, Buffalo, NY	2009
Earthquake, Haiti	2010
Tornados, Joplin, MO	2011
COVID, New York City	2020

with the earthquake that devastated the island country of Haiti. DMORT was deployed but ostensibly to assist only with the identification of American victims. This illustrates another feature of DMORT, flexibility in responding to a disaster. Like the situation following Hurricane Katrina, Haiti presented an extremely austere environment with little standing infrastructure. In contrast, for most DMORT deployments team members have been housed locally in hotels with most amenities readily available. Despite being volunteers, or perhaps because being a volunteer creates a deeper sense of dedication, DMORT teams respond to assist with DVI regardless of locale and conditions. This level of dedication is exemplified in the most recent DMORT deployment to New York City to assist with the processing of COVID deaths. In some ways this was perhaps the most hazardous DMORT deployment to date. DMORT deployments are never hazard-free, but this is the first deployment into an MFI with potentially fatal conditions.

4.5 Transportation Disaster Response

Prior to 1996 transportation disasters resulting in a major loss of life were variously handled, either locally or with varying degrees of federal support. In the aftermath of the crashes of TWA Flight 800 and Value Jet Flight 592 Congress responded with the enactment of the Aviation Disaster Family Assistance Act of 1996 (ADFAA) (NTSB 2008). The function of this legislation was to coordinate local, state, and federal resources and assets in the timely processing and identification of airline crash fatalities. The Family Assistance Center (including the VIC) is a key element of this federal response to aviation disasters. This legislation also led to an interagency agreement with DMORT and the NTSB (National Transportation Safety Board) when there is a major loss of life in an aviation disaster. As always, DMORT functions at the behest of the local medicolegal jurisdiction. The earliest example of this arrangement came in August 1997 with the crash of Korean Airlines Flight 801 on the island of Guam. DMORT deployed to Guam with the first, and at that time only, DPMU and FAC. Since then, DMORT and the NTSB have worked together on a number of airline accidents resulting in the timely and respectful identification and processing of victims. Although less visible in the public eye passenger rail service (AMTRAK) has also been involved in several deadly accidents. In 2008 the Rail Passenger Disaster Family Assistance Act was enacted. This legislation mirrored the ADFAA in requiring, among other things, an FAC to be set up following a rail passenger accident (NTSB 2010).

4.6 State Reponses to Mass Fatalities

The Stafford Act and later the NRP and NRF placed an emphasis on the role that each state should play in both disaster preparedness and disaster response. Like that of the ME/C jurisdictions, state efforts toward mass fatality preparedness vary. A recent survey conducted of state health departments and their degree of preparation for a mass fatality incident found a substantial range of preparedness and capabilities (Merrill et al. 2017). Most states lack a budgetary commitment to MFI and disasters in general. Major disasters are sporadic and MFI extremely uncommon, so fiscally planning for them is difficult. State responses to disasters and MFI usually take the ad hoc or early federal response format. Florida stands out as an exception. Burdened by annual hurricane impacts Florida has not only created but funded its own SMORT (State/Special Mortuary Operational Response Team) team, FEMORS (Florida Emergency Mortuary Operations Response System). Like Florida, Texas has a formal mass fatality team that is integrated into the state's emergency management system. Most states, like Alabama, fall back on the NFMC/NFDA model of volunteer teams. SMORT training and preparedness, like state responses in general, vary considerably from non-existent to realistic. SMORTs, as in the case of FEMORS, have deployed on several occasions without federal support (FEMORS 2013). As with DMORT, population size and frequency of mass fatality disasters play a role in the level at which each state plans for mass fatalities. SMORTs also have to cope with limited resources, financially and personnel-wise, that individual states have at their disposal for mass fatality response.

4.7 The Private Sector

Given the federal government's role in mass disaster planning and response the private sector finds itself in an ancillary position. A glance through the 15 ESFs finds that nongovernmental assets play a part in each, including ESF #8. The placement of private sector assets is usually one of support for federal, state, and local responses. For example, refrigerator trucks are often needed following a mass fatality incident to properly store victims until they can enter the morgue (local or DPMU). These trucks, in turn, need fuel and maintenance while in use. Morgue workers need to be housed and fed, another supplementary function outside of the government's direct response. Volunteers (e.g., urban search and recovery teams) and volunteer agencies, both secular and faith-based, such as the American Red Cross and the Salvation Army, typically provide support outside of direct governmental channels. Whether DMORT is deployed or not the funeral industry will almost always be involved in mass fatality responses. This may occur in the FAC/VIC or at the conclusion in funeral preparations for the victims.

4.8 Summary

Regardless of the nature of a mass fatality event, the ME/C medico-legal jurisdiction is always the lead agency in DVI. As mass fatality events continue and evolve, federal and state responses will continue and evolve in their scope as well (see Chapter 11). The financial contribution of the federal government, and to a lesser extent each state, in responding to mass fatalities is no small matter. The value of the MFI response to the American people cannot be measured in dollars, however.

Governmental responses to disasters and MFIs began as individual mitigations progressing over time to the current NRF framework. Along with changes in federal and state responses, mass fatality incidents have also changed. DMORT was designed to respond to well-contained short-term events (e.g., transportation accidents). But, as COVID and the annual onslaught of hurricanes and tornados have taught us, the medicolegal jurisdiction response to DVI in the twenty-first century requires a degree of preparedness and readiness for any and all future events.

References

ASPR (2020) HHS office of the assistant secretary for preparedness and response [online]. Available at: https://www.phe.gov/about/aspr/Pages/default.aspx (Accessed 21 August 2020)

Carroll, E., Johnson, A., DePaolo, F., Adams, B.J., Mazone, D. and Sampson, B. (2017). Trends in United States mass fatality incidents and recommendations for medical examiners and coroners. *American Forensic Pathology* 7 (3): 318–329. [online]. Available at: https://doi.org/10.23907/2017.029 (Accessed 20 August 2020).

DHS (2004) *National response plan* [online]. Available at: https://www.hsdl.org/?view&did=450766 (Accessed 21 August 2020)

FEMA (2008) *Emergency support function annexes: introduction* [online]. Available at: https://www.fema.gov/media-library-data/20130726-1825-25045-0604/emergency_support_function_annexes_introduction_2008_.pdf (Accessed 21 August 2020)

FEMA (2016) *Emergency support function #8 – public health and medical services annex* [online]. Available at: https://www.fema.gov/media-library-data/1470149644671-642ccad05d19449d2d13b1b0952328ed/ESF_8_Public_Health_Medical_20160705_508.pdf(Accessed 24 August 2020)

FEMA (2019a) *The Federal emergency management agency publication 1* [online]. Available at: https://www.fema.gov/sites/default/files/2020-03/publication-one_english_2019.pdf (Accessed 21 August 2020)

FEMA (2019b) *Stafford act* [online]. Available at: https://www.fema.gov/disasters/stafford-act (Accessed 21 August 2020)

FEMA (2019c) *National response framework, fourth edition* [online]. Available at: https://www.fema.gov/sites/default/files/2020-04/NRF_FINALApproved_2011028.pdf (Accessed 21 August 2020)

FEMORS (2013) Florida emergency mortuary operations response system FEMORS fog field operations guide, sixth edition [online]. Available at: https://femors.org/files/2013/05/FEMORS-FOG-6th-Edition-2013.pdf (Accessed 21 August 2020)

Fierro, M. (2003). Comparing medical examiner and coroner systems. In: *Medicolegal Death Investigation System: Workshop Summary* 2328. Washington: National Academies Press. [online]. Available at: https://www.ncbi.nlm.nih.gov/books/NBK221913 (Accessed 21 August 2020).

Gershon, R., Orr, M.G., Zhi, Q., Merrill, J.A., Chen, D.Y., Riley, H. and Sherman, M.F. (2014). Mass fatality preparedness among medical examiner/

coroners in the United States: a cross-sectional study. *BMC Public Health* 14: 1275. [online]. Available at: https://bmcpublichealth.biomedcentral.com/articles/10.1186/1471-2458-14-1275 (Accessed 20 August 2020).

Hanzlick, R. (2003). Overview of the medicolegal death investigation system in the United States. In: *Medicolegal Death Investigation System: Workshop Summary* Washington: National Academies Press. [online]. Available at: https://www.ncbi.nlm.nih.gov/books/NBK221926 (Accessed 21 August 2020).

Hanzlick, R. and Combs, D. (1998). Medical examiner and coroner systems: history and trends. *Journal of the American Medical Association* 279 (11): 870–874.

HHS (2017) *Disaster mortuary operational response teams* [online]. Available at: https://www.phe.gov/Preparedness/responders/ndms/ndms-teams/Pages/dmort.aspx (Accessed: 22 August 2020)

Jensen, R.A. (2000). *Mass Fatality and Casualty Incidents: A Field Guide*. Boca Raton: CRC Press.

Merrill, J.A., Orr, M., Chen, D.Y., Zhi, Q. and Gerson, R.R. (2016). Are we ready for mass fatality incidents? Preparedness of the US mass fatality infrastructure. *Disaster Medicine and Public Health Preparedness* 10 (1): 87–97. [online]. Available at: https://www.cambridge.org/core/journals/disaster-medicine-and-public-health-preparedness/article/are-we-ready-for-mass-fatality-incidents-preparedness-of-the-us-mass-fatality-infrastructure/4F63B3DD1AF64B563994786DCC353AB6 (Accessed: 20 August 2020).

Merrill, J., Zhi, Q. and Gershon, R.R. (2017). Self-reported preparedness to respond to mass fatality incidents in 38 state health departments. *Journal of Public Health Management and Practice* 23 (1): 64–72. [online]. Available at: https://journals.lww.com/jphmp/Abstract/2017/01000/Self_reported_Preparedness_toRespond_to_Mass.10.aspx (Accessed: 20 August 2020).

NAME (2010) *National association of medical examiners standard operating procedures for mass fatality management* [online]. Available at: https://www.thename.org/assets/docs/31434c24-8be0-4d2c-942a-8afde79ec1e7.pdf (Accessed: 22 August 2020)

NIJ (2005). *Mass Fatality Incidents: A Guide for Human Forensic Identification*. Washington: Office of Justice Programs.

NTSB (2008) Federal family assistance plan for aviation disasters. US National Transportation Safety Board Office of Transportation Disaster Assistance, Washington [online] Available at: https://www.ntsb.gov/tda/TDADocuments/Federal-Family-Plan-Aviation-Disasters-rev-12-2008.pdf (Accessed: 21 August 2020)

NTSB (2010) Federal family assistance plan for rail passenger disasters. US National Transportation Safety Board Office of Transportation Disaster Assistance, Washington [online] Available at: https://www.ntsb.gov/tda/TDADocuments/NTSB%20Federal%20Family%20Assistance%20Plan%20for%20Rail%20Passenger%20Accident.pdf (Accessed: 21 August 2020)

CHAPTER 5
DVI Morgue Operations

John A.Williams

Department of Anthropology and Sociology, Western Carolina University, Cullowhee, NC, USA

5.1 Introduction

Disaster victim identification (DVI) begins and ends in the morgue. This may be the local morgue or a DPMU (Disaster Portable Morgue Unit) (see Chapter 4). This chapter will describe the functions of a DVI morgue from the perspective of full operations and a DPMU deployment, remembering that the DVI morgue will be tailored to the specifics of the MFI mission.

5.2 DVI Morgue Considerations

The physical setting for the morgue is dependent on several variables. The first is the extent of the mass fatality incident (MFI). A large medical examiner/coroner (ME/C) office may be able to handle a small number of deaths without compromising routine morgue activities and therefore the need for a DPMU. The scope of the MFI is another factor. If the local infrastructure has been impacted severely (e.g., a Category 5 hurricane with a loss of basic local infrastructure functions) a DPMU would be the likely option. State or federal involvement also plays a role in the decision as to where to place morgue operations.

Disaster Victim Identification in the 21st Century: A US Perspective, First Edition.
Edited by John A Williams and Victor W Weedn.

The federal asset DMORT (Disaster Mortuary Operational Response Team) has an MOU with the NTSB (National Transportation Safety Board) to be the DVI presence in transportation accidents. DMORT typically deploys with one of its three DPMUs. Some states like Florida have a well-funded and established mass fatality unit (e.g. FEMORS). Each MFI is unique even if causality is the same (e.g., a transportation accident). A full morgue (DPMU or local) might be necessary where there is large loss of life, as in the World Trade Center terrorist attack or in a transportation accident. Conversely, the displacement of caskets in a flooded cemetery would dictate the need for a truncated morgue presence.

Regardless of the morgue deployment or use, the medical examiner/coroner is legally responsible for DVI (NAME 2010; NIJ 2005). This is a fundamental element of DVI in the United States, regardless of whether there is a state or federal presence at the MFI. The ME/C's role in the morgue, as in all else, will vary from jurisdiction to jurisdiction, and more likely from one MFI to the next. A short-term, small-scale MFI might find the ME/C directly involved, especially if the local morgue is the DVI operational morgue. A large MFI with substantial fatalities requiring a DPMU might find the ME/C in a more peripheral role, permitting morgue operations to function without a daily presence by the ME/C.

5.2.1 Morgue Site Selection

This discussion assumes that the DVI morgue will be located away from the local ME/C morgue. This may be due to the size of the MFI or to disruptions in the local infrastructure, necessitating that morgue operations be elsewhere. The details of morgue site selection have been covered previously (Jensen 2000; NAME 2010; NIJ 2005). The morgue does not need to be at the MFI scene but should have easy accessibility for transportation flow into and out of the morgue location. Overriding this need is the nature of the MFI. If it involves a major regional disruption (e.g., a wildfire or a Class 5 Hurricane) there may be no suitable locations in close proximity to the MFI. If at all possible, the morgue should be located in a physical structure (i.e., a warehouse) where the morgue workers and the deceased are protected from the elements and have some degree of climate control.

For obvious reasons, good airflow ventilation is a must. COVID has been a stark reminder of the need to maintain stringent biohazard protocols. The morgue structure should be chosen with safety in mind.

One important site choice is the presence of utilities, in particular water and electricity. The latter may require the allocation of external generators, an absolute if the local infrastructure is down. The size of the morgue building will vary with the size of the MFI, but a good morgue plan should permit ease of logical workflow as remains travel from one station to the next (see Section 5.3). The building should also be large enough to permit some degree of isolation for hazardous morgue stations (e.g., radiology and embalming). This brings us to the question of storage. Refrigeration is an absolute necessity. The routine and easiest form of refrigerated storage is the use of refrigerated truck trailers. One reason a DPMU may be used, even if the local morgue is adequate, may be a lack of storage. This need for added refrigerated storage was demonstrated recently in New York City during the height of the 2020 COVID epidemic there, and later in the summer of 2020 as the pandemic peaked in Texas (Rose 2020). Refrigerated trucks must be located adjacent to the morgue for ease of access during morgue operations, but not situated in such a way that the general public can observe trailer activities. Security is an absolute: think "what goes on in the morgue stays in the morgue." Any choice for a morgue location must be securable.

5.2.2 Incident Command System

Shortly after the formation of the Department of Homeland Security in late 2001 came the establishment of the National Response Plan (NRP) and the National Incident Management System (NIMS) (DHS, 2004). Relying on the Incident Command System (ICS), the NRP and NIMS provided for a coordination of efforts across state and federal jurisdictions and private agencies to prepare for, prevent, and react to the variety of hazards the country faces.

The ICS originated in the 1970s as a means of coordinating wildfire firefighting efforts in the state of California (FEMA 2018; Irwin 2004). The principle is simple: create an organizational hierarchy of personnel, assets (equipment, supplies, and facilities), and, importantly, procedures to respond to a disaster incident. A critical feature of ICS is the Incident Commander (IC), under whom the organizational hierarchy expands via a Chain of Command (COC). At any point in time during an incident (disaster) response there will be only one IC. The actual person staffing the IC can and will change over time (as do other positions under the IC). But there will be only one position (person) conducting the overall incident response. This is critically important when multiple agencies, each with their own protocols, are responding to a disaster. This was one of the reasons for the formation of ICS, warring interests and conflicting procedures. By its definition, a mass disaster will be a multiagency response. When one occurs, the IC becomes part of what is referred to by NIMS as "Unified Command." Efforts by individual responding agencies, instead of being duplicated or inefficiently used, are coordinated to respond to the disaster, sometimes at a level as simple as using the same radio frequency to communicate.

An MFI will, in all likelihood, be one component of a multiagency, governmental (state and/or federal) incident response. The DVI morgue becomes part of the Unified Command. The morgue itself, like the larger incident response, should be organized using the ICS. DMORT, when mobilized, functions under the ICS as a matter of course. While the morgue is a much smaller and self-contained unit it can easily suffer from a lack of coordinating effort. The ICS functions on a well-established chain of command. Decisions may initiate with the individual morgue staff member, but they must flow through the appropriate COC to be carried out. For example, if a morgue station runs low on PPE (personal protective equipment) a request is made through the established logistic supply channel. This allows the logistics personnel to stay abreast of PPE use, something they would not be able to do if each morgue station simply picked up PPE whenever it was needed. ICS ensures that the morgue functions smoothly. This in turn means that DVI will be completed in a timely manner and with proper results (i.e., correct identifications).

In the DVI morgue there will be a single Morgue Commander (MC) under whom the various functions of the morgue will occur. The MC, in turn, is part of the larger incident ICS framework and maintains an upward COC. As DVI is legally a function of the ME/C the MC maintains close communication with the ME/C. Within the DVI morgue each major morgue station (see Section 5.4) will have a supervisory Team Leader through which the COC will flow to and from the team/station to the Morgue Commander.

5.3 Workflow in the DVI Morgue

The purpose and function of the DVI morgue is to facilitate the identification of victims of a mass fatality incident in a timely and accurate manner, with no incorrect identifications. To this end, there is, in any DVI morgue, a workflow from the moment human remains enter the morgue complex until they are identified and discharged. Figure 5.1 is generic diagram of the workflow of human remains into and through a typical DVI morgue. It is based on a DMORT/NIJ (Disaster Mortuary Operational Response Team/National Institute of Justice) model of operations (DMORT 2008; NIJ 2005). Although the DVI morgue is a single unit, there are two functional divisions of morgue "stations": non-forensic and forensic (Table 5.1). The function of each individual morgue station will be described in Section 5.4. The non-forensic activities incorporate those not directly involved in the identification process and procedures. This includes admitting and

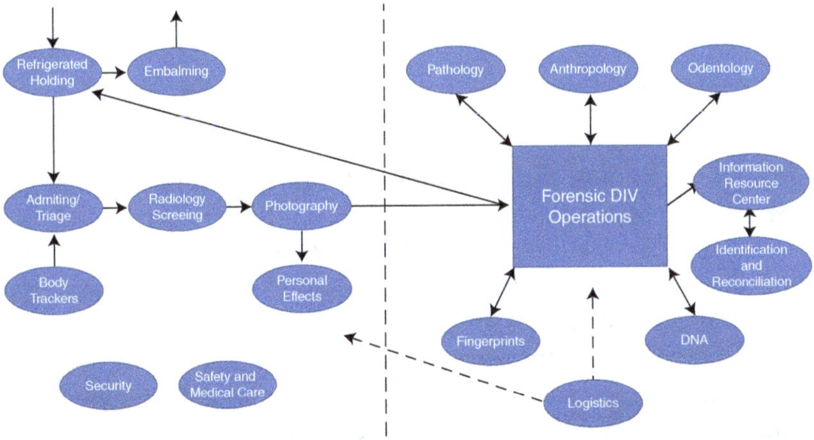

Figure 5.1 Operational workflow in the DVI morgue. The vertical dashed line separates the non-forensic from the forensic morgue activities.

Table 5.1 Typical DVI morgue stations.

Non-forensic
Refrigerated holding
Admitting and Triage
Body trackers
Radiology
Photography
Personal effects
Embalming
Forensic
Anthropology
DNA
Fingerprints
Information resource center
Identification and reconciliation
Odontology
Pathology
Morgue Utility
Security
Safety
Logistics

triage at the beginning and embalming at the end, after identification has been made and authorized by the ME/C. The forensic side of the DVI morgue focuses specifically on those procedures which lead to an identification (e.g., odontology and DNA). The functional separation of the morgue activities does not preclude interaction between stations during the flow of remains through the morgue. It is not uncommon for the anthropology station to request additional radiographs from radiology to examine a feature on a bone. In other words, while there is a functional separation of morgue stations they work together as an interrelated unit whose goal is the identification of MFI victims. As each MFI is different in terms of DVI requirements (see Chapter 4), the DVI morgue is flexible by design. Unneeded stations can be removed or reduced in size while those under greater need can be enhanced (i.e., in an MFI involving coffin displacement at a cemetery, a pathology station is unlikely to be required).

If you examine the flowchart, you'll see that there are three outliers, three stations that are not directly connected to either the nonforensic or forensic functions of the DVI morgue. They function in a broader, behind-the-scenes, role of morgue utility, serving all aspects of the morgue. The first of these is security. The DVI morgue, whether it is a function of a federal or state deployment and whether it is a DPMU or a permanent morgue within a large metropolitan area, requires a secure setting. The respectful treatment of human remains necessitates accountability, both within the morgue and in regard to outside entities (e.g., the funeral industry). MFIs are typically in the public spotlight and so the news media and other agencies feel that they have an obligation to know what is taking place within the morgue. It is in the best interest of all parties that access to the morgue be restricted, and that there be a significant level of security. Who provides security will depend on where the DVI morgue is located and under whose immediate control it is functioning. If, for example, a military base is used then security comes with the facility. If the DVI morgue is located in a less secure area then security will need to be provided, perhaps by local law enforcement, or perhaps by a private security agency. In any event, access to and from the DVI morgue must be controlled. This function easily fits into the ICS framework.

As anyone who has ever worked in a DVI morgue can attest, the morgue is by its nature prone to hazards. A safety officer is a required component of the ICS and the DVI morgue. The safety officer monitors work conditions within the morgue, and also outside the morgue during downtime, to ensure the safety of the morgue workers. Undetected human biohazards (e.g., infectious agents like HIV and hepatitis) and physical hazards (e.g., chemicals and sharp objects) make the handling of human remains at all times a dangerous activity. It goes without saying that PPE is mandatory. A location for donning and doffing PPE should be established that creates both a biohazard zone and a clean zone. The latter is needed for ease of movement around the morgue without entering a "hot" zone (e.g., a break room and the IRC [see 5.5]). Morgue activities involving remains should be clearly and functionally separated. There should be no inadvertent crossing from a clean zone into the biohazard zone without first donning proper PPE.

Instruments like scalpels and saws are routinely used in the morgue and accidents can and do happen. A medical unit should be attached to a DVI morgue, or at a minimum be easily accessed, should an injury occur. This includes unanticipated organic medical conditions (i.e., a heart attack or allergic reaction). In a large-scale federal deployment, a DMAT (Disaster Medical Assistance Team) will likely have to be deployed and may be available locally to serve in this capacity. Working in an MFI response is a stressful activity, enhanced by the frenetic pace of morgue activities, compounded by being billeted away from home and in unfamiliar surroundings. Even those who routinely work with the dead are affected by the sheer immensity of an MFI. Another component of morgue safety is so-called psychological first aid. Employing therapists skilled in the human response to death, as well as training morgue workers in the signs of a negative mental response to an MFI, is a necessary component of a safe morgue environment. The morgue is not the only location where hazards can occur in an MFI response. Climate, geography, and the conditions that may have led to the MFI are hazards that the morgue and those working in it must also contend. For example, the National Disaster Medical Service (NDMS) creates an annual HASP (Health and Safety Plan) to cover anticipated risks for NDMS employees during deployments (HHS 2016). Each deployment will generate a HERA (Hazard Evaluation and Risk Assessment) outlining incident-specific risks (e.g., daily temperatures and humidity, dangerous storm potential, as well as possible disease conditions). The safety officer should ensure that morgue staff take regular "breaks" and stay hydrated (as PPE is notorious for water loss through sweating). A clean zone breakroom should be located away from the morgue proper to provide a physical place of relative safety (physical and mental) for the morgue workers.

While people staffing the morgue stations may be the backbone of the DVI morgue, the morgue does not function without a support team. Logistics functions behind the scene, so to speak, to keep the morgue operating at peak efficiency. All morgue stations use PPE, especially the forensic stations. Logistic personnel ensure that each station has the consumables it needs. Equipment sometimes fails in use, so repairs and replacements are a logistic responsibility. Keeping refrigeration functioning as well as lighting and ventilation in the morgue structure, especially troublesome if the local infrastructure has been compromised by the MFI, is a key activity of morgue logistics. One element of twenty-first-century DVI is a reliance on computers and router connectivity. Morgue stations can enter data and connect in real-time. Stations can check on the status of remains and cross-check findings with other stations. Information technology is an integral part of morgue logistics to keep the morgue "connected."

5.4 DVI Morgue Stations

As previously stated, the number of morgue stations and how extensively they are staffed will vary with each MFI and the needs of the individual response. Also, as the MFI mission progresses the morgue will likely change with no-longer-necessary stations phased out. Variations in morgue composition are more likely to be seen on the forensic side of the morgue, as these stations more closely match the needs of the MFI DVI requirements. This is not to say that the non-forensic stations are always needed regardless of the MFI, but that they are more central to the morgue backbone.

5.4.1 Non-forensic Stations

The non-forensic stations handle and process the remains prior to, and at times during, forensic identification. Some stations, like admitting, are in play each and every time a set of remains is physically in the morgue space. Personal effects, on the other hand, should only be active the first time a set of remains enters the morgue proper.

Refrigerated Holding While human remains may come directly to the morgue from recovery at the MFI location, it is more likely that remains will first arrive at a refrigerated holding area prior to initial admitting (see "Admitting and Triage"). Here, the remains are kept segregated with other recovered remains that have not yet been given formal morgue tracking. Once admitted to the morgue, the now-tracked remains are placed in a separate refrigerated storage. A chain of evidence must be maintained at all times showing the location of all tracked remains until they are released after identification. In the DVI morgue, chain of evidence means that human remains can be accounted for at all times; where they are located in the morgue (i.e., which station or in refrigerated holding) and status in the identification workflow (i.e., which stations have been the remains been processed through).

The form that refrigerated holding takes will vary with the size and nature of the MFI. In a large jurisdiction and a small number of fatalities the local morgue may have sufficient capacity to handle storage in-house. If the number of fatalities is substantial, refrigerated trucks are the logical and best choice for storage. Each truck should be labeled such that the location of tracked remains in a specific truck will always be known. Access to the holding area should be limited to reduce the possibility of errors and disruption of chain of evidence. At the end of a DVI morgue shift all remains should be returned to their assigned refrigerated holding area (i.e., their assigned truck or location).

Admitting and Triage When recovered remains are first brought into the DVI morgue, usually in a disaster pouch and typically from the refrigerated holding area, they come to the admitting triage station. Note that the reference was to remains, and not "human" remains. The recovery process, which is outside the scope of this volume, is variably staffed and trained. In some locales search and recovery personnel have undergone detailed training in the recognition and recovery of human remains, while in other jurisdictions law enforcement or the National Guard may be "drafted" to carry out this function. The result then ranges from properly recovered and documented human remains to a collection of items that appear to be human regardless of whether they are or not.

Triage establishes whether the contents of the disaster pouch (body bag) are human. Inanimate material is removed as well as nonhuman animal remains. In an MFI it is not unexpected that nonhuman animals will also perish. It is also possible in disasters where structures have collapsed that restaurant food stuffs may be commingled with human remains. An anthropologist, capable of distinguishing human and nonhuman remains, as well as inanimate objects, is a key presence at the triage station. Another function of triage is to determine, if possible, the presence of commingled human remains. If this is the case, separating them is required.

Once the remains have been identified as human and separated, if commingled, they are assigned a morgue identification number (MIN) or similar identifier. This number *must be unique* to this set of remains for the duration of its time in the DVI morgue. If, for example, during forensic examination it should be determined that commingling has taken place the remains should return to Admitting/Triage and the remains segregated, and a new MIN created for the additionally discovered remains. All documentation, paper and electronic, will be associated with this MIN and this set of remains (whole body, body parts, bone(s)). At this time the remains should be placed in a clean body bag, clearly labeled with the MIN in such a manner that the MIN cannot be removed or lost (i.e., not only on a tag!). A gurney is a convenient and proper means of conveying the remains through the morgue stations. Depending on the ME/C and other jurisdictions involved a documentation packet should be created. The contents will vary, but minimally will include a checklist to show the progress and movement of the remains through the DVI morgue. As each station is "visited" the station leader must sign off as the remains enter and exit the station. This maintains the chain of evidence as well as provides a means to referring back to the station should a question arise at a later date. When the remains are returned to secure storage, paper documentation for that MIN is maintained at the Admitting Station to be reunited with the remains should they be removed from secure storage to the morgue for continued/additional examination.

Body Trackers At the time remains are given an MIN, a body tracker will be assigned to the remains for the duration that they outside of the secured storage area. The purpose of the body tracker is to maintain chain of evidence, ensuring the integrity of the remains. This individual will physically stay with the remains (e.g., the gurney) while they are being examined. The body tracker is usually responsible for maintaining any documentation, including required signatures, that accompanies the remains as they progress through morgue stations.

Radiology Screening Radiographs provide an internal view of the remains. Using portable (DPMU) or permanent X-ray equipment, radiology can perform everything from a whole-body radiograph to scans of individual bones. When there is a commingled mass of remains and inanimate matter (e.g., a transportation accident where remains and vehicle structure may be combined due to the force of the accident), an X-ray can provide a clarifying view. Full autopsies are not routinely performed. And, antemortem and perimortem trauma and the presence of orthopedic devices may not be detected without a radiographic assessment. Today's digital radiography permits forensic stations like Pathology and Anthropology to view radiographs at their individual stations with the remains at hand.

Photography Just as radiography documents the internal, photography documents the external, directly visible view of the remains. Whole-body photographs are taken clothed and unclothed in various orientations. Special attention is paid to tattoos and other features of the external remains that may be of special interest in matching antemortem and postmortem features (see Chapter 9). Digital cameras permit rapid image processing and storage.

Personal Effects Usually connected to the photography station is personal effects. Unless remains are lacking in clothing and adornments, personal effects are removed, physically documented using non-specific language (e.g., yellow-colored instead of gold), and photographed. The personal effects are then securely stored separately from the remains using the same unique MIN associated with those remains.

Embalming After a set of remains have been identified and the ME/C concurs with the identification the remains will be processed for final disposition and release. This may involve/require embalming. At a minimum, the remains will be casketed, or, if requested, prepared for cremation, before release to next of kin or other responsible party. Release will take place only with proper authorization and all efforts made to ensure that the MIN associated with those remains is to be released.

5.4.2 Forensic Stations

Once the remains have moved through initial processing, been assigned an MIN and body tracker, radiographed, and photographed, they will progress through the forensic stations. Each station should examine the remains even if the station has no specific reason to do so (i.e., a single human bone should still pass through the dental station even if no teeth are present). This ensures the integrity of the forensic identification, should questions arise at a later date. The morgue leader can be assured that no steps were ignored in the process of identifying the remains. During the last quarter century record keeping and DVI have evolved from a strictly paper-based system to live entry at each morgue station via router interconnected laptop terminals. Live entry enhances the speed at which identifications can be made as hand data entry in the IRC (see below) is no longer necessary. That said, a paper backup is a prudent precaution. Sole reliance on digital data storage opens up the potential for catastrophic loss should a server fail. Specialists thrive on jargon, but station workers should use, if at all possible, regular wording that any person regardless of training can understand (e.g., fracture instead of the acronym fx). While pathology is the station of choice to begin the forensic workflow, there is no set path for how remains should travel through the forensic stations. In a practical setting, to have remains follow a specific path through workstations would unnecessarily result in a backup within the morgue and a reduction of throughput efficiency. Possible exceptions to this include the DNA station and the possible need to remove tissue. Tissue removal, without guidance from the other forensic stations, might inadvertently remove valuable identification information. The DNA station should, whenever possible, be the last forensic station the remains pass through.

Pathology This station is staffed by forensic pathologists, MDs with discipline-specific training and licensure. Duties of this station vary. Although the autopsy is the norm for most morgues, it is generally the exception in DVI. It is time consuming and generally does not yield much useful information that will result in an identification. In most MFIs the cause and manner of death is already apparent (e.g., trauma from a transportation accident), which is the primary reason to conduct an autopsy. The one exception may be in some transportation accidents where federal dictates may require that crew members be autopsied. Additionally, if the DVI morgue is a DPMU the physical setup is not optimal for conducting a full autopsy. Most often, pathologists will examine the external body and radiographs noting evidence of prior surgical procedures (e.g., joint replacements and surgical scars), anatomical defects, deficits, and anomalies, and external identifying traits (e.g., tattoos). Identifiable medical devices, such as pacemakers, may be removed from the body as these have traceable manufacturer's serial numbers.

Anthropology Forensic anthropologists are human osteologists trained in the analysis and forensic identification of human skeletal remains. While board certification (a PhD and a certification examination) is preferred, a master's degree in forensic anthropology is recognized as the minimum needed to work in the DVI morgue. Dependent on how much of the skeleton is present and observable, anthropologists can assess the age, sex, ancestry, and stature of skeletal remains. Depending on the norms of the ME/C, skeletal features (i.e., the pubic symphysis) that can be age-assessed may be dissected from a fleshed body. Skeletal anomalies, which might aid in identification, may also be noted by the anthropology station. An anthropologist is commonly placed in admitting/triage to answer questions regarding human vs nonhuman vs inanimate and the commingling of human remains.

Odontology Currently, assuming teeth are present, odontology is responsible for the majority of MFI identifications. Forensic odontologists are licensed dentists with training in forensic identification procedures. Further DVI training or experience is preferred due to the conditions under which MFIs occur. Chapter 6 describes in detail the tools and methods forensic odontologists employ in the DVI morgue. In simple terms, antemortem dental records are compared with postmortem dental records created in the DVI morgue. Antemortem dental records are retrieved through the VIC (see Chapter 9). Odontology operations in the DVI morgue, like DVI procedures in general, rely heavily on computer applications in making antemortem and postmortem dental comparisons (e.g., WinID, see Section 6.15). This includes the use of digital imaging in the DVI morgue.

Fingerprints Unlike staffing at other forensic DVI stations there are no discipline-specific requirements to collect fingerprints (see Chapter 7). Morgue staff may collect fingerprints, if available, or the task may fall on law enforcement (local, state, federal). Collection methods vary from paper and ink to the use of a cell phone to digitally capture images of ridge patterns. Comparison of antemortem and postmortem patterns follows collection. This is now mostly done through digital comparison using various online databases. Unlike dental records, and lacking a governmental mandate for universal collection, antemortem fingerprint records are far less common and the nature of the MFI may reduce postmortem availability (i.e., severe burns and decomposition).

DNA For the present time, the DNA morgue station is almost exclusively for the proper collection and storage of postmortem DNA samples. As new technologies emerge and become practical and fiscally feasible in a DVI morgue, DNA routinely may be analyzed on-site. Some large urban ME/Cs may have the capability for in-house processing. For now, samples are almost always processed off-site at a private or governmental laboratory. Chapter 8 covers the various methods for recovery and analysis. Although the DNA station is located in the DVI morgue, there should be a coordination of effort with antemortem DNA collected at the Victim information Center (VIC) (see Chapter 9).

5.5 Information Resource Center

As the remains flow through each forensic morgue station information is collected. Some of it is basic (e.g., age and sex), and some will be more specific and highly individual (e.g., prior surgery or tattoos). All of these data collectively work toward an identification. In the DVI morgue of the twenty-first century, data should be entered live, or electronically. The repository of the electronic and paper (see 5.4.1) data collection is the IRC or Information Resource Center.

If forensic station data are entered real-time, it is likely that the computer application VIP, or Victim Information Program, will be used. This software was developed in cooperation with DMORT at the time DMORT was organized in the mid-1990s. It is available for use and modification by other agencies (FEMORS, n.d.). It has data entry portals for antemortem information (see 9.4.1) collected at the VIC and postmortem information collected at each DVI morgue station. In its initial DVI applications, data were entered at each station and the VIC via paper forms. Staff at the IRC then hand entered information from the paper forms into VIP. This can still be performed if necessary. But, with a server or servers and Wi-Fi, data can be entered real-time at each DVI station, greatly accelerating the speed at which possible matches can be made (see 5.6). For this reason, the IRC should be staffed by at least one IT-savvy person. Software glitches occur and servers can "crash." Due to the highly sensitive nature of the IRC database, and that alterations to the database may impact a correct accurate identification, IRC security is paramount. Access to VIP, or the software application in use in the DVI morgue, should be restricted to a limited number of authorized persons. As VIP can be used for real-time data entry it is designed with unrestricted ease of revision (i.e., entered changes occur instantly across all terminals connected to the server). For this reason, physical access to the master VIP terminal should not be left unattended as unauthorized changes could easily take place with no record.

5.6 Identification and Reconciliation

With real-time data entry VIP (or other software) can, once both antemortem and postmortem information have been entered, immediately begin to find possible matches. Typically, those working in the identification station (IRC staff) first go for the so-called low hanging fruit. These would be matches made based on odontological or other "hard" criteria. As the MFI mission progresses "easy" matches usually decrease in frequency, leading to matches based on less firm criteria. These matches may have to wait for DNA, if available, before submission to the ME/C. Because these matches are not as clear, a reconciliation team works together to resolve these cases. Their task is made more difficult if there are less than perfect correlations between antemortem and postmortem information and multiple unmatched (i.e., unidentified) processed remains in the morgue.

5.7 Summary

The DVI morgue is designed to efficiently process human remains from an MFI. While the DVI morgue can function inside of an ME/C morgue facility, the nature of an MFI usually dictates that the morgue is located near the MFI locale but at a separate facility. The DVI morgue is composed of stations, divided between non-forensic and forensic, the latter focused on the identification process. As no two MFIs are ever the same, even if of similar origins (i.e., a transportation accident), no two DVI morgues will be the same. This is one of the valuable features of the DVI morgue, its flexible, scalable design. A morgue can be created with a full complement of stations, or only a handful needed to complete the mission. With few exceptions, the twenty-first-century DVI morgue is "wired" and data entry is real-time. This necessitates a greater attention to detail while yielding faster and more accurate results.

References

DHS (2004). National response plan [online]. Available at: https://www.hsdl.org/?view&did=450766 (Accessed 21 August 2020).

DMORT (2008). Disaster Mortuary Operational Response Team (DMORT) Standard Operating Procedures 2008 [online]. Available at: https://pdf4pro.com/view/disaster-mortuary-operational-response-team-a72a4.html (Accessed 3 September 2020).

FEMA (2018). ICS review document, ICS 300 [online]. Available at: https://training.fema.gov/emiweb/is/icsresource/assets/ics%20review%20document.pdf (Accessed 29 August 2020).

FEMORS (n.d.). Florida emergency mortuary operations response system downloads [online]. Available at: https://femors.org/downloads (Accessed 16 September 2020).

HHS (2016). 2016 Force protection: Health and safety plan [HASP] [online]. Available at: https://files.asprtracie.hhs.gov/documents/ndms-health-and-safety-plan.pdf (Accessed 9 September 2020).

Irwin, R.L. (2004). Chapter 7: the incident command system (ICS) [online]. Available at: https://web.archive.org/web/20080423021922/http://orgmail2.coe-dmha.org/dr/DisasterResponse.nsf/section/07?opendocument&home=html (Accessed 29 August 2020).

Jensen, R.A. (2000). *Mass Fatality and Casualty Incidents: A Field Guide*. Boca Raton: CRC Press.

NAME (2010). National association of medical examiners standard operating procedures for mass fatality management [online]. Available at: https://www.thename.org/assets/docs/31434c24-8be0-4d2c-942a-8afde79ec1e7.pdf (Accessed: 22 August 2020).

NIJ (2005). *Mass Fatality Incidents: A Guide for Human Forensic Identification*. Washington D.C: Office of Justice Programs.

Rose, J. (2020). As an ER doctor, I fear our era's defining symbol will be the refrigerator truck. Washington Post, 11 April [online]. Available at: https://www.washingtonpost.com/outlook/2020/04/11/refrigerated-truck-morgue-coronavirus (Accessed: 28 August 2020).

CHAPTER 6

Forensic Odontology and Disaster Victim Identification

Kenneth W. Aschheim
Office of the Chief Medical Examiner, New York, NY, USA

6.1 Introduction

Uniting a decedent with their loved ones is an essential component of disaster management and is often the most important metric by which the public judges the competency of the government's response to a multiple fatality incident. Victim identification is the part of fatality management involved in the scientific identification of human remains. Identification is essential for family members to complete the grieving process and provide closure. In the United States, the statutory judicial authority for identifying human remains is the local Medical Examiner or Coroner (ME/C).

6.2 Methods of Identification of an Individual

6.2.1 Non-Dental Methods of Identification

Numerous methods of human identification exist. The most common method is visual identification. However, this requires a viewable body and the participation of an individual familiar with the descendant. Ridgeology, based on the comparison of fingerprints and, to a lesser extent, palm and footprints, has seen tremendous advances due

Disaster Victim Identification in the 21st Century: A US Perspective, First Edition.
Edited by John A Williams and Victor W Weedn.

to the expansion of national and international databases. However, an obvious limitation is that it cannot be used in cases where fingers or other potential body parts are absent. Radiological identification is based on the comparison of historical radiological images and is especially useful in cases where a unique skeletal characteristic, such as a medical device, is present. Unfortunately, the biometric uniqueness of a pathological condition or an image of an implanted medical device cannot be quantified. Anthropological identification, which is based on examination of the skeletal structure of the decedent, can be helpful in estimating an age range interval, skeletal gender, and skeletal ancestry of the victim. However, unless a unique medical device is present, anthropological identification is only helpful in determining the appropriateness of a presumptive identification. Medical device identification depends on the use of the product numbers or serial numbers of implantable medical devices. US federal law requires the registration of a unique series of numbers in the internet-based Global Unique Device Identification Database (GUDID), which contains essential device identification information ("track and trace"). When a Unique Device Identification (UDI) is present, it can be an extremely useful method of identifying an individual.

The use of deoxyribonucleic acid (DNA) has revolutionized disaster victim identification and forensic science in general. The ability to identify an individual is based on the uniqueness of an individual's DNA (except in the case of identical siblings) and on the genetics of inheritance to correlate an individual ancestry. In the past, DNA identification was considered the most time-consuming and costly method of identification; however, with the advent of rapid DNA, the method has proved extremely useful, especially in smaller-scale mass fatality incidents (Page 2019). As technology improves, governmental (CODIS) and private DNA databases expand, and costs are reduced, it will replace most other methods of identification.

6.2.2 Dental Identification

Historically, dental identification was one of the first scientific methods used for human identification. The first recorded case of human identification by dental means occurred in 49 AD when Nero's mother, Agrippina, ordered the execution of Lollia Paulina (Bowers 2011).

She confirmed that the assassins had killed the correct individual based on distinctive features of the anterior maxillary teeth. The first recorded case in the United States involved Major General Joseph Warren, who was killed in the battle of Bunker Hill. Following his exhumation, Warren was identified by his dentist, Paul Revere, based on previous dental work. The first use of dental identification in a mass fatality incident was on May 4, 1897, following the Bazar de la Charité fire. Dr. Oscar Amoedo, a Cuban dentist who is considered the "father of forensic odontology," identified 30 victims based on their dental restorations. He is also the author of the first textbook on the subject titled *L'Art dentaire en Médecine Légale* (Bowers 2011).

Dental identification of human remains is still considered one of the most cost-efficient methods of identifying decedents, especially in cases of burning, decomposition, skeletonization, or fragmentation. Human teeth are resistant to heat and crushing and are easily found in debris. Their ceramic casing (i.e., enamel and dentin) which protects the pulp and the fact that dental pulp is highly vascular also makes them a good source of DNA.

6.3 Theoretical Basis for Comparative Dental Analysis

6.3.1 Basic Theory

Human identification by comparative dental analysis is based on recording specific properties of the human dentition and surrounding dental structures and dental restorations. In addition, the dental record information is used to determine the likelihood that patient information and decedent information are from similar sources.

Numerous biometric markers for comparing antemortem and postmortem dentition exist; however, the most common is detail coding. This involves determining; if a tooth is present, if it is a primary or permanent tooth, and if a tooth is virgin (unrestored) or restored, and if the later, if any of the five surfaces (mesial, occlusal, distal, facial, and lingual surfaces) is restored (Figure 6.1). In addition, an alteration in the development or anatomy of the tooth can *also* be used as a biometric marker.

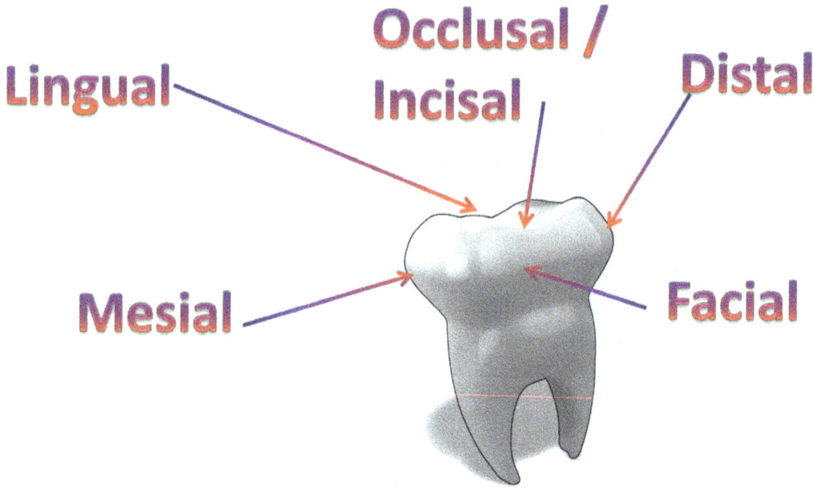

Figure 6.1 Surfaces of a tooth.

Data granularity refers to the level of detail of the dental data collected. A high degree of granularity would involve specifying each individual restoration and material separately. A moderate degree of granularity would aggregate data, such as recording restored surfaces as a single data field and material utilized as a second combined data field. The level of granularity of collected information is often determined by the data entry format requirements of the specific dental forensic software. This coding style is the basis for all computerized comparison algorithms.

An alternative system, simple or generic coding, used by the NamUS (www.namus.gov) national database, involves recording whether a tooth is present, missing, or restored. Recent studies have shown that for the majority of mass fatality incidents, there is a little variation in computer ranking algorithms between detailed and simplified coding systems (Adams and Aschheim 2016). However, there may be some benefit to recording greater detail, especially when searching for specific unique characteristics of an individual.

Although specific pathologies, such as fractures, caries, developmental grooves, or curved roots may be significant, the pervasiveness within a population may make their usefulness as an identification marker questionable. Therefore, they are often considered contextual data and may be helpful to support or exclude a presumptive identification.

6.3.2 The 32 Teeth Concept

It is impossible to conclusively prove the uniqueness of any human characteristic, only the lack of uniqueness. This limitation exists for all scientific methods of identification, including DNA which is reported as a probability. However, as the number of distinctive dental restorations increases, the likelihood of uniqueness also increases.

Historically, dental identification is based on a theory of the number of opportunities for restoration placement. Since there are 32 teeth and each tooth had one of 32 permutations of surface restoration combinations "of equal weight and validity," the theoretical number of possible permutations is 32^{32} (CAPMI 1989). However, population studies have shown that dental restorations have a far higher probability of occurring in certain anatomical areas of the mouth and therefore are not random events. Data from these studies show that an upper-right first molar is unrestored 57.5% of the time and is coded V (Virgin meaning no restoration), or O, OL, MODFL, MO, OD almost 94% of the time (Figure 6.2) (Table 6.1). In fact, almost 85% of all restorations and 73% of all extraction in a sample US population occur on posterior teeth (Figure 6.3).

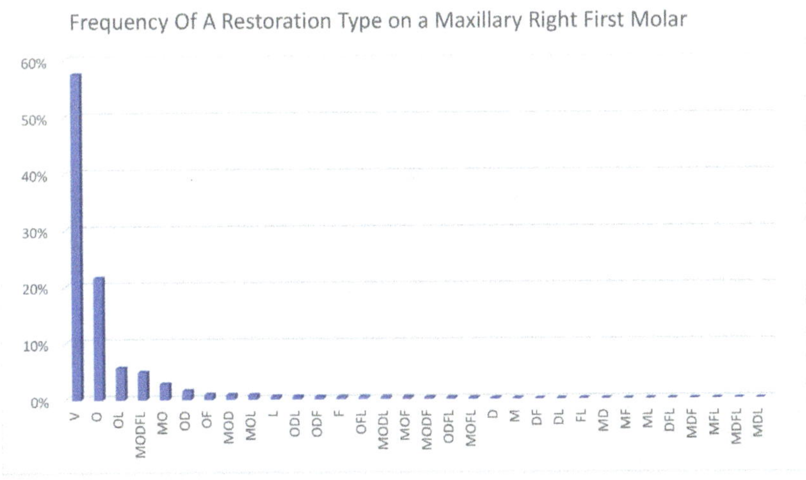

Figure 6.2 Frequency of a Restoration Type on a Maxillary Right First Molar.

Table 6.1 Frequency of a restoration type on a maxillary right first molar.

Restored Surface	Frequency	Restored Surface	Frequency	Restored Surface	Frequency
V	57.499%	ODF	0.404%	DL	0.016%
O	21.524%	F	0.354%	FL	0.014%
OL	5.616%	OFL	0.350%	MD	0.010%
MODFL	4.850%	MODL	0.328%	MF	0.006%
MO	2.780%	MOF	0.314%	ML	0.003%
OD	1.542%	MODF	0.283%	DFL	0.003%
OF	0.887%	ODFL	0.253%	MDF	0.002%
MOD	0.801%	MOFL	0.176%	MFL	0.001%
MOL	0.778%	D	0.142%	MDFL	0.001%
L	0.485%	M	0.093%	MDL	0.000%
ODL	0.467%	DF	0.016%		

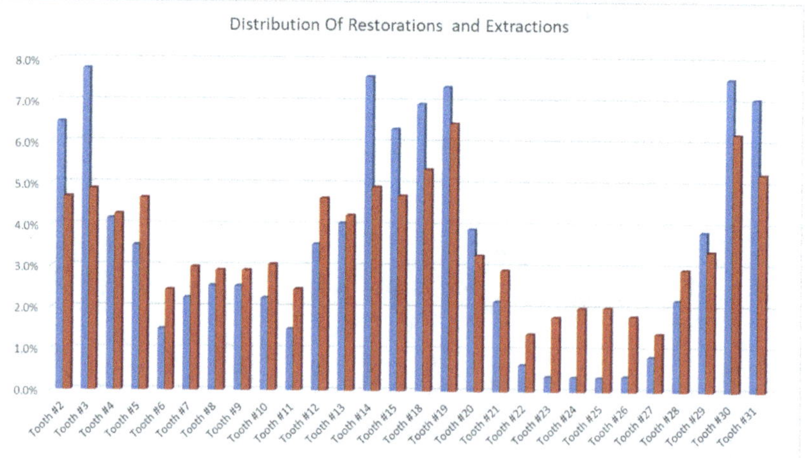

Figure 6.3 Distribution of Restorations and Extractions.

Although the number of possible restored surface combinations is far more limited than initially believed, the success rate of dental identifications has been well established by the concurrent use of DNA analysis (NYC OCME 2003). Even in cases where restorations are not present, the absence of teeth, the placement of dental implants, and a range of surgical treatments can aid in decedent identification. The use of numerous anatomical and anthropological landmarks further increases the likelihood that a successful dental identification can be made.

6.3.3 Logical Direction of Change

Unlike other scientific modalities of identification, one unique issue of dental biomarkers (restorations) is their ability to change over time, especially when deterioration of a tooth or restoration requires physical alteration of the biomarker by the dental provider. However, these changes can only occur in a predictable manner, referred to as a logical direction of change (e.g., restorations can only become more extensive; after a tooth is extracted, it can no longer be present). The logical direction of change, and irreconcilable discrepancies (illogical directions of change) between antemortem and postmortem situations are critical components of matching algorithms.

6.3.4 Comparison Discrepancies

Discrepancies due to alteration of biomarkers need to be accounted for before a conclusion can be determined. Explainable discrepancies are changes in dental data due to dental treatment. Irreconcilable discrepancies are disparities that cannot be explained by the logical progression of treatment changes. While a dental identification can have multiple explainable discrepancies, a single irreconcilable discrepancy will eliminate a record as a candidate for an identification (Figure 6.4).

6.3.5 Concordant Features

A concordant feature is a single tooth characteristic, restoration, anatomical structure, or pathological process that has an individually distinct, biometrically measurable, describable characteristic. In addition, certain concordant features, such as a dental restoration, can exhibit more uniqueness than many morphological features. There is no

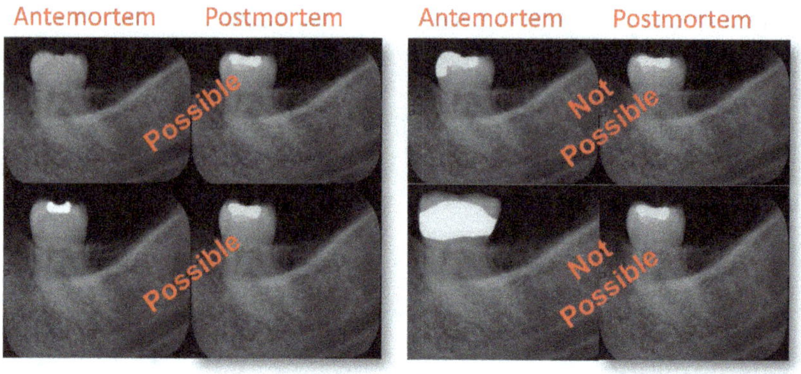

Figure 6.4 Examples of explainable discrepancies showing a logical direction of change (A) and irreconcilable discrepancies showing illogical directions of change (B).

standard as to the minimum number of concordant features (points of concordance) necessary to assign a qualitative assessment of identity (Figure 6.5).

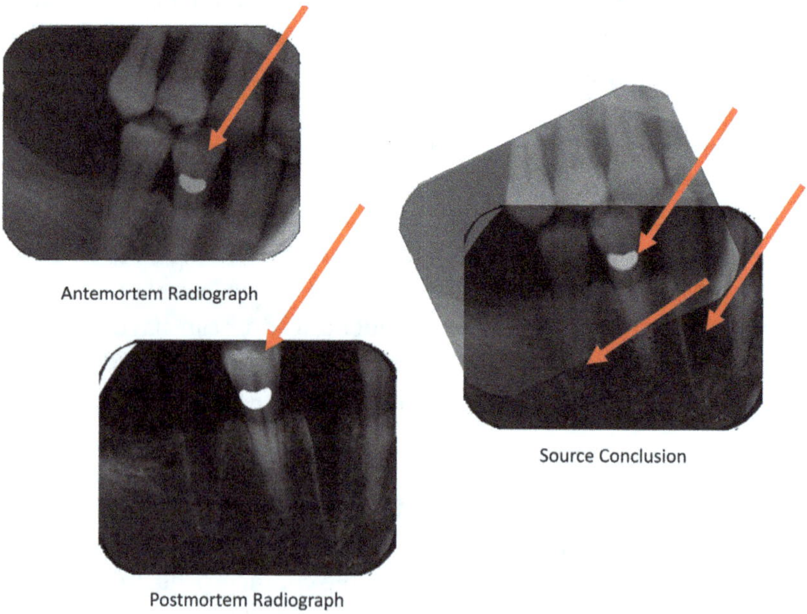

Figure 6.5 An example of a human identification by dental means utilizing a single restoration but multiple concordant features.

6.4 The Antemortem Dental Record

An essential component for performing a human identification by dental means is the need for dental information of all individuals that may have been involved in the incident. Every effort must be made by the Victim Information Center (see Chapter 9) to obtain an up-to-date presumed victims list. Since no national dental database exists, useful antemortem data requires presumptive dental identification information.

Antemortem dental data consist of all the historical dental information on an individual and should include their treatment record, radiographic and photographic information, and, if available, dental casts. This information, which is part of an individual's personal health information (PHI), may also be in electronic format (ePHI). Ideally, it should contain a complete clinical charting of the patient's status when first examined by the dental professional, radiographic and photographic examination of the oral cavity, and a treatment record of all procedures and changes that occurred while the patient was under the care of the dental professional including other dental providers including specialists (Figure 6.6). Since this information can come from multiple sources, it must be consolidated into a single coherent record in order to establish the entire dental condition of an individual before the time of an incident. Therefore, whenever possible, standardized terminology such as ISO/DIS 1942(en) Dentistry – Vocabulary or ANSI/ADA Standard 1058 Forensic Dental Data Set should be used to describe common dental terms (ANSI/ADA 2015; ISO 2009).

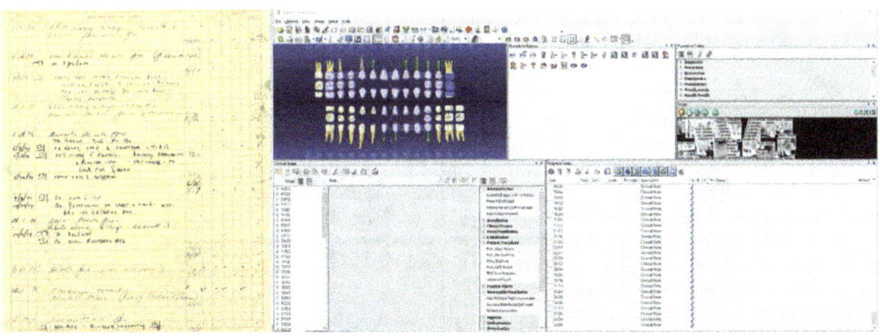

Figure 6.6 Examples of written and digital dental records.

6.4.1 Tooth Numbering Systems

A vital component of the dental record is the recording of characteristics of individual teeth. Typically, this information is recorded using a specialized dental notation system that associates a specific number or letter to a specific tooth. The assignment of these numbers is based on the anatomy of the tooth regardless of its location or area in the mouth (ISO 2016).

Currently, there are two commonly used numbering systems the American Dental Association's (ADA) Universal/National Tooth Designation System (United States) (Box 6.1, Box 6.2) assigns the letters A to T to the primary teeth, 1 to 32 to permanent teeth and 51 to 82 to supernumerary (anomalous extra) teeth ADA (2007). The ISO (FDI) numbering system (other countries), formally known as ISO 3950 – 2016 Dentistry – Designation System for Teeth and Areas of the Oral Cavity, not only includes tooth numbers but also enumerates the mouth (00), maxilla (01) mandible (02) as well as sextants (03-08) and quadrants (10,20,30,40) (ISO 2016).

One common source of error is the failure to recognize which tooth numbering system is used. Whenever possible, the transfer of a

Box 6.1 ISO FDI Numbering System

Maxillary Permanent Teeth

Right 3rd Molar	Right 2nd Molar	Right 1st Molar	Right 2nd Premolar	Right 1st Premolar	Right Canine	Right Lateral Incisor	Right Central Incisor	Left Central Incisor	Left Lateral Incisor	Left Canine	Left 1st Premolar	Left 2nd Premolar	Left 1st Molar	Left 2nd Molar	Left 3rd Molar
18	17	16	15	14	13	12	11	21	22	23	24	25	26	27	28
48	**47**	**46**	**45**	**44**	**43**	**42**	**41**	**31**	**32**	**33**	**34**	**35**	**36**	**37**	**38**
Right 3rd Molar	Right 2nd Molar	Right 1st Molar	Right 2nd Premolar	Right 1st Premolar	Right Canine	Right Lateral Incisor	Right Central Incisor	Left Central Incisor	Left Lateral Incisor	Left Canine	Left 1st Premolar	Left 2nd Premolar	Left 1st Molar	Left 2nd Molar	Left 3rd Molar

Mandibular Permanent Teeth

MaxillaryPrimary Teeth

Right 2nd Molar	Right 1st Molar	Right Canine	Right Lateral Incisor	Right Central Incisor	Left Central Incisor	Left Central Incisor	Left Central Incisor	Left Central Incisor	Left Central Incisor
55	54	53	52	51	61	62	63	64	65
85	**84**	**83**	**82**	**81**	**71**	**72**	**73**	**74**	**75**
Right 2nd Molar	Right 1st Molar	Right Canine	Right Lateral Incisor	Right Central Incisor	Left Central Incisor	Left Lateral Incisor	Left Canine	Left 1st Molar	Left 2nd Molar

MandibularPrimaryTeeth

Box 6.2 Universal numbering system

Maxillary Permanent Teeth

Right 2nd Premolar	Right 1st Premolar	Right Canine	Right Lateral Incisor	Right Central Incisor	Left Central Incisor	Left Central Incisor	Left Central Incisor	Left Central Incisor	Left Central Incisor
4	5	6	7	8	9	10	11	12	13
29	**28**	**27**	**26**	**25**	**24**	**23**	**22**	**21**	**20**
Right 2nd Premolar	Right 1st Premolar	Right Canine	Right Lateral Incisor	Right Central Incisor	Left Central Incisor	Left Lateral Incisor	Left Canine	Left 1st Premolar	Left 2nd Premolar

Mandibular Permanent Teeth

Maxillary Primary Teeth

Right 2nd Molar	Right 1st Molar	Right Canine	Right Lateral Incisor	Right Central Incisor	Left Central Incisor	Left Central Incisor	Left Central Incisor	Left Central Incisor	Left Central Incisor
A	B	C	D	E	F	G	H	I	J
T	**S**	**R**	**Q**	**P**	**O**	**N**	**M**	**L**	**K**
Right 2nd Molar	Right 1st Molar	Right Canine	Right Lateral Incisor	Right Central Incisor	Left Central Incisor	Left Lateral Incisor	Left Canine	Left 1st Molar	Left 2nd Molar

Mandibular Primary Teeth

decedent's ePHI should follow protocols outlined in ANSI/ADA Standard No. 1067–2013 Electronic Dental Record System Standard Functional Requirement, ANSI/ADA Technical Report No. 1085 Implementation Guidelines for the Secure Transmission of Protected Health Information in Dentistry and ANSI-NIST ITL Type 12 Dental Data Set (ANSI/ADA 2013a, 2013b; ANSI/NIST 2015).

6.5 Laws Governing the Transfer of Protected Dental Information

In the United States, regulations concerning the transfer of personal health information (PHI), or electronic formatted PHI (ePHI), is managed by the Office of Civil Rights and Centers for Medicare and Medicaid Services and are collectively known as "HIPAA regulations." To overcome concerns about releasing PHI information and to expedite a forensic identification, these agencies have codified an exemption under 45 CFR (Code of Federal Regulations) 164.512 that allows offices to comply with authorized agency requests.

Section (g) of 45 CFR states:

> A covered entity may disclose protected health information to a coroner or medical examiner for the purpose of identifying a deceased person, determining a cause of death, or other duties authorized by the law. A covered entity that also performs the duties of the coroner or medical examiner may use protected health information for the purpose described in this paragraph.

6.5.1 Electronic Dental Record

In order to reduce the possibility of misinterpreting an illegible chart, an electronic dental record (EDR) should be requested. If this information is transferred electronically, a security transfer protocol should be used. Unfortunately, because of a lack of adoption of standardized methods of data transfer, the EDR data is typically transferred in a paper format or as an Adobe PDF document. Care should especially be taken to ensure that the forensic odontologist is familiar with the EDR's odontogram so that it is interpreted correctly.

6.5.2 Issues Concerning Dental Data

Although the antemortem record is the critical source of dental information, the data itself may sometimes be inaccessible or unreliable. In addition, human error in charting, liberal use of billing codes, and simple misnumbering of teeth may be issues in obtaining reliable information. Therefore, merely transferring the information without the review of a trained forensic odontologist is strongly discouraged. Finally, the disaster that caused the multiple fatality incident may also impact the availability of dental records (Acharya et al. 2017).

6.6 The Postmortem Dental Record

The postmortem dental record should reflect the findings of a dental autopsy and should include the presence or absence of teeth, dental restorations, dental prostheses, dental orthoses, bone and soft tissue anomalies, and other identifiable conditions (Figure 6.7). A critical difference between the antemortem and the postmortem collection of data is that the information concerning antemortem restored surfaces

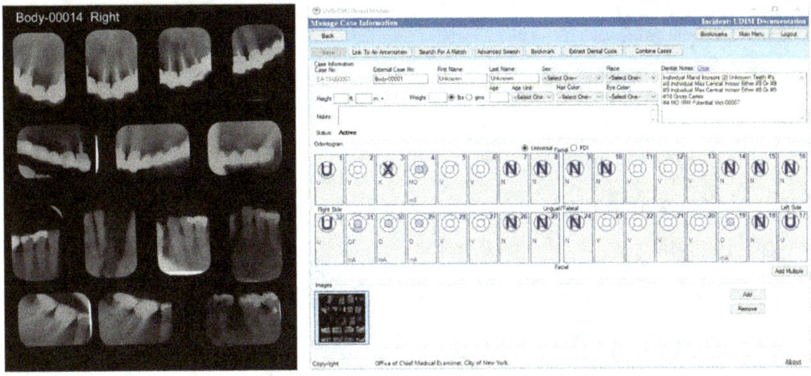

Figure 6.7 An example of the UDIM postmortem dental record showing a the dental radiograph as well as an odontogram of the findings of a dental autopsy.

is indirectly inferred from radiographs and charts, while postmortem data reflects an actual visual confirmation by direct examination of the decedent.

6.7 The Dental Autopsy

The dental autopsy records information from radiographic imaging and visual examination of the oral cavity (Table 6.2) (Charan Gowda et al. 2016). Often the remains are in a poor state of conservation, may exhibit varying degrees of fragmentation or decomposition, and various degrees of taphonomic (how organisms decay and become fossilized) degradation. During the decaying process, rigor mortis may set in, making visualization difficult, if not impossible. Although the goal of the dental autopsy is to record sufficient dental data for comparison with the antemortem data, out of respect for the decedent, it still should be as minimally invasive as possible.

A typical dental autopsy may include:

i. Missing and present teeth.
ii. Location and materials used for all existing restorations, dental prostheses and dental orthoses.
iii. All endodontic therapy, intra-coronal posts, implants, and any notable treatments.

Table 6.2 Basic information recorded in the forensic dental record.

Demographic Information	
Name of individual (if known)	Case Number
Date and time of examination	Jurisdiction
Location of the examination	
Antemortem Data	
Age (if known)	Gender (if known)
Ancestry (if known)	Any other relevant demographic data (if known)
Reporter information (if known	Source of data information (if known
Date of data (if known)	Content of data (if known)
Postmortem Data	
Description of remains	Estimated age of decedent (optional)
Estimated gender (optional)	Estimated ancestry (optional)
Other Significant Postmortem Findings	
Oro-dental Information	
Oro-dental structures examined (decedent, jaw or fragment)	Tooth numbering system used
Presence or absence of teeth	Presence or absence of restorations
Presence or absence of prostheses	Presence or absence of orthoses
Anomalous teeth	Traumatized teeth
Supernumerary teeth	Malposed teeth
Specific metric data concerning the dental restorations, dental prostheses, caries, fractures, anomalies, abrasions, implants, erosions or other features for all teeth (based on the granularity of software)	
Materials used in dental restorations and prosthetic devices, when known (based on the granularity of software)	

(*Continued*)

Table 6.2 (Continued)

Lab prescriptions	Dental casts
Digital imagery	3-D scans
An odontogram (graphic chart of the condition of the teeth) should illustrate as graphically as possible the following:	
Periodontal conditions, calculus, stain (optional)	
Occlusal relationships (optional)	
Medical records showing oro-dental structures	
Additional oral features (e.g., tattoo, dental jewelry, scars, tori, etc.)	

iv. All fixed, removable and implant-based prostheses, and when possible their material composition.
v. Occlusal relationships and pathological positions of individual teeth.
vi. Other anomalies, fractures, soft tissue, extraoral clinical findings and other potential dental identifiers.

6.7.1 Visible Light Fluorescence

Advances in esthetic dentistry and restorative materials have made it far more difficult to visualize some restorations. Fluorescence is a property of esthetic dental materials to emit a longer wavelength light when a specific lower-wavelength light illuminates the object. During the dental autopsy procedure, the use of ultraviolet light in the 365 to 395 nm range may help to delineate the size and extent of a tooth-colored restoration (Figure 6.8).

6.7.2 Craniofacial Dissection

Although craniofacial dissection can improve visibility into the oral cavity, its invasive nature makes its use less than desirable. It is forbidden to be used by some religions. Before performing a craniofacial dissection, it should be determined if adequate information can be obtained without the procedure. In addition, the procedure must conform with local jurisdiction guidelines, applicable laws and regulations, and receive preapproval by the medical examiner, coroner, or incident commander.

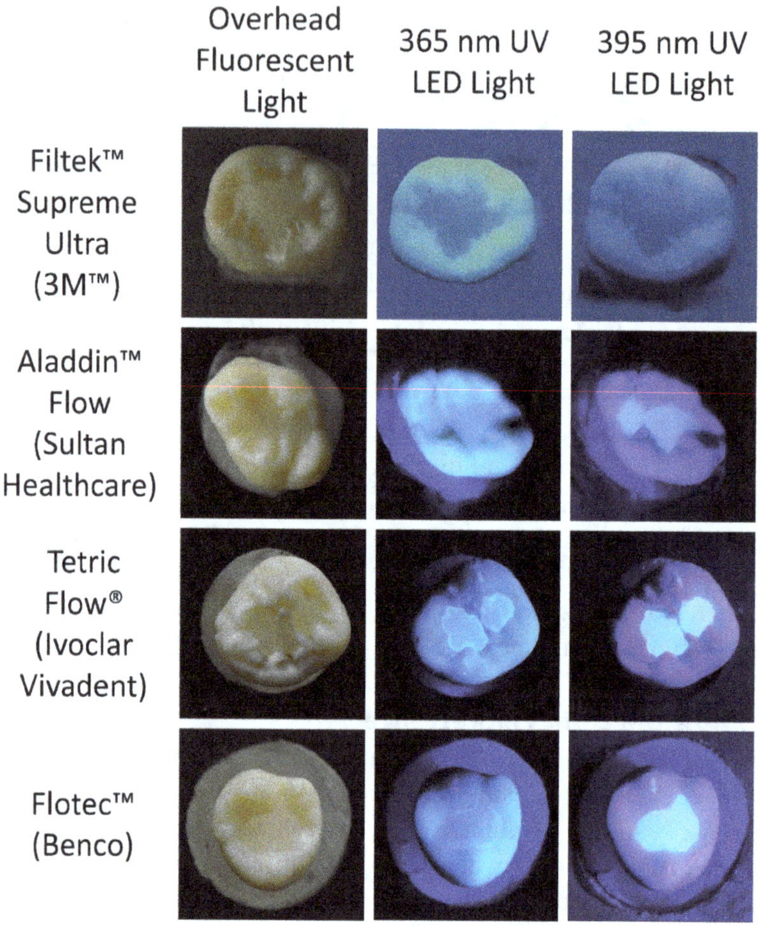

Figure 6.8 Examples of Fluorescence properties of different composite resin material at various visible and ultraviolet light ranges (courtesy of Dr. Gerald Guzy).

6.7.3 Antemortem Radiographs

Human identification by dental means depends on an accurate comparison of antemortem and postmortem radiographs. The lack of forensically useful radiographic information can make a determination difficult. Dental radiographs may be the only method to verify the existence of numerous dental conditions such as endodontic pathology or treatment, retained roots, impacted teeth, or an odontological or osseous pathology. Radiographs are the only objective method of substantiating the accuracy of the dental record. Since the quality of the antemortem radiographs will affect the ability to make a positive dental identification, the original antemortem radiographic images should be requested from the missing person's dental provider. However, the missing person's dental provider must still keep a duplicate set within the patient's record.

6.7.4 Postmortem Radiographs

It is mandatory that the postmortem dental autopsy include a complete set of radiographs in order to assess dental characteristics. The radiographic set should include ideally angulated periapical dental images of the teeth and surrounding structures. Edentulous areas must also be imaged to verify the presence or absence of retained roots, oral pathology, fractures, or impacted teeth. In cases of poorly angulated antemortem radiograph, the forensic odontologist may attempt to duplicate those imaging errors in order to aid in the reconciliation process. Unlike an antemortem radiographic exam, any postmortem images of poor forensic value can be retaken since radiation exposure is not a consideration. Postmortem imaging equipment must be adjusted to compensate for the fact that skeletal remains often require less radiation due to the lack of soft tissue absorption.

6.7.5 Types of Imaging Devices

Numerous types of image recording devices exist for forensic dental radiography, and each device has advantages and disadvantages (ANSI/ADA 2017).

6.7.5.1 Film

Since its introduction in 1896 by Dr. C. Edmund Kells, recording dental images on photographic film has revolutionized clinical dentistry. Although digital technologies have largely replaced film, it is still used throughout the world and can be an important historical source of dental information. The ability to quickly assemble a film processing station, especially in a morgue area where computer usage would be challenging, makes it a useful alternative in certain situations. If possible, film images should be converted to an electronic format using a specialized scanner capable of transmissive scanning at a suitable resolution.

6.7.5.2 Phosphorus Storage Plates (PSP)

Phosphorus storage plates function similarly to photographic film. The images are recorded on specialized flexible phosphor-backed thin plastic sensors, which are considered wireless since they are not directly connected to a computer. After exposure, the PSP is placed in a digital scanner, and the latent image is processed, digitized, and transferred via specialized imaging software and ultimately displayed on the computer. Although the process of image acquisition is slower than a digital sensor, a significant advantage of PSP technology is that a single scanner can serve multiple autopsy stations, thereby making it a less costly alternative to digital sensors. The flexibility of PSPs simplifies the imaging of decedents when compared to digital sensors, especially in cases of rigor mortis. Because image quality diminishes with PSP usage, some consider the radiographic quality to be inferior to those of solid-state digital sensors (Anas et al. 2010).

6.7.6 Digital Sensors

The current gold standard of dental radiographic imaging is the digital sensor. These solid-state devices are directly connected to a computer, typically through a USB port, and the image is immediately viewable. However, digital sensors are more costly than PSPs and their bulkiness causes them to be more challenging to use in cases where access to the oral cavity is limited. Digital sensors produce high diagnostic quality and are more durable than PSPs, which makes them an ideal choice for use in a morgue environment.

6.7.7 Radiographic Sources

Numerous dental radiographic sources are available for forensic dental imaging. Radiographic sources can be wall-mounted or handheld, with the former preferred for antemortem imaging and the latter for postmortem imaging. In both cases, the radiographic source is used extraorally, and both give diagnostic quality radiographs (Pittayapat et al. 2010). It is vital that the forensic odontologist is familiar with the proper operation and settings for the device used, including radiation safety protocol and the protection of the operator and nearby personnel. This is especially important when handheld devices are utilized (Figure 6.9).

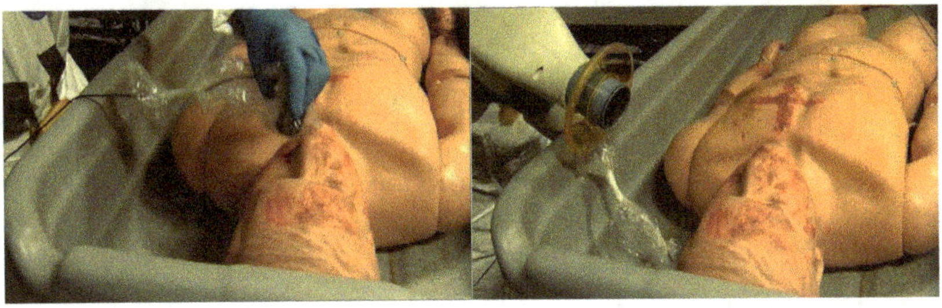

Figure 6.9 Examples of digital intraoral sensors and handheld radiation Source.

6.7.8 Types of Dental Radiographs

Dental radiography consists of two types of dental radiographs: intraoral radiographs, where the imaging film or sensor is placed within the mouth, and extraoral radiographs, where the film or sensor is placed outside the mouth.

6.7.8.1 Intraoral Radiographs

Intraoral radiographs are the most common type of dental image recorded. Several types of intraoral radiographs are used, each designed to image a different part of the oral cavity.

Periapical radiographs are images that include the tooth crown and root of the surrounding bone structures. They provide the best representation of individual teeth; however, the tooth/sensor (or phosphor plate or film) angulation and the angulation of the external radiation beam can distort the size and shape of restorations. Periapical restorations are also the most sensitive to operator error, and only a small portion of the surrounding structures are imaged because of their small size.

Bitewing radiographs are ideal for imaging the crown portion of posterior teeth in a less-distorted manner than periapical images. They provide a more accurate comparison of restoration morphology. Although common in antemortem records, the ability to take this type of image in the postmortem environment is somewhat limited because they require precise manipulation of both the maxilla and mandible in order to place the imaging device in the appropriate intraoral position.

Theoretical concerns have been raised that antemortem bitewing radiographs may represent an insufficient number of points of concordance to make a positive identification. However, population studies have shown that 70% of all restorations are placed in the posterior region of the mouth. Therefore these radiographs have a high yield for forensically useful information (ANSI/ADA 2015).

Occlusal radiographs are intraoral images that require a large film packet or digital phosphor plate (~5.7 × 7.6 cm), which is placed parallel to the occlusal plane and are used to image the anterior teeth. Occlusal radiographs are rarely used antemortemly, which makes their direct comparison with postmortem images difficult. However, they are well suited for imaging when rigor mortis is present and surgical exposure of the jaws is contraindicated. There is currently no suitable solid-state digital sensor available for this type of radiographic image.

6.7.8.2 Extraoral Radiographs

Although less common than intraoral radiographs, antemortem extraoral radiographs are gaining popularity with the use of 3-D radiographic imaging. It is expected that these images will not only become more common but will allow for a more accurate comparison of antemortem and postmortem radiographic data. However, few medical examiners and coroner offices have these devices because of their cost. An additional disadvantage is that most devices are designed for imaging in the prone position, although newer supine positioning devices are slowly entering the market.

Panoramic radiographs are the most common type of extraoral radiographs. They image the entire intraoral cavity and surrounding structures. This includes the maxillary and mandibular teeth, the entire maxilla and mandible, maxillary sinuses, nasal passages, the inferior orbital structures, and adjacent bone structures can be visualized in a single radiograph. This image is particularly useful in diagnosing previous jaw fractures, as well as the development of the tooth buds within the jaw for dental age assessment. It is also useful for detecting impacted teeth and any hard tissue pathologies within the jaws. However, individual teeth and supporting structures may overlap or be distorted, especially in the anterior region, making a comparison with intraoral images difficult.

Cephalometric radiographs are a standardized lateral radiographic view of the skull used for craniofacial metric analysis. These images are commonly used for orthodontic diagnostic purposes and can easily be obtained postmortem when a survey radiograph of the entire body is performed. Because of the superimposition of the right and left teeth, it has limited value for comparing dental restorations. However, it may be useful in obtaining diagnostic information to support a presumptive identification from non-dental other methods.

Dental Cone Beam Computed Tomography (CBCT) is a specialized type of radiographic equipment used to produce a three-dimensional image of the skull. Unlike medical CT units where the X-rays diverge in a fan-shaped configuration, CBCT units use a cone beam–shaped radiation source. The CBCT scanner rotates 360° around the patient's head and can create a 3-D rendition of not only the dentition but a pseudo-cephalometric radiograph of surrounding structures. However, the images are not as high resolution as intraoral radiographs and are similar to cephalometric radiographs. Metallic objects tend to create a metal artifact, making imaging near metallic restorations difficult. However, unlike cephalometric radiographs, CBCT scanners can correct for geometric distortion and create views that will prevent the superimposition of anatomical structures. When using CBCT images, care must be taken when comparing its thin slices of images against a two-dimensional image, which superimposes multiple structures onto a single radiograph.

Although CBCT use in clinical dentistry has become far more common, it may be cost-prohibitive for postmortem disaster victim identification (DVI) deployments. However, should CBCT antemortem and postmortem images be available, a three-dimensional virtual superimposition of the images can assist in the matching, and therefore the identification, of an individual.

Other medical radiographs – An experienced forensic odontologist may be able to use other medical radiographs for inclusionary/exclusionary comparison when antemortem dental radiographs are not available. Anatomical features such as the maxillary and frontal sinuses, and numerous other bones of the skull, can be used for comparison. However, unless a medical device or a unique skeletal landmark is present, their use for a definitive finding may be questionable. Standard medical radiographs often exhibit superimposition of the right and left dental structures. Medical-grade computerized tomography (CT) imaging of the head may also be helpful, but unless the scan used specialized dental upgraded software, the resolution of the teeth and jaws may be insufficient to make an adequate comparison.

6.7.9 Radiographic Guidelines

Dental imaging guidelines should be standardized within the DVI environment. A protocol should recommend a modified dental complete mouth series radiographic survey including at least two periapical images of each tooth. For the adult dentition, three maxillary and three mandibular anterior periapical and eight posterior periapical radiographs (two in each quadrant) should be imaged. For the pediatric dentition, one to two maxillary and one to two mandibular anterior periapical and eight posterior periapical radiographs (two in each quadrant) should be obtained. Sometimes, an occlusal view can be substituted for an anterior periapical radiograph in pediatric cases. Should conventional bitewing radiographs be needed, a "simulated bitewing projection" can be made by placing the teeth out of occlusion and placing the imaging device perpendicular to the dentition. Edentulous regions should also be imaged to determine perimortem tooth loss, impacted teeth, healing fractures, implanted medical or dental devices in the region, or any dental pathology that may be useful in assisting in a dental identification.

Because a dental identification depends on the quality of the radiographs, it is vital that the antemortem radiographs are of the highest quality possible. Unfortunately, the forensic odontologist has little control over the quality of these radiographs. In cases where film was used, the dental provider must send the original radiographs and maintain a duplicate copy. The name, birth date, and the date the original radiographs were taken must be clearly annotated. In addition, the orientation of the films should be clearly marked, and, if they are not present, the forensic odontologist should use the rules concerning the "dot" present on the film. For horizontally oriented films, the dot must be on the upper-left or lower-right-hand corners of the film. The dot must be on the upper right, or lower left for vertically oriented films. This rule is valid for both original films and duplicate films regardless of the orientation of any of the films when the duplication process took place (Gibson and Aschheim 2003). When PSP plates are used, extra caution should be taken since they lack a herringbone lead backing necessary to verify the film was in the correct orientation (Weems 2013).

Ideally, digital dental radiographs should be transferred in a Digital Imaging and Communication in Medicine (DICOM) format, via an encrypting storage device or following the American Dental Association recommendations, by a secure messaging system (ADA 2015; Farman 2005). Whenever possible, DICOM structured display information should be included (http://dicom.nema.org/medical/dicom/current/output/chtml/part03/sect_C.11.16.html).

If the forensic dental management software cannot import DICOM information, intermediate software should be used to convert the images to a compatible, lossless or at least minimally lossy graphics format such as Tagged Image File (TIF) or Joint Photographic Expert Group (JPG) file format. If the sender uses a generic image format, the images should be annotated to prevent the possibility that the images are misassigned to another individual (Hyatt 2008). Regardless of the format, there must be sufficient resolution (300 to 600 dpi) to guarantee proper visualization of dental details. Paper printouts or fax copies of digital radiographs should be used with caution since they rarely provide sufficient detail to support the number of points of concordance necessary to make an appropriate dental identification.

6.8 Intraoral and Extraoral Photographs

The use of photographs of the teeth may also be helpful in the dental identification process, especially when there are unique dental features that provide points of concordance for comparison. Ideally, the comparison should be performed using photographs taken at similar angulation and magnification (Figure 6.10). However, many of these features are difficult to describe, and since there is no way to assess

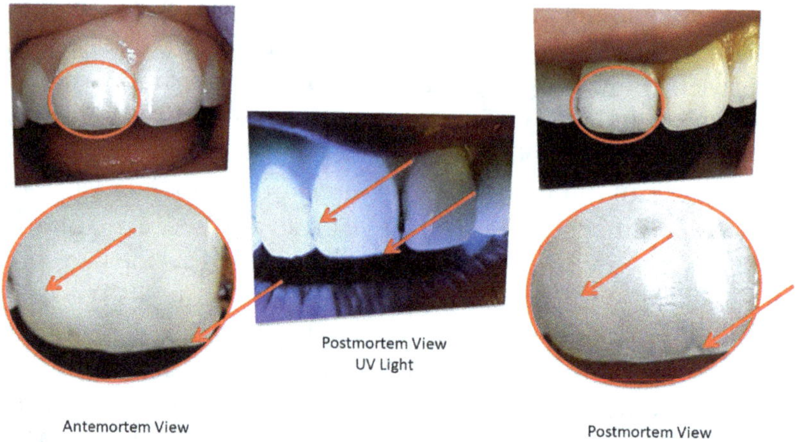

Figure 6.10 An example of the use of intraoral imaging and alternative lighting to assist in the dental identification process (courtesy of Dr. James Hudson).

the uniqueness of a characteristic in a given population they should be used with caution. Finally, orthodontic or restorative intervention may make a visual comparison of photographs ineffective.

6.8.1 Postmortem Photographs

Incident commanders must create specific rules regarding the photographing of human remains during a mass fatality incident. A standardized protocol for the types of recorded images will significantly assist the dental forensic team. Images should be recorded using digital equipment, with cameras capable of sufficient image resolution and appropriate flash attachments to record human dentition accurately. It is recommended that the American Board of Orthodontics (ABO) Case Submission Display (ABO-01) be followed for defining appropriate, photographic views (Table 6.3) (ABO 2018).

Before photography commences, oro-dental structures and prostheses should be clean and debris-free. Images should clearly show the facial, lingual, and occlusal surfaces. In addition, a survey image displaying the case number identification tag should be made to allow for future verification that those images are from the decedent. If necessary, an American Board of Forensic Odontology (ABFO) #2 ruler should be included in at least one image.

Table 6.3 Oro-dental photographic views.

Photographic Views
Full face, lips retracted
Close-up view of anterior teeth
Lateral views of teeth in a slightly open position, and in occlusion
Occlusal views, maxillary and mandibular teeth
Removable dental prostheses

6.9 Study Casts

Dental casts can also be used as valuable comparison tools. The direct comparison of tooth morphology and oral landmarks, such as arch form, tooth position, and even rugae anatomy, may be used to support a positive dental identification. Occlusal relationships and comparisons can also be used in determining if there is a relationship between the antemortem and postmortem models (Figure 6.11). If the 3-D antemortem dental information is in a digital format, a 3-D printer can be used to create a physical model.

Care should be taken in the handling of all study casts. The forensic odontologist should be aware that family members may request an antemortem cast be returned to the family, and therefore a duplicate should be used in cases where the model may become damaged or

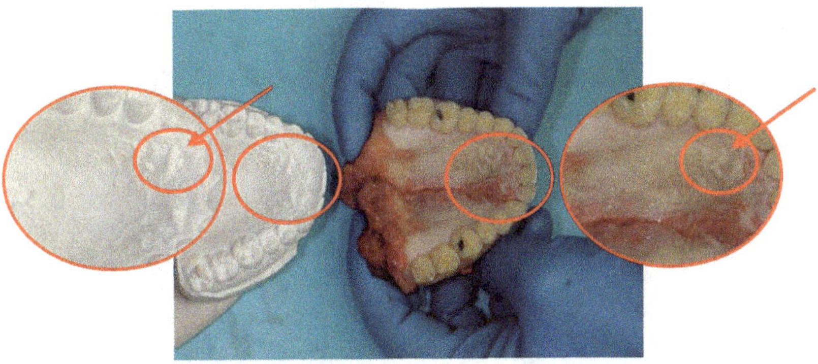

Figure 6.11 An example of the use of study casts and as well as rugae morphology to lighting to assist in the dental identification process.

discolored. In addition, when making impressions of the decedent, extra care should be taken due to the possibility of postmortem fragility of the teeth, especially in skeletonized situations, and decomposition of the soft tissue.

6.10 Denture Labeling

The placement of identifying information on or in a dental prosthetic device can serve as an essential tool for the forensic odontologist. Often there is a legal mandate to place, or at least to offer to place, this information. Identification markings can be one of two types: surface markings and inclusion markings. Surface markings consist of carving or engraving patient identifier information into the denture base (Figure 6.12). Inclusion markings consist of placing an identification

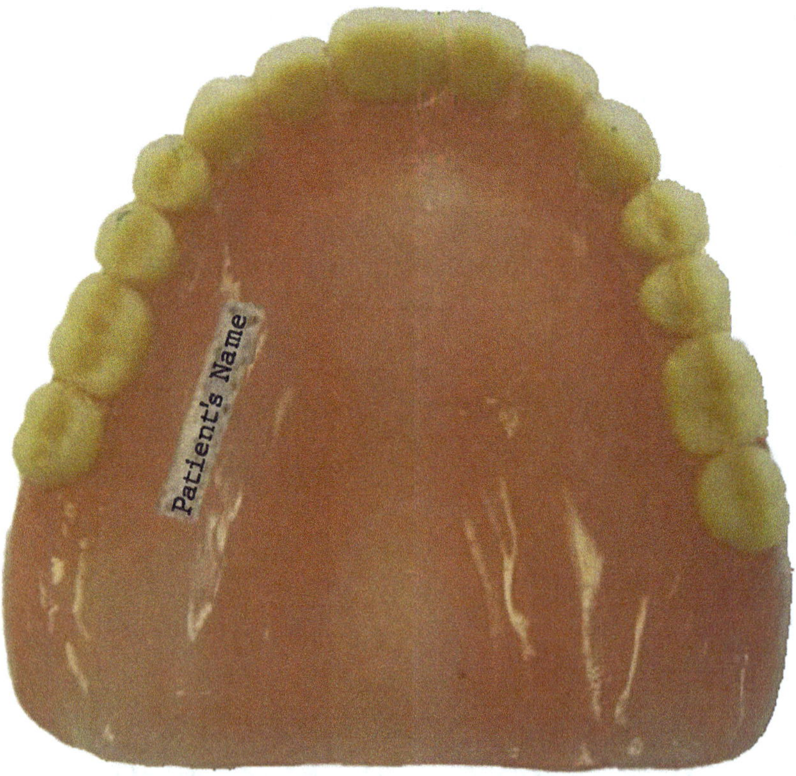

Figure 6.12 An example of the use of denture label study to assist in the dental identification process.

label within the denture acrylic base, either using an auto polymerizing acrylic resin following processing or directly into the base during the processing of the prosthesis. Newer technologies such as the inclusion of Radio Frequency Identification (RFID) chips, barcodes, and microchips further aid in the identification process. A labeled denture should be considered contextual evidence, and the uniqueness of the denture and the specificity of its fit to the dentition will determine the degree of certainty in the identification process.

6.11 Dental Age Assessment

Dental age assessment is the process of determining the individual's age range based on the development of tooth buds (Figure 6.13). Like other age estimation techniques, it does not provide a definitive source conclusion; however, especially in cases of a small closed population, it can be used as a confirmatory or exclusionary tool. It is especially useful in incidents that involve a limited number of infants, children, and sub-adults whose age ranges do not overlap. However, this technique should be performed by forensic odontologists trained in selecting the correct age-assessment methodology and reference database. It is important to note that development rates vary between individuals.

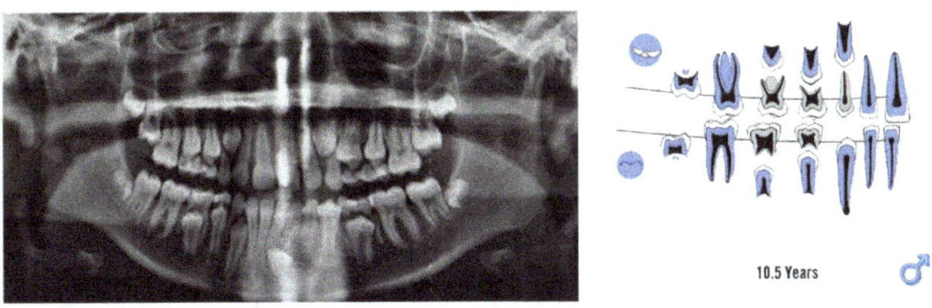

Figure 6.13 An example of the use of the London Atlas for estimating an age range to assist in the dental identification process. (Table Image from the Atlas of tooth development and eruption (https://www.qmul.ac.uk/dentistry/atlas).

6.12 Characterization of Dental Materials

Although considered contextual evidence, the analysis of the microstructure and composition of dental materials can aid in establishing a victim's identity. Dental materials, especially filler particles and chemical binders, are unaffected by extremely high temperatures and even cremation. Therefore, knowing the manufacturer-specific composition of these materials and their location of the restoration to correlate it with the dental record can assist in the identification process (Bush et al. 2006, 2008). This technique involves the use of Scanning Electron Microscopy (SEM provides structural detail of the restorative material) and Energy Dispersive X-ray Spectroscopy (EDS provides quantitative elemental composition information about the restoration). Similar results can be obtained with X-Ray Fluorescence (XRF). A significant shortcoming of these techniques is that there are no reference databases; therefore, local reference samples must be obtained to perform a comparison.

6.13 Reconciliation

Comparison and reconciliation are the processes by which the antemortem and postmortem dental information is compared, and a determination is made as to whether the two data sets are from the same source. This conclusion is typically referred to as an identification and comes with varying degrees of certainty.

6.13.1 Source Conclusions

Although forensic odontologists commonly report conclusions based on levels of identification, in reality, they are deciding whether two sets of data have come from the same source. In order to do this, it is necessary to determine if there is enough information to make a comparison. Since this is often based on a qualitative assessment of the information provided, there is currently no standard for making this determination. In addition, there are no official guidelines on making what could be considered a subjective decision as to whether the two sets of data being compared have enough evidentiary value and whether a determination of insufficient information should be made. In reaching this determination, the forensic odontologist must evaluate the quality, quantity, clarity, and specificity of the two data sets before comparing the extent of similarities and dissimilarities.

There is currently no agreed-upon standard for the qualitative reporting of whether the observed characteristics of the two data sets are sufficiently similar to determine that they came from the same source. The forensic odontologist must report a qualitative assessment and also delineate specific similarities, referred to as points of concordance. Exclusionary determinations must include reporting characteristics that are suggestive of different sources.

6.13.2 Serial Unmasking

Although a holistic approach is sometimes advocated wherein the forensic odontologist is provided all available scientific and contextual evidence to facilitate identification, concerns have been raised that this method can introduce cognitive biases. To prevent a deviation in judgment based on a preexisting perception of an identification, it is recommended that the odontologist have limited access to external information during the review. Should additional information be needed, serial unmasking, the sequential release of limited additional information, should be performed if the evidence remains inconclusive. The withholding of non-dental information could serve as a quality assurance method in the entire forensic identification process, especially if irreconcilable discrepancies between the dental and non-dental findings are noted. It is recommended that the Identification Review Board (see Section 6.14.10) should verify that the preliminary dental identification is based solely on the dental evidence.

6.13.3 Criteria for Comparison and Reconciliation

The fundamental theory behind human identification is that each individual has a sufficient number of biometrically measurable, unique sets of features to allow for comparison to exclude all others. Unfortunately, uniqueness cannot be proven; it can only be disproven. Therefore, all dental identifications may be assumed to be a qualitative assessment and cannot be defined with a known error rate. However, historical studies of dental identifications with follow-up verification incorporating DNA comparison have shown that this process has a high degree of reliability (NYC OCME, n.d.). In addition, since dental identification often uses physical alterations of the dentition by individual dental providers, there is an additional level of uniqueness.

6.13.4 Reporting

It is important to note that most jurisdictions require the medical examiner or coroner to make the final determination of identification, but typically it is based on the recommendations of forensic specialists. Therefore, although reporting is expressed as levels of identification, in reality, the forensic specialist is making a source comparison (see **6.13.1 Source Conclusions**). Unfortunately, there is no approved suggested ISO standard terminology for qualitative source conclusions between forensic science disciplines. However, suggested standards from ISO Technical Committee 272 Forensic Sciences are currently being circulated.

Numerous dental organizations have attempted to establish guidelines for levels of reconciliation (e.g., INTERPOL, IOFOS). The forensic odontologist should be aware of the terminology used in the current DVI operation so that their conclusions will be consistent with those of other forensic science teams.

6.13.5 Terminology

In the United States, forensic odontologists primarily use terminology defined by the American Board of Forensic Odontology (ABFO) (Table 6.4). Interpol DVI operations commonly use International Organization for Forensic Odonto-Stomatology (IOFOS) terminology (Table 6.5).

6.14 Assembling the Forensic Odontology Team

Although most medical examiners offices use a trained forensic odontologist for daily operations, the DVI forensic odontology team members require additional specialized training. This includes the handling of fragmented, commingled, heat, and fire-altered remains and remains that have the potential to be contaminated by chemical, biological, or nuclear means. In addition, in cases where outside forensic odontology consultants will be used, the DVI team must verify credentials and ensure compliance with any applicable local, state, or federal regulations.

Table 6.4 I.O.F.O.S. Levels of identification (IOFOS 2020).

Terminology	Definition
Identity Established	There is enough PM and AM dental comparison information with several specific characteristics that are identical. Any discrepancies are compatible with the time difference between the AM dental records and the PM dental investigation. Nothing refutes identity.
Identity Probable	There is limited PM and AM dental comparison information with at least one specific characteristic that is identical between AM and PM. Any discrepancies are compatible with the time difference between the AM dental records and the PM dental investigation. Nothing refutes identity
Identity Possible	There is limited PM and AM dental comparison information with no specific characteristic that is identical between AM and PM. Any discrepancies are compatible with the time difference between the AM dental records and the PM dental investigation. Nothing refutes identity. In this case, identity cannot be excluded.
Identity Excluded	At least one special characteristic refutes identity

Table 6.5 ABFO categories & terminology for body identification (ABFO 2020).

Terminology	Definition
Positive Identification	The antemortem and postmortem data match in sufficient detail to establish that they are from the same individual. In addition, there are no irreconcilable discrepancies.
Possible Identification	The antemortem and postmortem data have consistent features, but, due to the quality of either the postmortem remains or the antemortem evidence, it is not possible to positively establish dental identification.
Insufficient Evidence	The available information is insufficient to form the basis for a conclusion.
Exclusion	The antemortem and postmortem data are clearly inconsistent. However, it should be understood that identification by exclusion is a valid technique in certain circumstances.

The number of necessary forensic odontology team members varies with the size of the incident. For more minor incidents, one or ideally at least two individuals may perform multiple team member tasks. More significant incidents may require multiple team members to be assigned to an individual team task. When determining the necessary number of forensic odontology team members in a particular situation, it is essential to ensure their mental and physical health by providing adequate time away from the incident.

6.14.1 Leadership Team

The leadership team is responsible for the overall organization and deployment of the overall team. For minor incidents, only a chief forensic odontologist is necessary; however, for more complex mass fatality incidents (MFI), an assistant chief and deputy chiefs (tour commanders) may be required. Whenever multiple forensic odontologists are involved, a single individual must be assigned the chief leadership position to adjudicate any issues. In addition, when multiple supervisors are necessary, there must be an overlap of their work assignments to allow for the orderly passing of information between work tours. Team meetings should be conducted at regular intervals to address any issues arising during the investigation. In cases where teams are operating on a 24/7 basis, these meetings should be scheduled at a time when as many individuals as possible can attend. Online web participation should be considered to maximize the number of leadership members participating in these meetings.

6.14.2 Administration Team

The administration team is responsible for scheduling and credentialing professionals participating in DVI operations. This includes verifying educational and licensing credentials and ensuring appropriate liability and malpractice insurance coverage. Verification must include establishing that their generic dental professional malpractice insurance coverage includes the practice of forensic odontology. The team is also responsible for creating a mechanism for decredential individuals should it be deemed necessary.

6.14.3 Site Assessment Team

There is a difference of opinion as to whether forensic odontology team members should assist at the disaster site to identify, collect, and preserve dental evidence or whether exposure to this environment poses an unnecessary health risk. The DVI management team must evaluate this risk before deploying a dental team for site assessment, and, if deployment is deemed necessary, the individuals must be adequately trained in functioning in a contaminated environment using the appropriate personal protective equipment (PPE). Medical follow-up may be necessary for an extended time to confirm that the individuals did not sustain any injuries due to hazards in the on-site environment (Yip et al. 2016).

6.14.4 Antemortem Team

The antemortem team should be staffed by dental professionals with training and experience in determining what data is necessary from an antemortem perspective to perform a dental reconciliation. Their function is to procure, analyze, and consolidate the dental data into a single standardized dental record. A key to this process is consolidating multiple missing person reports into a single missing person record. Algorithms should be incorporated in the forensic dental management software to prevent the duplication of entries when this information is retrieved electronically. It is also critical that the interviewer know the appropriate data formats and annotation of the information received. Antemortem radiographs are a vital component of the dental record. The antemortem team should attempt to collect the highest quality attainable radiographs possible (see Section 6.7.3).

The antemortem team should be present at the victim identification center to directly interact with family members when dental information is obtained; therefore, they must be trained in appropriate methods of interactions with grieving individuals. They must also be trained in acquiring valuable antemortem dental data from other dental or medical professionals, employers, insurance companies, government agencies, or military agencies. They should be knowledgeable in the use of social media for data collection. It is strongly recommended that the team be composed of a minimum of two members to avoid errors.

6.14.5 Postmortem Team

The postmortem team should be staffed by dental professionals with training and experience in determining what data is necessary from a postmortem perspective to perform a dental reconciliation. Team members must be trained in the intricacies of performing a dental autopsy and must be licensed by the state to perform this autopsy. They should also have training in photographic documentation of the remains, especially if no photographic team is available. The postmortem team is also responsible for verifying the readiness of the dental autopsy suite.

6.14.6 Coding Team

The coding team is responsible for ensuring that the forensic odontology data is entered into the forensic dental management system precisely and consistently. Codes must be entered consistently to allow the software algorithms to function properly; therefore, only a single individual should be responsible for determining the appropriate dental codes for ambiguous clinical situations. This team must understand the fundamental algorithms used by the software to make appropriate coding decisions. The use of standardized terminology is strongly encouraged (ANSI/ADA (2015), ISO (2020)(

6.14.7 Information Technology Team

The information technology team ensures that computer systems and software function correctly. This requires complete knowledge of forensic odontology operations and a high degree of computer literacy to interact with the information technology group operating the DVI operation. In addition, team members should be authorized to communicate with the hardware and software vendors whose products are used during the operation to troubleshoot issues.

6.14.8 Photographic Team

The photographic team is responsible for the capture and preservation of visual images of the decedent. They must use equipment capable of capturing both intraoral and extraoral detailed images for future reviewing of this information. Protocols should be in place to allow for prompt information transfer, secure storage, and prompt retrieval from an appropriate database.

6.14.9 Reconciliation (Comparison) Team

The reconciliation team should be staffed by dental professionals with training and experience in understanding what data is necessary to perform and justify a dental reconciliation. Team members must be adequately trained in reporting their source conclusions in a consistent and precise manner so that others can interpret their analysis and conclusions appropriately (see Section 6.13). Discrepancies must be reviewed and, if unexplainable, be justified and corrected before issuing a report.

6.14.10 Identification Review Board (IRB)

Ideally, the identification review board should review the preliminary reports from forensic disciplines and any other antemortem and postmortem contextual information before a final report is issued. The IRB should consist of specialists in each discipline involved in the identification process and include members of forensic pathology, forensic odontology, friction ridge analysis, DNA, and forensic anthropology. The forensic odontologist is responsible for justifying the conclusions drawn by the dental reconciliation team. A protocol should be established to resolve any irreconcilable discrepancies between the forensic specialists. When there is insufficient evidence to support a single identification modality, the team should determine if the weight of the conclusions from multiple teams supports the identification. The IRB ultimately reports to the medicolegal authorities responsible for issuing the death certificate.

6.15 Computer-Assisted Dental Identification

Dental identification has been available for many years. Initial systems were used to catalog data, but current systems include ranking algorithms that prioritize the likelihood of an antemortem and postmortem data match (Lorton and Langley 1986; Siegel et al. 1977). The data and images on the comparison list are reviewed, analyzed, and compared by a forensic odontologist for points of concordance to determine a data match.

6.15.1 Computer Assisted Post-Mortem Identification (CAPMI)

One of the first computer-assisted dental identification software programs, Computer Assisted Postmortem Identification (CAPMI), was developed by Lorton, Langley, and Weed (Figures 6.14-Figure 6.15) (Lorton et al. 1988, 1989). It was used for the Oklahoma City bombing incident in 1995 and the TWA Flight 800 crash in 1996. This DOS-based system was one of the first to standardize the coding of restorations and used simple ranking algorithms to produce a list of the most probable antemortem to postmortem record matches. CAPMI eliminated implausible records from immediate consideration and identified the most probably correct records for review using the concept of numerical ranking based on "Matches," "Mismatches" (exclusions), and "Possible" (non-matching restorations that exhibit a logical direction of change) (see Section 6.3.3). Coding consists of primary codes representing the presence or condition of a tooth and the restored surfaces. Additional modifier codes assign numeric values for materials and alphabetical values for modifications of a tooth (i.e., root canal, etc.). Version 3 exhibited codes in a tabular form, while Version 4 used a text-based version of an odontogram.

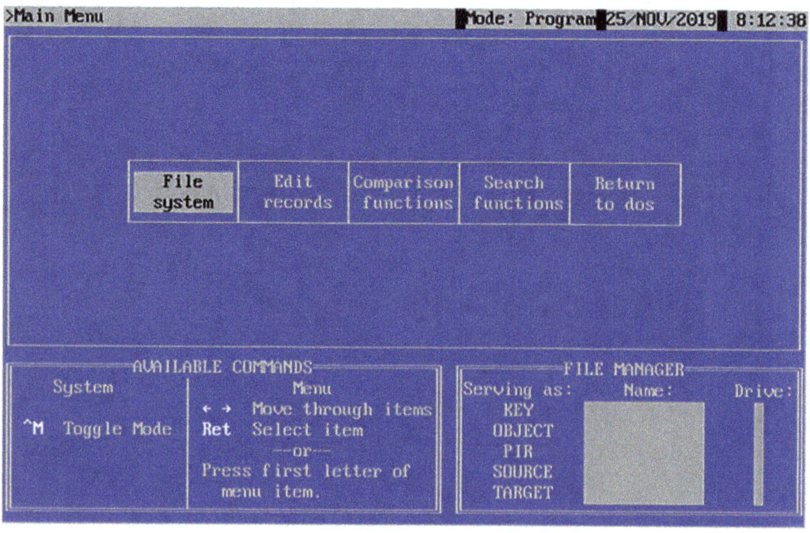

Figure 6.14 CAPMI 3 Opening Screen (Courtesy of Richard Fioxett).

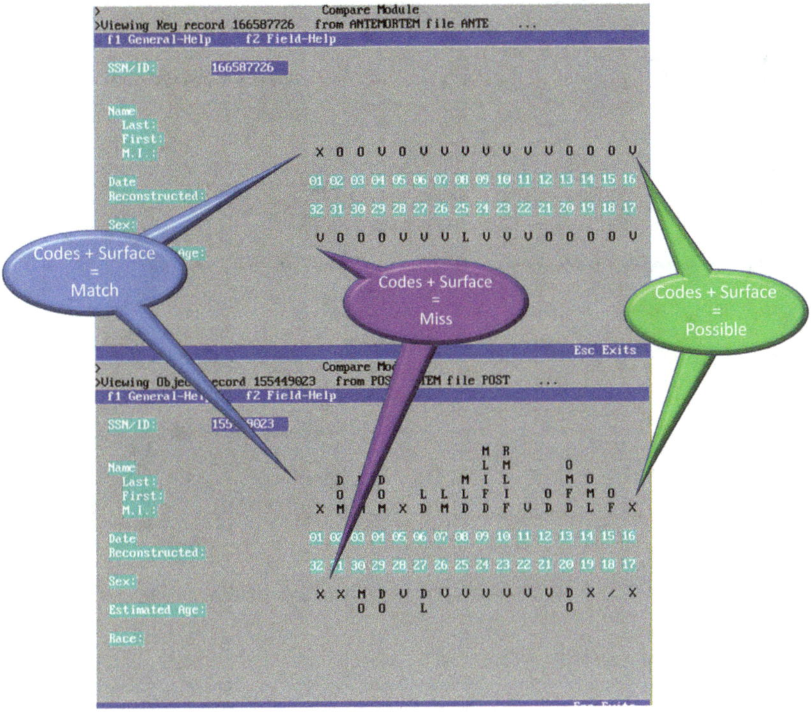

Figure 6.15 CAPMI 4 Screens showing comparison (2 screens) (Courtesy of Richard Fioxett).

6.15.2 WinID3

In the late 1990s, Dr. James McGivney introduced WinID, one of the first Windows-based software packages, which remains one of the most popular forensic odontology software packages in the United States (Figures 6.16–Figure 6.18). It uses Microsoft Visual Basic 6 programming language and Microsoft access database. Unlike CAPMI, it can import a single image of a radiograph and can also record some anthropological information concerning the missing person or decedent. WinID ranking algorithms calculate "Hits" (matches), "Misses" (mismatches), and "Possible" (comparisons with a logical direction of change). It offers three standard methods of ranking lists: "Most Dental Hits," "Least Dental Mismatches," "Most Restoration Hits." WinID also offers an additional "Fuzzy Logic" ranking that combines "Hits," "Misses," and "Possible" and a ranking based on biometric and

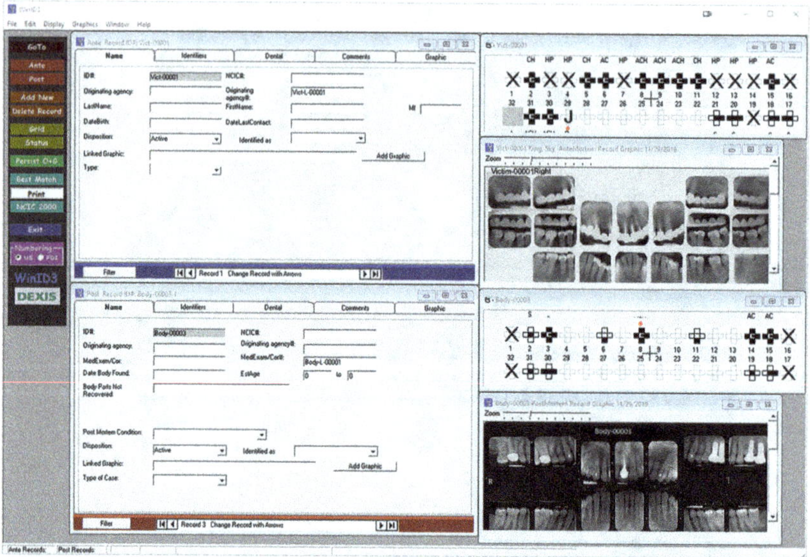

Figure 6.16 WinID3 Showing Antemortem and Postmortem Data Entry.

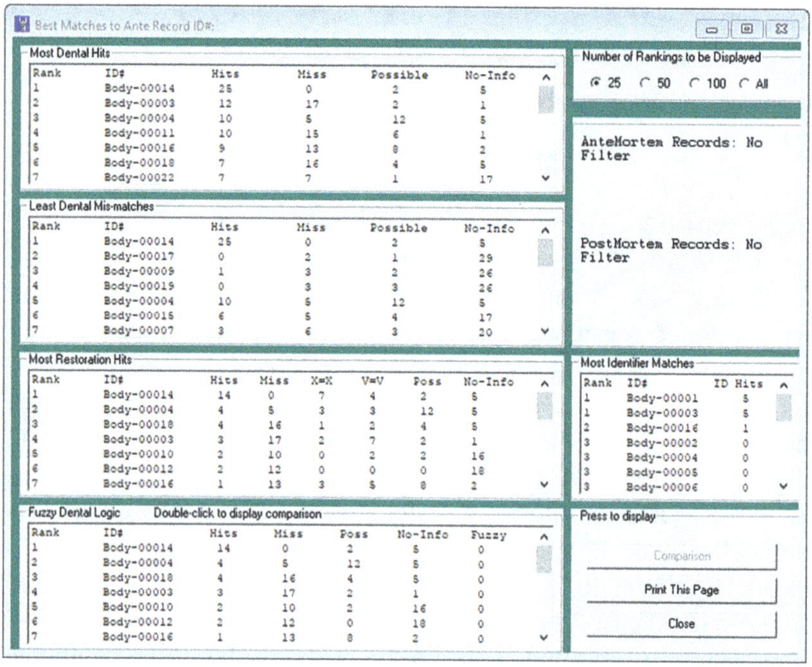

Figure 6.17 WinID3 Comparison Options.

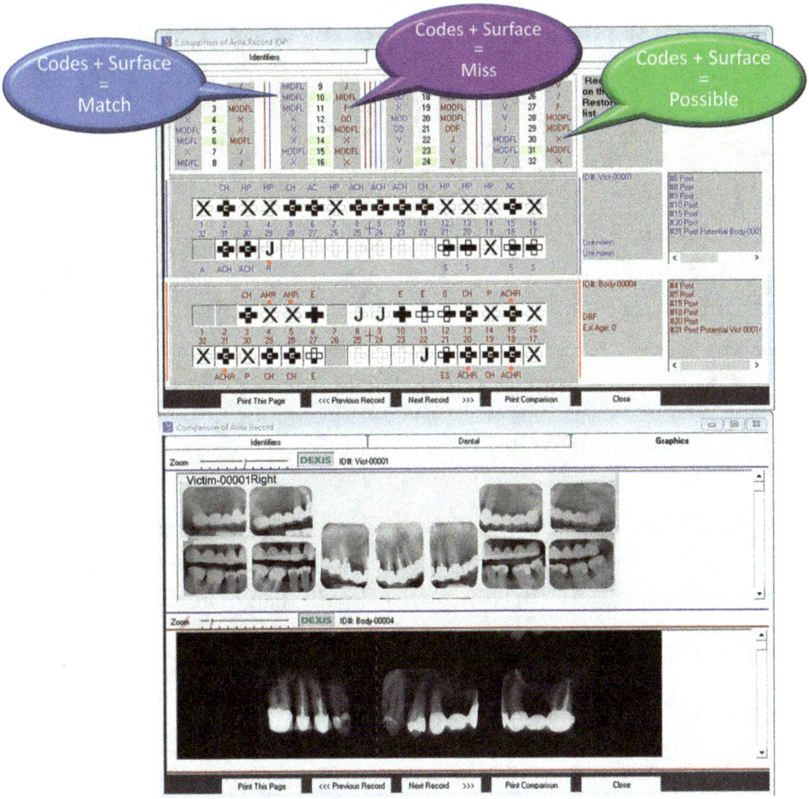

Figure 6.18 WinID Comparison Screens.

anthropological information ("Most Identifier Matches"). WinID is capable of interfacing with Dexis radiographic imaging software. A web version of WinID is currently under development by Dr. John Melville as part of his PhotoDoc Suite (https://www.drjohnmelville.com/WinIdForWeb/Production) (Figures 6.19).

6.15.3 UVIS/UDIM

Following the September 11 attack in New York City, the office of the Chief Medical Examiner for the City of New York undertook a significant software development project for mass fatality management and created the Unified Victim Identification System (UVIS). This software was designed to manage and coordinate the cataloging of missing persons and disaster victims following a mass fatality incident. It

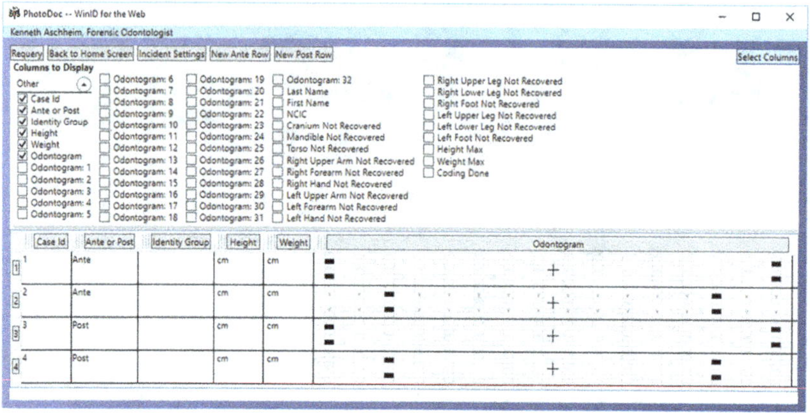

Figure 6.19 WinID for the Web.

included coordinating information and data from a centralized call center, family assistance center, field, and morgue operations. The software was designed for enterprise-level usage and used a SQL server backend and multiple levels of security.

The UVIS Dental Identification Module (UDIM) was developed based on research and software developed by Dr. Kenneth W. Aschheim. Initially designed as an add-on to WinID and originally called Query Analyzer for WinID (QA for WinID), it relied on an optimized single sorting algorithm (method), improved graphics handling, and a click-to-code (Codes can only be entered by clicking on icons) interface (http://www.dentisys.com/qaindex.html)(Aschheim 2005) (Figures 6.20-Figure 6.21). UDIM uses a mandatory core coding system of 10 tooth surface status codes and optional restorative codes, condition codes, and material codes. The user interface has been optimized to focus on irreconcilable discrepancies. There is a robust fragmentation management system (the ability to handle victims that have been fragmented into multiple specimens) to allow for the joining of multiple specimens. Next of kin interview questions are included in the software. UDIM has a direct bridge with Dexis, allowing for simplified accessing of dental radiographic images.

In 2010, it was decided that the UVIS disaster management system would be recoded as UVIS CMS (Case Management System) to allow

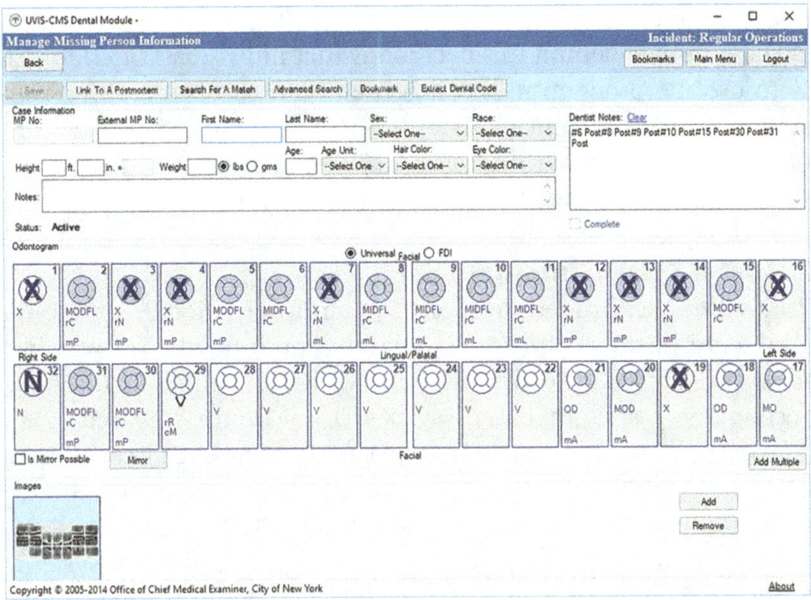

Figure 6.20 UDIM.

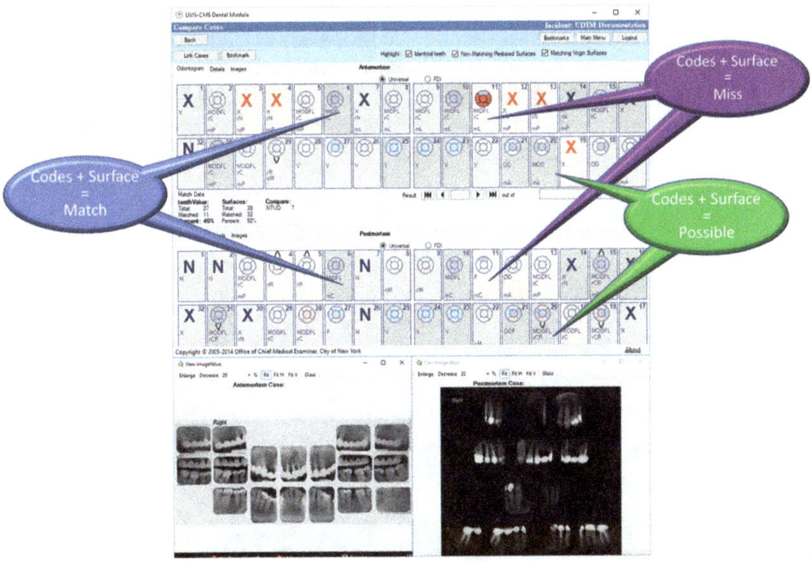

Figure 6.21 UDIM Comparison Screen.

its use as a complete morgue management software package for daily use. The rationale behind this decision is that individuals often forget how to use the program unless it is used on a consistent basis. This recoding included modifications to the UDIM module, which is currently being used for all forensic odontology operations at the New York City Office of Chief Medical Examiner (OCME).

6.15.4 DVI System International

DVI (Disaster Victim Identification) System International is the official software of Interpol for mass fatality management and was the product of Plass Data Software A/S of Holbaek, Denmark. In 2019, the company was purchased by KMD, a Denmark-based NEC Corporation subsidiary located in Ballerup, Denmark. Unlike CAPMI, WinID, or UVIS/UDIM, DVI International is a commercial product and requires purchasing a licensing agreement. The system is designed to work as either a paper-based or a computer-based entry system. The dental module uses an Interpol-specific coding system and is managed by forensic odontologists from INTERPOL DVI Standing Subcommittee's Forensic Odontology Subworking Group) (Figures 6.22, Figure 6.23).

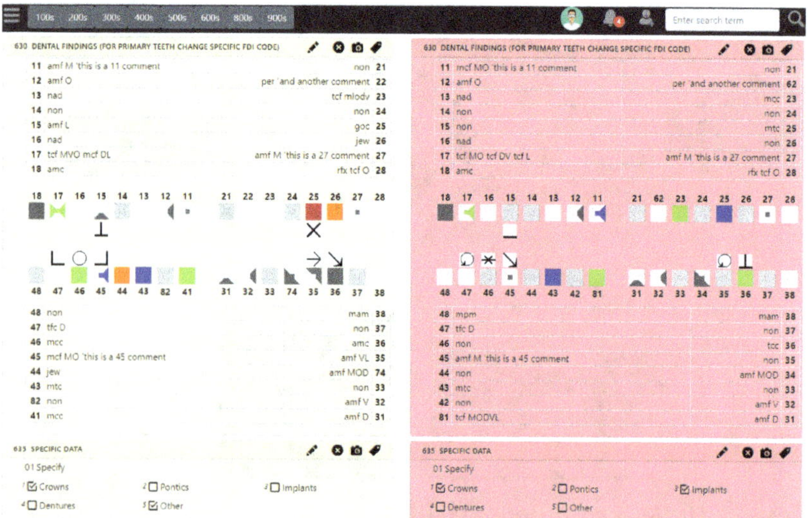

Figure 6.22 PLASS DVI Screens.

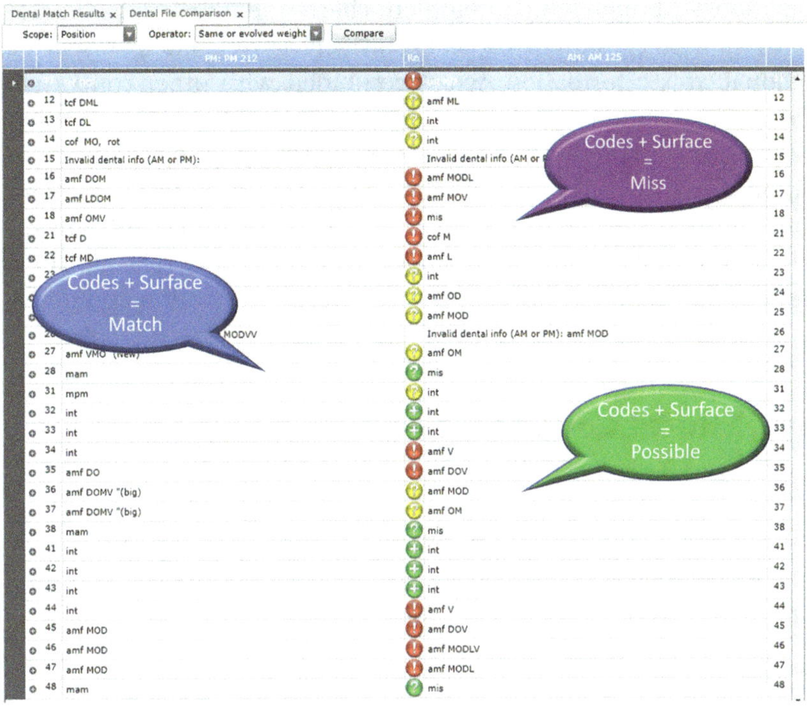

Figure 6.23 PLASS DVI Comparison Screen.

6.15.5 OdontoSearch

OdontoSearch, although not a forensic dental management software package, can serve as a valuable tool in helping to establish contextual evidence for a possible identification of an individual by dental means. Based on the work of Dr. Bradley Adams, this website, developed by Dr. Kenneth W. Aschheim in conjunction with Eric Zaidins and Gregory Renza, provides an objective means of assessing the frequency of occurrence of dental restoration patterns. When antemortem radiographs are not available, OdontoSearch can assess the weight of the dental comparison based only on written notes and charts obtained from a missing individual's medical/dental records. The methodology and rationale behind the OdontoSearch program are very similar to the procedures that have been established for mitochondrial DNA comparisons. The program compares an individual's pattern of missing, filled, and unrestored teeth to a large, representative sample of the US population. Although dental treatment charts and notes, unlike radiographs, cannot be shown to be exclusively correlated to a specific individual, this information, when combined with other contextual information, is often sufficient to determine an identification, especially in non-fragmented cases (Adams and Aschheim 2016). In addition, the software allows for the coding of restoration in either a detailed format specifying the involved surfaces of the teeth; mesial (incisal), occlusal, distal, facial (buccal/labial), lingual (palatal), or a less specific format that disregards the surface information and designates the tooth as restored (R) (Figures 6.24).

6.16 Ethical Considerations

Forensic odontologists have legal and ethical obligations to make every effort to identify and return the remains of a mass fatality incident to

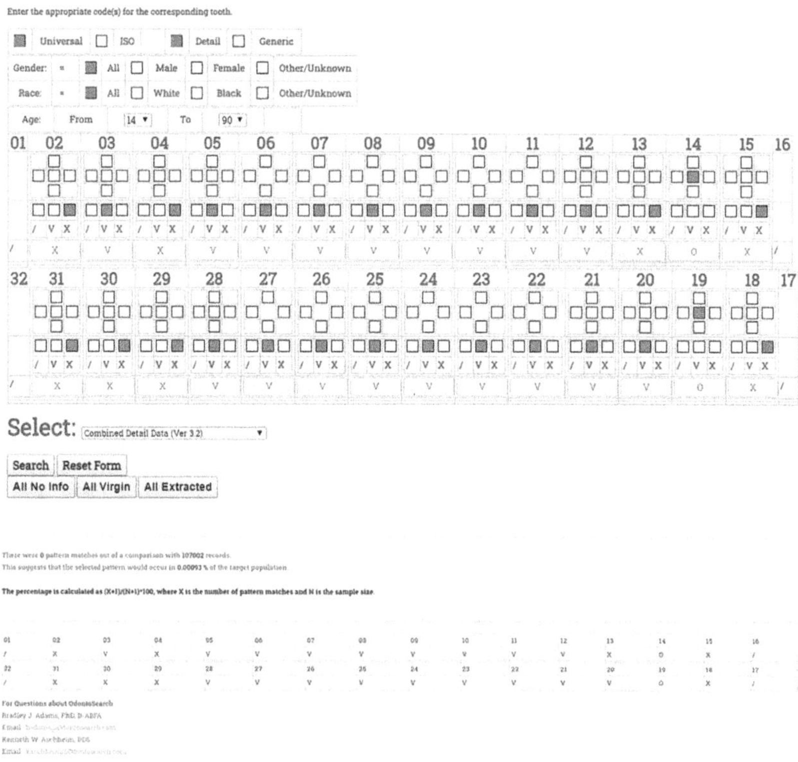

Figure 6.24 Odon to Search.

the next of kin. Therefore, the forensic odontology team must be trained to manage the deceased in a dignified and respectful manner. The forensic odontology team should follow generally accepted standards of scientific competency and must respect the rights and welfare of both the victims and the next of kin, particularly during the postmortem examination where the procedure's degree of invasiveness must be carefully considered regarding community and family wishes. If surgical access is required for the proper documentation of all oral cavity structures, forensic odontologists must always consider the degree of disfigurement that occurs during this process. Disaster victim identification is considered a human right (ICRC 2006).

6.17 Demobilization and After-Action Reports

6.17.1 Demobilization

Demobilization occurs after the incident command determines that the disaster victim identification operation should terminate. The leadership team must confirm that all postmortem examination reports have been completed, all antemortem records were reviewed, and all data was entered into the forensic dental management software. Protocols for the archiving and storing of all physical, printed, and electronic information and data from the DVI operation should be established. The forensic odontology leadership should complete an after-action report before demobilizing the dental identification team.

6.17.2 Preservation of Dental Data

6.17.2.1 Preservation of Antemortem Dental Data

All antemortem dental data, including exclusions, should be preserved once the identification operation is completed. In exclusion situations, and if policy allows, uploading the information into a missing person database (NamUS, National Crime Information Center [NCIC], etc.) should be considered to allow for the comparison of the unknown decedent in the future. If the original records are to be stored, they must follow the evidence retention policies of the local medical examiner/coroner or law enforcement agencies. If the original medical/dental record has been suitably copied or digitized, and if local policies allow, the record should be returned to the provider if requested.

6.17.2.2 Preservation of Postmortem Dental Data

All postmortem dental data, including unidentified individuals, should be preserved once the operation is completed. Although formal disaster victim identification operations are terminated, new information may subsequently become available. A policy regarding the disposition of unidentified human remains should be in place. It is critical to retain the software used to archive the information to allow for retrieval of that information in the future.

6.17.3 Post-Action Follow-Up

When formal DVI operations are completed, a policy must be in place to monitor the psychological well-being of the forensic odontology team. Monitoring physiological and psychological health-related issues following the operation is an essential component of the DVI operation. In addition, debriefing meetings during and after the incident and follow-up assessment of personnel can reduce the possibility of adverse sequelae. Therefore, a policy requiring mandatory debriefing of each team member is highly recommended.

6.17.4 Planning and Training

Successful forensic odontology DVI operations require that resources are in place for the adequate planning and training of these operations before an incident occurs. All dental equipment required to perform a dental autopsy, especially computer equipment, must be in a deployable state at all times. The use of software for daily operations that can also be used in disaster victim identification operations and daily operations will enable rapid and efficient deployment of forensic odontology personnel when an incident occurs. A written organizational plan which includes contact information for the dental identification team, standardized participation agreements, remuneration information, job protocols, and responsibilities should be in place. Documentation concerning necessary vaccinations and immunizations, training documentation, and jurisdictional and licensing verification should be readily available. Mandatory continued education training and familiarity with equipment and software used in DVI deployment operations should be an ongoing consideration. A just-in-time training protocol (teaching available when the learner needs it) should be readily available and should be implemented before the deployment of the forensic odontology team.

6.18 Conclusion

Human comparison by dental means is a vital component of the disaster victim identification process. Dental identification is both a rapid and a cost-effective method of identifying a victim and should be considered an essential component for ensuring the success of an identification operation. Preparation, training, and, most importantly, understanding of the capabilities and limitations of forensic odontology in the disaster victim identification process will lead to successful outcomes and allow for the rapid repatriation of human decedents to the next of kin.

References

ABFO (2020). ABFO body identification information and guidelines (revised February 2017) [online]. Available at: http://abfo.org/wp-content/uploads/2012/08/ABFO-Body-ID-Information-Guidelines-Feb-2017.pdf (Accessed 2 September 2020).

ABO (2018). American Board of Orthodontics (ABO) case submission display DICOM correction proposal – DICOM [online]. ftp://medical.nema.org/medical/dicom/cp/cp1571_14_OrthoVL.pdf (Accessed 14 December 2019).

Acharya, J., Shrestha, R., Shrestha, P.K., Kanchan, T. and Krishan, K. (2017). When protocol become fairy tales and gods remain buried under: Excerpts from the diary of forensic experts at ground zero during the mega quake that hit Nepal. *American Journal of Forensic Medicine and Pathology* 38 (1): 5–8.

ADA (2007). *American Dental Association Current Dental Terminology 2007–2008, Tooth Numbering and the Oral Cavity, 109*. American Dental Association.

ADA (2015). *The Secure Exchange and Utilization of Digital Images in Dentistry: (Technical Report No. 1060)*. American Dental Association. (2011, Reaffirmed 2015).

Adams, B.J. and Aschheim, K.W. (2016). Computerized dental comparison: A critical review of dental coding and ranking algorithms used in victim identification. *Journal of Forensic Sciences* 61 (1): 76–86.

Anas, A., Asaad, J. and Tarboush, K. (2010). A Comparison of intra-oral digital imaging modalities: Charged couple device versus storage phosphor plate. *International Journal of Health Science (Qassim)* 4 (2): 156–167.

ANSI/ADA (2013a). *Electronic Dental Record System Standard Functional Requirement (Standard No. 1067)*. American National Standards Institute/American Dental Association.

ANSI/ADA (2013b). *Implementation Guidelines for the Secure Transmission of Protected Health Information Health Information in Dentistry.* American National Standards Institute/American Dental Association. Technical Report No. 1085.

ANSI/ADA (2015). *Forensic Dental Data Set.* American National Standards Institute/American Dental Association Standard. 1058.

ANSI/ADA (2017). *Human Identification by Comparative Dental Analysis.* American National Standards Institute/American Dental Association. Technical Report No. 1088.

ANSI/NIST (2015). *Data Format for the Interchange of Fingerprint, Facial and Other Biometric Information (NIST Special Publication 500-290e3).* American National Standards Institute/ National Institute of Standards and Technology – Standard. (ANSI/NIST-ITL 1-2011 Update: 2015).

Aschheim, K.W.A. (2005) New method to assist in the rapid identification of unknown bodies utilizing a nationwide database of specialized forensic data. In: *Proceedings of the American Academy of Forensic Sciences* 191–192.New Orleans, LA: The American Academy of Forensic Sciences.

Bowers, C. (2011). *Forensic Dental Evidence: An Investigator's Handbook,* 2nd ed. Boston: Academic Press.

Bush, M.A., Bush, P.J. and Miller, R.G. (2006). Detection and classification of composite resins in incinerated teeth for forensic purposes. *Journal of Forensic Sciences* 51 (3): 636–642.

Bush, M.A., Miller, R.G., Norrlander, A.L. and Bush, P.J. (2008). Analytical survey of restorative resins by SEM/EDS and XRF: Databases for forensic purposes. *Journal of Forensic Sciences* 53 (2): 419–425.

CAPMI (1989) 3-*0 Tutorial documentation.*

Charan Gowda, B.K., Mohan, C.V. and Hemavathi, (2016). Oral autopsy: A simple, faster procedure for total visualization of oral cavity. *Journal of Forensic Dental Sciences* 8 (2): 103–107.

Farman, A.G. (2005). Applying DICOM to dentistry. *Journal of Digital Imaging* 18 (1): 23–27.

Gibson, B. and Aschheim, K.W. (2003). A consistent and accurate method of interpretation of duplicate dental films in mass fatality incidents. In: *55th Annual Meeting of the American Academy of Forensic Sciences* 20 February. Illinois, Chicago, IL: The American Academy of Forensic Sciences.

Hyatt, J. (2008). Digital imaging. *Journal of the American Dental Association* 139(9): 2.

IOFOS (2020) I.O.F.O.S. Recommendations for Quality Assurance: body Identification Mass Disaster, International Organization for Forensic Odonto-Stomatology [online]. Available at: http://www.iofos.eu/Quality-Ass/QA_2018_final/Identification_disaster_final.pdf (Accessed 2 September 2020).

ICRC (2006). *The Missing: ICRC Progress Report.* International Committee of the Red Cross. www.icrc.org.

ISO (2009). *Dentistry – Vocabulary.* International Organization for Standardization. (ISO/DIS Standard No. 1942).

ISO (2016). *3950:2016 Dentistry – Designation System for Teeth and Areas of the Oral Cavity.* International Organization for Standardization.

ISO (2020). ISO 20888:2020 Dentistry -Vocabulary and designation system for forensic oro-dental data.

Lorton, L. and Langley, W.H. (1986). Decision-making concepts in postmortem identification. *Journal of Forensic Sciences* 31 (1): 190–196.

Lorton, L., Rethman, M. and Friedman, R. (1988). The Computer-Assisted Postmortem Identification (CAPMI) System: a computer-based identification program. *Journal of Forensic Sciences* 33 (4): 977–984.

Lorton, L., Rethman, M. and Friedman, R. (1989). The Computer-Assisted Postmortem Identification (CAPMI) system: sorting algorithm improvements. *Journal of Forensic Sciences* 34 (4): 996–1002.

NYC OCME (2003). *Unpublished Data: World Trade Center Dental Identification Team.* Office of Chief Medical Examiner for the City of New York.

NYC OCME (n.d.). *Ongoing World Trade Center Dental Identification Team Results (Unpublished), Office of Chief Medical Examiner for the City of New York, 2001-2019.* Office of Chief Medical Examiner for the City of New York.

Page, A.W. (2019). What is rapid DNA? [online]. Available at: https://www.ande.com/what-israpid-dna (Accessed 8 December 2019).

Pittayapat, P., Thevissen, P., Fieuws, S., Jacobs, R. and Willems, G. (2010). Forensic oral imaging quality of handheld dental X-ray devices: Comparison of two image receptors and two devices. *Forensic Science International* 194 (1-3): 20–27.

Siegel, R., Sperber, N.D. and Trieglaff, A. (1977). Identification through the computerization of dental records. *Journal of Forensic Sciences* 22 (2): 434–442.

Weems, R.A. (2013). Critical effects of improper exposure of digital dental radiographs derived from PSP plates. In: *65th Annual Meeting of the American Academy of Forensic Sciences* 20 February. Washington DS: The American Academy of Forensic Sciences.

Yip, J., Zeig-Owens, R., Webber, M.P., Kablanian, A., Hall, C.B., Vossbrinck, M., Liu X., Weakley J., Schwartz T., Kelly K.J., and Prezant, D.J. (2016, Jan). World Trade Center-related physical and mental health burden among New York City Fire Department emergency medical service workers. *Occupational and Environmental Medicine* 73 (1): 13–20.

CHAPTER 7

Fingerprints and DVI

Bryan Johnson[1]

[1] *Federal Bureau of Investigation, Quantico, VA, USA*

Names of commercial manufacturers are provided for identification purposes only, and inclusion does not imply endorsement of the manufacturer or its product or services by the FBI. Any reproduction, or other use of these presentation materials without the express written consent of the FBI, is prohibited. The views are those of the author(s) and do not necessarily reflect the official policy or position of the FBI or the US government.

7.1 Introduction

The primary goal of Disaster Victim Identification (DVI) is to ensure that the victims of a tragic event are identified as quickly and efficiently as possible, using valid, scientific means. In any mass fatality event, regardless of the number of persons impacted, there will inherently be competing priorities amongst agencies, investigators, and families. The twenty-first century has seen a significant paradigm shift dictating the socially acceptable timeframe for resolving these events. The media, politicians, and even the victims' families define the expectations and social tolerance for the identification process. Regardless of whether the disaster event has a criminal nexus, all decedent identification work must withstand the scrutiny of the legal system, as the ramifications of certifying someone as deceased have a significant impact on the survivors and vital statistics.

In traditional US death investigations, the case is initiated when the decedent is discovered. A standard medico-legal death investigation follows, with autopsy and postmortem (PM) identification. Each case is typically treated with a cradle-to-grave mentality. The investigator assigned to the case will follow standard operating procedures and exhaust each step within the required processes until that

Disaster Victim Identification in the 21st Century: A US Perspective, First Edition.
Edited by John A Williams and Victor W Weedn.

case is resolved, and another one begins. In DVI, this simply cannot be the standard methodology as it will not allow for swift and accurate identification of all the victims.

Friction ridge skin covers the palmar surface of the hand and the plantar surface of the feet (Holder et al. 2011). It is utilitarian for grip, unique and persistent, and functional as a means for identification. Friction ridge skin is extremely resilient throughout life, maintaining its arrangement through trauma and scarring. The skin also maintains its integrity through PM trauma, including exposure to fire and water, until decomposition takes place. Friction ridge skin has been used as a reliable method of identification for over a hundred years (Ashbaugh 1999). It continues to serve as the fastest and easiest means of decedent identification, given that the friction ridge skin is still present PM. Typically, fingerprints are used for identification of live and deceased persons on a day-to-day basis, and many people refer to the whole process as fingerprint identification rather than friction ridge print identification. This is not wrong if using the fingers to make the identification; however, palm prints and footprints are also utilized for PM identification just as easily and must be referred to as such. Palm prints and foot prints are typically less readily available as antemortem (AM) records and may require additional investigative work to recover possible purported prints of the deceased from their living accommodations or workplaces.

Due to the different causes and manners of death that attribute to a mass fatality, it is important to understand not only the capabilities of using postmortem friction ridge impressions for victim identification, but also how-to best capture and record high-quality prints in a timely manner. With abundant advancements in technology, there are now high-quality mobile scanners that attach to cell phones and tablets for on-scene identification needs. There are vast resources of AM fingerprint databases all over the world, and it is imperative that the practitioner know how to properly search and submit prints to the appropriate agencies to effect an identification. This chapter will outline many of the methods of postmortem fingerprint capture, including those encountered in more challenging circumstances, and address how to use these prints to achieve the primary DVI goal of timely victim identification to allow proper closure for the families of those affected.

7.2 Role of Fingerprints in DVI

Friction ridge prints, more specifically fingerprints, are the most readily usable primary identifier for victim identification (INTERPOL 2014). The terms "primary" and "secondary" identifiers are more readily used internationally, but effectively convey the weighted value of the information. Primary identifiers are those which are meant to establish a scientific identification of the deceased, typically referring to ridgeology (study of friction ridge skin), odontology (study of teeth), and DNA analysis. Unlike DNA and dental identifications, which require some notion of the AM identity of the deceased, the prevalent use of fingerprints in everyday life allows vast databases to be searched and identifications to be made without knowing anything about who the person was prior to the incident. Information may be provided through a commercial manifest or through a family member coming forward to report their loved one missing, whereas AM dental records or DNA family reference samples are not typically available, and comparisons cannot be made without the tentative biographic information. Rapid DNA analysis is a relatively new technology which can expedite the DNA collection and profile development, but still requires a known AM reference for comparison. Secondary identifiers such as medical devices may be serialized and be helpful for corroborating a tentative identification during pathological and anthropological examinations. Other secondary identifiers such as scars, marks, and tattoos that a family member or friend may recognize or may be correlated through social media photographs are very helpful, but rarely serve as the sole means of identification unless all other primary avenues have been exhausted. It is instead an identification matrix, a use of all available primary and secondary identifiers that will eventually establish the identity of the decedent.

Visual identifications, those in which a surviving relative identifies a decedent solely based on their opinion or by using a photograph of a possible match, have led to numerous false identifications. This practice is still in existence all over the world, especially within the United States, even though there are numerous examples of identifying the incorrect individual and a resultant plethora of lawsuits. It cannot be stressed enough that visual identification alone should not be acceptable as a *legal* means of identifying a decedent, especially within DVI. The sheer psychological stress and trauma caused by the thought of losing a loved one, or the disfigurement that may accompany the death, has shown to distort a person's ability to see the truth or accurately identify their family member. Unfortunately, it typically requires a false identification of someone that is later discovered and ends in civil litigation, before the responsible agency changes its methodology. If a person is found deceased alone in their home, with their identification card in their wallet and still on the body, then it can be considered strong circumstantial evidence to aide in the identification of that person. But for DVI events, where there is often an open population, or with people of similar age, sex, and race involved, visual identification alone is simply an unacceptable risk (Caplova et al. 2017).

7.3 The DVI Process and Fingerprints

The DVI process is unlike the traditional day-to-day function of PM identification, and does not necessarily encompass the same tasks. Most Medical Examiner and Coroner (ME/C) systems within the United States have a mortuary setup with individually dedicated stations for each body, in order to handle multiple cases daily. The number of stations is usually dictated by the locality and the anticipated number of deaths that occur on an average, daily basis. A large municipality may be able to handle ten or twenty bodies at a time, whereas a smaller jurisdiction may only have a few stations. This arrangement is functional for a typical workday, but it will not efficiently work for a DVI event. When a mass fatality is deemed a "disaster," it is due to the principle that the local jurisdiction may be overwhelmed, and the standard setup must be abandoned.

When a DVI event occurs, the daily caseload of a ME/C does not desist. These routine decedents must be processed with the same diligence and reverence as would prevail under normal constraints and should not be included within the mass fatality setup as the intermixing of data could be problematic. Funding, staffing, declarations of emergency, epidemiology, and even other political factors are determined based on the number of casualties and value of destroyed property from any given event. It is imperative that DVI and daily cases be tracked separately. For example, it may be helpful to have dedicated teams of pathologists, technicians, and other staff assigned to process the daily intake separate from the mass casualties. This allows for an easy transition when the other staff members from outside jurisdictions assist as a force multiplier. On the other hand, depending upon geography and capability, the standard cases may be able to be routed temporarily to another facility to minimize the chaos and logistical challenges of maintaining a separate standard caseload in one facility.

In the unfortunate event of a mass shooting, the bodies will most likely be intact. Specifically, the hands of the deceased will typically be unaltered. Alternatively, in a transportation incident such as a plane crash, there are typically high levels of fragmentation, which require the utilization of all primary identifiers for re-association of the remains. Once the remains are triaged, photographed, and cataloged, the workflow may be prioritized to obtain high-quality fingerprints from all the victims in the beginning stages of the DVI process. The order of work remains the same, but the amount of forensic and scientific specialties involved may increase. There is no perfect setup when it comes to a DVI morgue as no two facilities are alike, but it will most likely differ from the usual daily approach. The early stages of triaging the remains will indicate whether odontology, DNA, friction ridge prints, or a combination of all three will be the most effective way to quickly and efficiently identify the victims.

In an effective DVI workflow, there is an assembly-line progression, rather than a case-by-case process. The bodies will be triaged at the scene and cataloged with a field numbering system but may need to be re-numbered and re-inventoried at the mortuary using ME/C numbers or barcodes for tracking. It is imperative that these numbers stay correlated. After proper photography of the overall remains is complete, the next station should be fingerprints. Dental analysis, followed by DNA collection, imaging, and then autopsy, will conclude the exams. The only exception is when closed bag computerized tomography (CT) scans are being conducted on all remains, as this is usually done before triage. Finally, a quality assurance check should be performed on all remains to verify that all examinations were performed and that the PM records and samples collected are of sufficient quality. There is not always another opportunity to re-capture the PM data needed once the body has returned to storage, or in some cases gone onto preservation/embalming. Initial triage would indicate that a portion of the remains has no friction ridge skin or teeth and can therefore skip the respective station and be prioritized for further analysis better suited to aide in its identification.

While the goal of DVI is to quickly and validly identify deceased persons en masse, it is imperative to do this in a safe manner. It is essential to ensure that any remains being processed have been rendered safe from physical or respiratory hazards such as munitions, chemical contaminants, or obvious sharp objects comingled with the remains. If there will be hazards, they should be identified and addressed prior to the postmortem printing work commencing. It is just as important to know what personal protective equipment (PPE) is required to protect the workers at any given stage. Aside from the biological hazards associated with death, disease, and decomposition, there are often hazards associated with DVI work that must be considered. In a transportation incident, jet fuel, broken glass, or metal shrapnel may be imbedded into the remains. The practitioners should be outfitted with specialized cut-proof gloves under their disposable nitrile or latex gloves. After flight MH-17 was shot down over the Ukraine, all the remains were soaked in formaldehyde by the first responders to the scene to preserve the bodies, which rendered it a long-term chemical hazard that required respirators to conduct the DVI work. Not all chemical, biological, radiological, or nuclear events are the result of weaponized attacks, but the hazards associated with them require additional training and medical monitoring of the personnel working the DVI operation.

7.4 Postmortem Fingerprinting Station

No two car mechanic shops are alike. The tools they need to fix cars are customarily the same, but each person will have their preference for which tools are in which drawer, what brands of tools they prefer, and even simple oddities ranging from tool grip color to toolbox shape. The same can be said for a scientist at a lab bench or a pathologist working at a personalized autopsy station. People work best when they know where their tools are and have what is comfortable to them. With that in mind, there are the necessary tools to conduct PM fingerprinting, and there are conveniences. Each of the techniques outlined in this chapter will describe the required equipment needed to perform it, but at no time can it ever be considered an exhaustive list because one practitioner may do it slightly differently but obtain the same result. It is also anticipated that new techniques for faster and more efficient processes will continue to be published and should be employed when appropriately validated.

The fingerprint station setup should be primarily focused on high throughput. All of the standard, high-volume PM impression recording equipment should be at the forefront for the cases which are easily printed, and all of the advanced PM recording equipment should be located further back, out of the way where a second technician can diligently be reconditioning without hindering the flow of the processing line. All designs and layouts should be chosen to ensure that the station does not become a bottleneck for cases.

Cleanliness plays an equally important role as the ergonomics, and there is a need to have separate clean and dirty stations for the quality assurance and comparison of records. If digital scanners are not exclusively being used to collect the PM prints directly from the deceased, there should be a designated (dirty) table for the completed PM records to be scanned and reviewed. If space allows, this will enable the second team of practitioners to work in a (clean) area with lower level of PPE and therein be more suited for quality checking the work for longer periods of time. Rotation of these roles also allows for some practitioners to sit for a period while others stand, without anyone standing for the entirety of a work shift. If the technicians are unnecessarily and irrevocably fatigued on the first day with multiple days of processing ahead, inevitably there will be a backlog and a lack of personnel to complete the mission in a timely manner.

The equipment needed to print deceased persons can be divided into two categories: reconditioning and recording (Figure 7.1). Reconditioning tools may consist of items such as a boiling pot, hypodermic needles and tissue builder, scissors or a scalpel, or even chemicals and lotions. These items allow the practitioner to

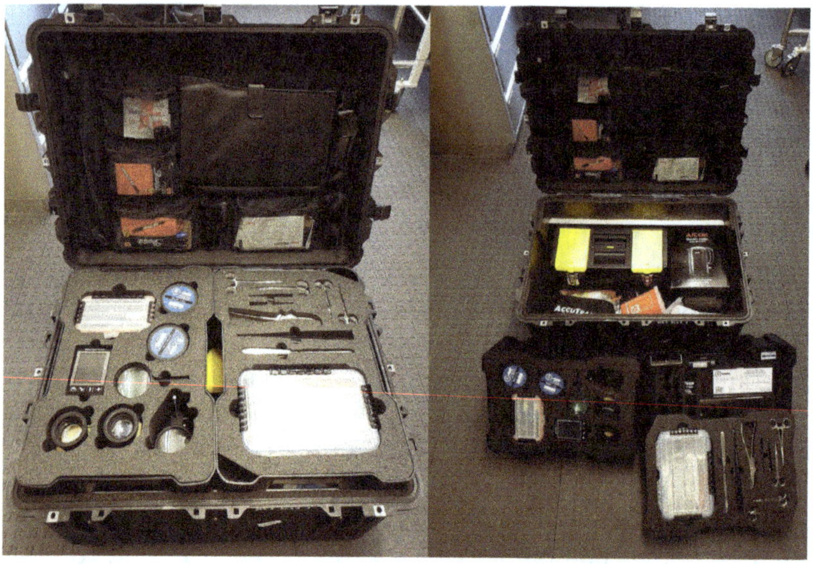

Figure 7.1 Example deployable PM Fingerprinting DVI kit.

recondition the skin to allow it to be printable. Recording tools consist of ink and paper, adhesive lifters and fingerprint powder/brushes, digital fingerprint scanners, casting materials, or a macro photographic capture setup, allowing for the friction ridge skin to be reproduced in a manner that permits it to be used for identification. These necessary items have different purposes, but all are useful in arming a technician with the capabilities needed for a variety of friction ridge skin conditions. Although it is not essential to have running water or electricity to be able to conduct PM printing, these are necessary components for the boiling method. Having a portable boiling pot that lifts off its base, rather than one that is tethered to a cord, greatly helps the technician avoid entanglement of wires and their contact with water during the printing process. If the infrastructure of the region where the work is being performed has been disrupted, the gear that is brought onsite should be appropriate to the limitations that will be encountered. A mobile or temporary mortuary setup in a Deployable Rapid Assembly Shelter (DRASH) tent on scene may not have all the helpful outlets and sinks that would be found in a standard mortuary. Anyone doing DVI work under unfavorable conditions will have to be resourceful regarding their equipment and rely on their experience and creativity. An outside-the-box mentality will be necessary to address unforeseen issues.

7.5 Personnel and Postmortem Fingerprinting

There are approximately 2,400 Medico-legal Death Investigation (MDI) systems in the United States. These comprise Medical Examiner systems, Coroner systems, and mixed Medical Examiner/Coroner (ME/C) systems. These apply to some states as a whole or to every county and parish in others (Hickman et al. 2007). There are accreditations that each system or facility may obtain, but federally there is no mandatory governing body that dictates how the work is done, or if certain forensic processes, such as fingerprinting the deceased, are even mandatory. Because DVI work is often conducted in the closest facility that is functionally available near the incident, there will always be jurisdictional expectations that will dictate the anticipated workflow. When multiple jurisdictions are involved in large events such as tornados or floods, there may even be conflict as to what work is required or allowed by law across state and county lines. As it relates to fingerprints, there are no certifications or formal trainings in *postmortem* fingerprinting in the United States, no required job qualifications, experience, or proficiency testing (NRC 2009). This may become crucial during DVI work, as two people assigned to a PM printing station may have completely different backgrounds, roles, experience levels, and/or expectations. In well-established mortuaries, the autopsy technicians will perform such printing along with a variety of other tasks for daily cases. In smaller jurisdictions, it may be handled by local law enforcement or even the pathologist. It is important to establish what the expectation of work is prior to processing any remains. It is just as important to understand the skillset of those expected to perform that work to ensure they are capable if advanced printing methods are warranted.

The majority of PM fingerprinting may be overwhelming for a layperson without formalized training and experience. If the casualties are unaltered and not exhibiting signs of PM change, the required training would be similar to learning to record prints of living individuals. Once PM changes set in, the experience level required to effectively do the work quickly escalates. Another key distinction among personnel is that the technician performing the work does not need to be able to conduct a comparison of the recorded prints. Having a person record PM prints that *can* also compare them is an added quality assurance step. A person who will later compare the prints would be able to determine sufficiency for use while still working with the remains. If the prints are determined to be insufficient after the remains have been released to other stations or even relocated to a different facility, there is little that can be done to recall the remains for re-printing. The potential for a quick identification may be lost. In some jurisdictions the embalming or preservation process is the last step of DVI work on the line and happens before the remains are placed back in storage. It can permanently inhibit the ability to re-record viable prints and does not always wait until the identification is made. Choosing the right personnel is important not only for the success of the mission, but also to ensure the work is done correctly and in a timely manner.

7.6 Postmortem Fingerprinting Process

In all postmortem fingerprinting, a simple protocol can be followed to achieve optimum results: inspect the remains, recondition the remains as needed, and record high-quality PM prints (Uhle 2010). The individual methods will be described in greater detail later in the chapter but having a road map of the process allows the practitioner to plan appropriately. Likewise, it is very helpful to have case knowledge of the incident. This may be obvious, but if there is a traumatic event, knowing if there was fire involved or even trauma from recovery machinery will aid the practitioner in preparing the necessary equipment. For example, if it is not anticipated that the remains will be mummified or dehydrated, stocking a large amount of chemicals for rehydration is an unnecessary hazard and poor use of space. Contrariwise, if a mass grave is being processed, rehydration techniques may be the most utilized process, and extra chemical storage must be considered.

7.6.1 Inspection and Cleansing

In the inspection phase, it is important to establish if friction ridge skin is present. Furthermore, it is important to attempt to discern where the skin originated from anatomically. This may not be necessary if a full body is present. However, where there are high levels of fragmentation, this information can speed up the preliminary identification potential. While triage is done at intake to sort fragmented remains, any dissociated fingers present should be prioritized over non-friction ridge skin, if possible. Depending upon the situation and jurisdiction, feet, toes, and palms may be flagged and separated for processing at a later time if all of the victims are unaccounted for. If all the missing persons (i.e., from a manifest) are identified through fingerprints, printing palms and feet may not be a good use of resources unless DNA is backlogged or unavailable due to limited corresponding AM familial references. Furthermore, it would also require AM palm and footprint records to be located and these are not commonly recorded or readily available. During inspection, the technician will look for trauma (thermal damage or wounds), postmortem changes (sloughing or mummification), or additional concerns that would require additional care and attention. This integral step of assessing the remains will ensure the best practices are utilized when recording PM prints and that no prints are rendered unobtainable due to skipping vital steps or using the same "standard" process on the fingers, regardless of condition. The final part of the inspection phase is gently cleaning the skin with water and soap, alcohol, or other mild cleaners. This will prepare it for reconditioning and recording, as in some cases simply cleaning the skin is all that is needed prior to printing.

7.6.2 Rehydration

Rehydration of remains refers to the process of hydrating and softening the skin in attempt to have the fingers bear as much resemblance as possible to their AM state. It is sometimes overlooked by technicians during the recovery process that any postmortem fingerprints obtained still must be compared to AM records. Obtaining a quick low-quality print for the sake of speed and process may lead to a possible manual identification. However, if the print must be searched in a database, the records will match only if there is limited distortion and sufficient minutiae present. Macerated remains may need to be boiled to rehydrate the remaining dermal layer, whereas mummified remains may require chemical rehydration. Remains with thermal damage may not warrant much hydration but may need the epidermis to be carefully removed to expose a usable surface of skin. Unless the bodies are pristine, most remains are in conditions that cannot simply be printed with ink and paper in a quick fashion. Not dedicating the necessary effort to photograph and obtain useable PM prints may destroy any chance of identifying that individual (Box 7.1).

Not all DVI work is completed on current events. In the case of mass graves or even plane crashes in remote locations, there is a strong possibility of mummification, given the right climate conditions and enough elapsed time after death. Mummification is seen frequently in morgues when the decedent is not discovered for some time after death either in their residence or in a remote location where they are exposed to the elements. Mummification is also seen in DVI but is not easily handled because it can be a tedious, slow process to obtain the resultant prints. Recent research has provided techniques that can rehydrate mummified fingers in a matter of hours or a few days (Cardenas 2010). Traditional practices of processing wrinkled or hardened mummified fingers involved removing the digits and soaking them for weeks or attempting to take casts or photograph the fingers. While there is nothing wrong with casting or photography, the resultant wrinkles are also captured and the gross distortion they cause will often prohibit a successful database search for truly unknown prints.

Some rehydration techniques are simply performed to restore the rigidity and three-dimensionality of the finger. During the decomposition process, fingers can shrivel and prune. Unless the whole hand warrants boiling, restoring the structure of the dermal skin may only involve a simple fluid injection to restore the shape of each digit. By doing these types of basic or advanced procedures, the PM prints will again resemble the AM prints as closely as possible and allow for their capture.

Box 7.1 Case Studies

Case Study in Rehydration:

Following the Thailand Tsunami in 2004, the bodies were exposed to water for long periods of time, and advanced decomposition was quickly evident, resulting from a combination of environmental conditions (humid heat) and a lack of infrastructure to refrigerate the remains. These two factors led to very few fingerprint identifications in the early days following the incident. The maceration of the remains was so extensive that without rehydration techniques such as boiling, useable fingerprints were not even being attempted to be lifted from the bodies. Bodies that have been in water for a substantial amount of time will bloat, thereby stretching out the skin. Macerated skin can stretch to as much as 150% larger than it was AM. Because fingerprint databases are built to store, search, and identify primarily living individuals, there is not enough tolerance built into the algorithms to effect an identification without first decreasing the print image dimensions by a factor to make it comparable to the AM records. When the US-deployed team from the FBI Disaster Squad started to implement the boiling method, the percentage of remains being successfully printed increased significantly [(16)]. Resultant searches of those prints after altering the image sizes further propagated fingerprints as a viable means of early identification. This methodology and experience-based knowledge was vastly helpful when utilized in the 2005 Hurricane Katrina mass casualty, where similar environmental conditions of heat and moisture were widespread and led to macerated remains. Presently, there are now digital calibration tools that allow for sizing prints based on the span of friction ridges over a distance, when the intention is to conduct Automated Fingerprint Identification System (AFIS) searches. This technological advancement is essential when no scale is present in an image, or when maceration or fire trauma has altered the natural size of the prints.

Box 7.2 Case Studies in Database Use:

Following the MH-17 plane crash in July of 2014, the majority of fingerprint matches were effected through the US-VISIT databases, despite only one US victim being involved. Once the PM prints were obtained using the Dutch fingerprint "dead-scan" capture system or scanned via a flatbed scanner, they were quickly and easily shared with DHS through a portal setup specifically to receive prints for this event. Nearly 50 matches were made within days from the collected PM prints, since their system captured in the shareable NIST EBTS file format. This cooperation, combined with the use of local fingerprint records, resulted in 243 total fingerprint matches to 151 victims [(7)].

In the 2019 Ethiopian Air ET302 plane crash, there were eight Americans aboard at the time of the crash. The FBI Disaster Victim Identification Squad deployed a team of fingerprint experts to Ethiopia to assist in identifying those decedents on board on behalf of INTERPOL, who presided over the event. Through the use of US databases, and four additional AM records provided by other countries, 48 identifications were made to the remains based off of fingerprints. One of the foreign decedents did not have an AM DNA familial reference sample to work from, as the possible next of kin declined to provide one. The fingerprint match effected through DHS records enabled the rest of this individual's dissociated remains to be reconciled and repatriated. This technique has proven useful in many high fragmentation DVI events.

7.6.2.1 Macerated Remains

Maceration (water exposure/damage) and wet decomposition occur in a variety of situations. Tissue that has been submerged in water, whether a lake, ocean, river, or even a bathtub, will quickly exhibit signs of maceration. Lesser considered conditions such as clandestine burials in water saturated soil, or post-accident scenes where copious amounts of water have been used by first responders and the bodies are not recovered right away may also result in maceration. There are several techniques to combat these effects to obtain the best possible PM prints to identify the victims.

7.6.2.1.1 Tissue Injection

A quick and effective method for reconditioning macerated digits to regain their three-dimensional structure is the use of liquid injections beneath the epidermis. This is most commonly done by using an embalming solution called tissue builder. Tissue builder is a viscous liquid originally designed for embalming purposes that can be injected into the fingertips or other friction ridge skin areas. It semi-hardens upon contact with the skin, so that when the finger is manipulated for printing, the liquid does not seep back out of the injection site. Tissue builder, or any other suitable liquid that will not cause direct damage to skin, can be injected into the end joint of the finger by passing the needle through the middle joint or medial phalange, up into the finger's volar pad on the end joint of the finger. This will result in the elevation of depressed areas in the fingertip, thus smoothing and filling any wrinkles that are present. Other liquids, such as acetone or alcohol, may also work and add a drying benefit to the finger. However, caution should be taken if not using a liquid as viscous or stable as tissue builder. The injection site will not only potentially leak when the finger is pressed against a printing medium, compromising the print, but it may also eject from the injection site if enough force is applied and end up on the practitioner. A rubber band, zip tie, gauze wrap, or a makeshift type of tourniquet above the injection site may prove useful in these situations to keep the fluid under the skin. More importantly, the technician should be cautious not to perforate the friction ridge skin surface with the needle as this may obliterate the comparable details of the friction ridges. Instead, the needle can be inserted from the sides or top of the finger under the fingernail bed. This is most effective when the epidermis is still present, as there will be little change when injecting only the dermal layer. (Figure 7.2)

7.6.2.1.2 Degloving

The later stages of decomposition in wet environments may result in a phenomenon referred to as "gloving" or "de-gloving" where the epidermal layer of skin separates from the dermal layer. During degloving, the epidermal skin can be sloughed off or gently cut from the dermis, dried, and worn over the PPE gloved finger of a technician to simulate the three-dimensional structure of intact tissue (Figure 7.3). If the epidermal layer is already completely separated from the dermal layer in a body bag or at a scene, recordings of the epidermis AND dermis should be taken as they must both be independently identified to be properly re-associated. This is extremely important in disaster situations where a commingling of remains often occurs accidentally because of first responders doing the collection and recovery without formal training.

7.6.2.1.3 Boiling Method

In instances where the epidermis is fully compromised, the dermis may continue to remain intact for an extended period of time and can be boiled to recondition it for printing. The boiling method was published by the FBI following its successful use in the aftermath of the Thai tsunami and Hurricane Katrina (Uhle and Leas 2007). It is a method that utilizes boiling water to visualize or elevate ridge detail on the dermis through osmotic rehydration and has become a staple in PM fingerprint recovery. This process involves raising water to a full boil in a hot pot or kettle and then submerging the hand (or finger) into the near-boiling water for 5- to 10 second intervals. The hand is removed from the water after each interval and examined for friction ridge detail, which will be visible on the surface of the dermis if it has been successful. If no detail is present, the hand can be placed back into the water for an additional 5 to 10 seconds. Upon drying, the friction ridges should be printable using standard techniques. Because the effects of the boiling technique typically last for only 3 to 5 minutes, the technician should be prepared to print the remains immediately. There is also a limit on the number of times tissue can successfully

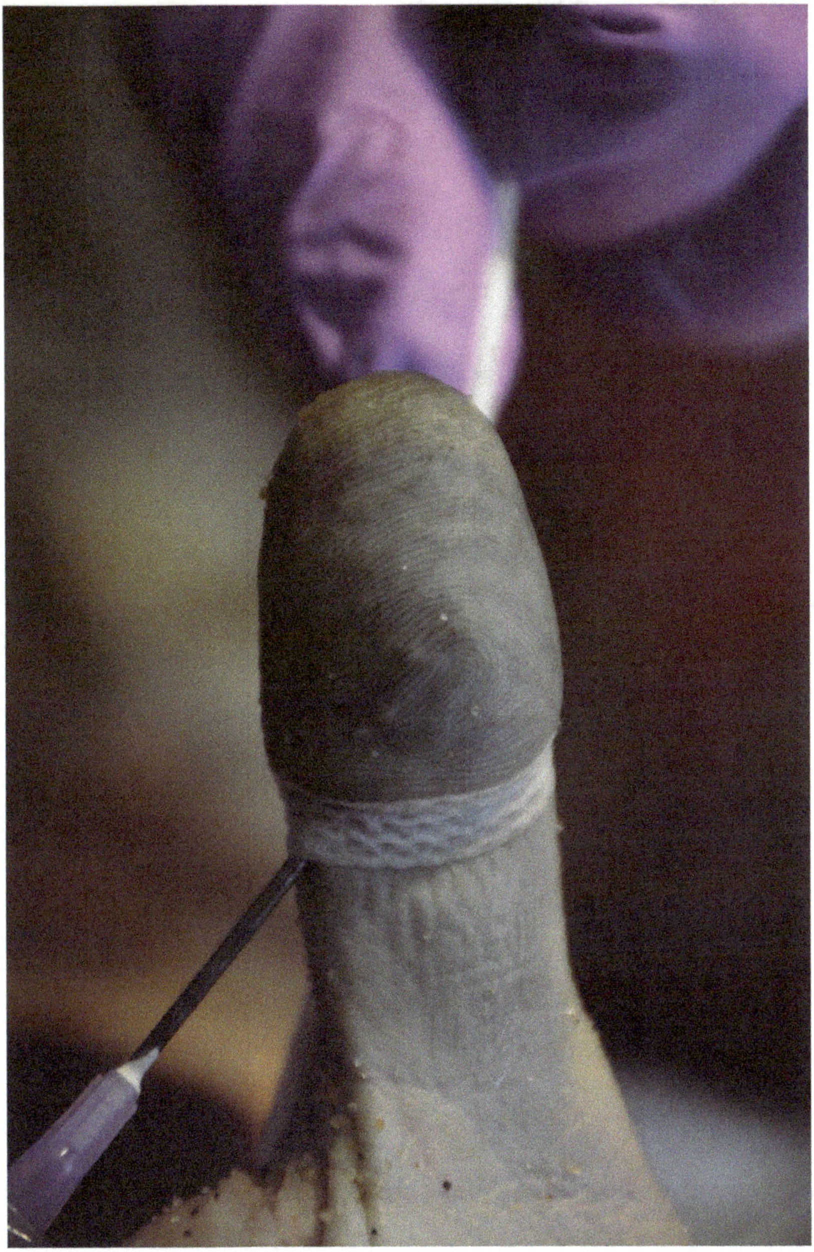

Figure 7.2 Photograph of a finger that has been injected for capture after the body was found floating in water. Good example of a gauze tourniquet and proper contrast in the photo.
Photo taken by and courtesy of MDI Selma Delic, Middlesex Regional Medical Examiner's Office, NJ.

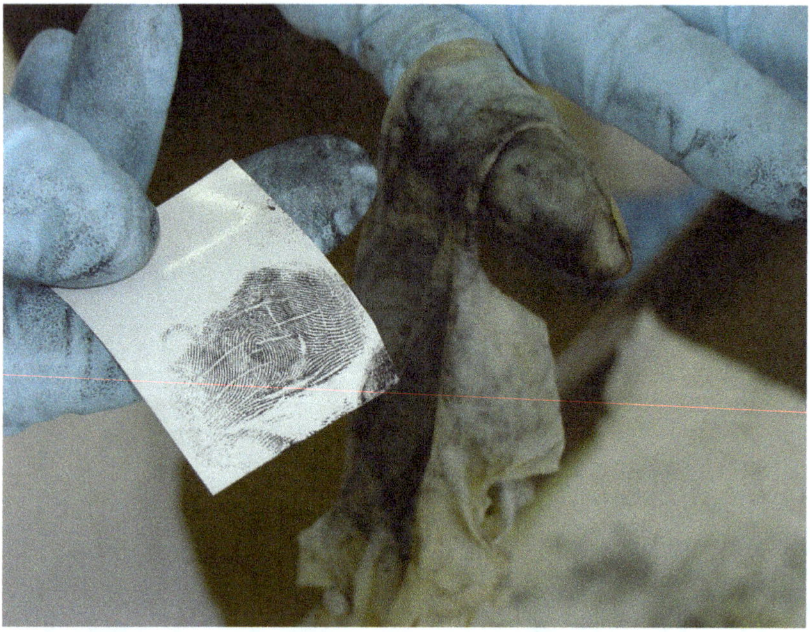

Figure 7.3 Example of degloved skin being printed by placing the skin on the technician's hand.

be boiled. Eventually the muscles in the hand will harden and contract, and the skin will start to shrink beyond use. Likewise, if there is any trauma present, care must be taken as the boiling water will greatly enhance cuts and tears. In the case of trauma, a sponge soaked in boiling water can be set on the hand or fingers to rehydrate them. When rehydrating the dermis, it should be noted that the dermal ridges are much finer than epidermal ridges. This may require the use of adhesive lifters and fingerprinting powder as opposed to ink/paper for the quality resolution to be usable (Figure 7.4). It is also possible to use certain digital capture systems after boiling and properly drying the skin. There is no defined total time limit or set number of times to boil a hand or friction ridge skin, as the composition of the tissue and deterioration of the cell structure will dictate how much is necessary. If the fingers start to contract too far, there is very little you can do to recondition them back to useable state, so multiple printing attempts are encouraged.

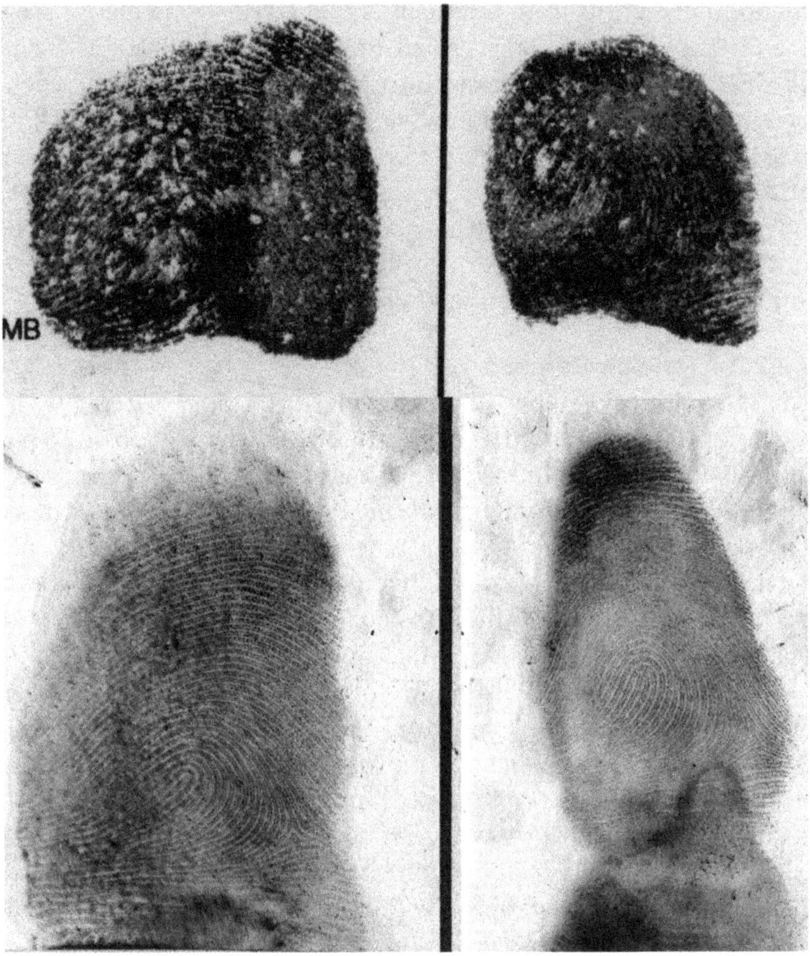

Figure 7.4 Ink prints of a macerated hand before boiling (top) and powder and adhesive lifter prints after boiling (bottom).

7.6.2.2 Thermal Modification (Charred/burned Skin)

Thermally damaged remains continue to be one of the most challenging scenarios for PM fingerprinting cases. The nature of thermal modification means there is good chance that the friction ridges will be burned completely off or otherwise damaged beyond recovery. However, just the mere appearance of burned skin on the outside should not be a deterrent from trying to obtain PM prints. The recovery of friction ridge prints from thermally modified skin is a delicate process and time should be taken to ensure the best technique is used. Entire bodies will usually contract into the pugilistic pose in fire, when the contraction and dehydration of all the body's tissue cause the fingers to be inaccessible for printing without physical manipulation. The contraction often also causes the hands to clench into fists, where the removal of the digits surgically may be necessary. However, this position may also protect the volar pads of the fingers allowing for a PM identification with the remaining protected friction ridge skin.

7.6.2.2.1 Tendon Release

A common difficulty when handling thermally altered remains is accessing the end joints of the fingers enough both to assess the damage to the skin and to record the fingerprints. In these scenarios, the palms are often badly burned, and the focus should be on end joints on the fingers, which may have been more protected due to the clenching. While the fingers of the hand may be forced open, there is a risk of damaging the brittle skin left behind. The flexor tendons which run through the hands are thick and tough. Once they are contracted from heat, they will likely not be able to be loosened or stretched back out like one could with a hand in rigor mortis. Care should always be taken to avoid removing fingers or hands by default to protect the dignity of the deceased. Instead, one option to "break" free the fingers is to perform what has been named the "Siwek slice." This technique involves making an incision in the wrist such that the three flexor tendons are severed without removing the hand or the digits. This allows the severed tendons to be able to slide up into the hand, potentially allowing the fingers to bend open again. While not always successful in significantly burned cases, it can be an easy way to access the fingers without having to remove, label, and track dissociated digits throughout the process (Siwek and Reinecke 2014).

7.6.2.2.2 Break and Twist Method

If severing the wrist tendons is not feasible or fails, or the remains are burned extensively so that all palmar tissue is contracted, the alternate method to expose and access the friction skin is referred to as the "Break and Twist method." This technique involves manual manipulation of the finger to free the epidermal skin and expose the dermal skin below. "Breaking" free the epidermal skin enables it to be printed more effectively, as the skin will likely be hardened and brittle from the heat. Likewise, the epidermis often protects the dermal layer from fire damage which can be accessed and printed only once the epidermis is removed. When trying to access the finger(s), it is possible to bend the finger(s) back with consistent gentle force until the muscles and tendons "break" free and the volar pad on the tip of the finger is accessible. This process is similar to "breaking" the effects of rigor mortis. When the skin is heavily burned or damaged, it may need to be cut with a scalpel at the base of the finger near the palm to release the tendons to avoid rendering the skin unusable. Once the finger is broken free or cut, a twisting motion can be used to remove the epidermis by twisting the skin as it is pulled away from the finger to slide it off. Once the dermal layer of skin is exposed on the finger, the practitioner may print or photograph either the dermis, or the underside of the epidermis once it has been turned inside out (Figure 7.5). Depending on the level of damage to the dermal skin, it may be boiled similarly to macerated remains in an attempt to reconstitute the dermal ridges. The epidermis, the underside of the epidermis, and the dermis all have the same friction ridge arrangement on them. It is important to keep this in mind as the remaining skin is assessed to best target the surface of skin most likely to have survived thermal trauma.

7.6.2.3 Desiccation (Mummification)

Remains that are in a mummified or hardened state from desiccation are traditionally difficult to quickly obtain PM prints from, which is problematic in DVI work. Desiccated remains often exhibit visual ridge detail, yet most practitioners in the field either deem them as "unprintable" if the friction ridge details do not transfer with ink and paper, or they resort to photography in attempt at collecting something usable so the next case can be addressed. While the use of photography provides some hope, most AFIS systems cannot use photographs of fingers to directly ingest and search. Photographs of fingers typically will need to be searched by a crime lab as a latent print or compared manually in order to effect an identification. Fortunately, recent research into rehydrating desiccated tissue has provided

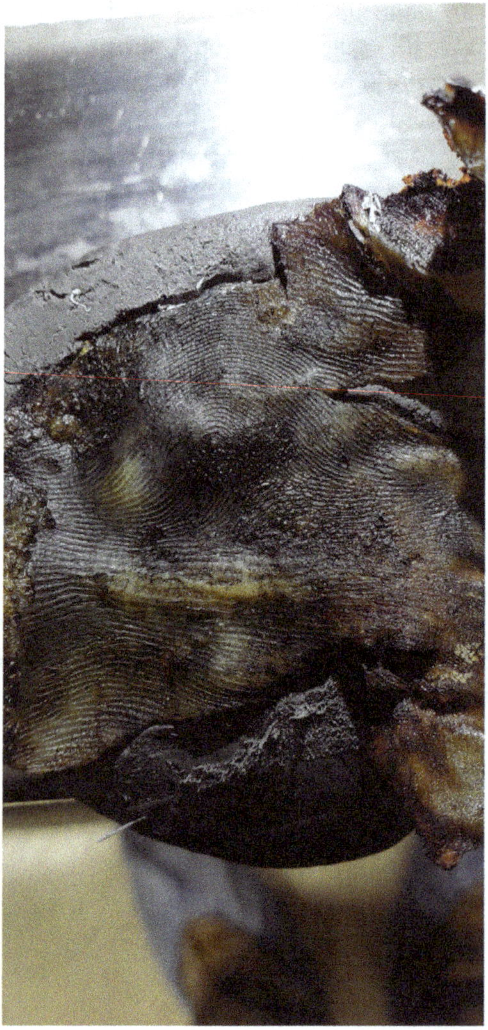

Figure 7.5 Example of burned epidermis following a car fire. The skin was removed, turned inside out, and then placed in duct seal putty to be photographed.

chemical solutions that may rehydrate digits in a matter of hours or days as opposed to weeks or months.

In 1977 the FBI published *The Science of Fingerprints* which contained basic references on fingerprinting the deceased (FBI 1977). The FBI suggested using dilute solutions of sodium hydroxide or potassium hydroxide as a way to rehydrate mummified tissues. These solutions were combined with water rinses and acetone for drying to attempt to print the tissue. Due to the destructive nature of the processes and lack of empirical experience, most practitioners shied away from their use. The method was republished by the Pima County Office of the Medical Examiner following their great success with bodies that had been extensively mummified from exposure to the elements in the desert (Hernandez and Hess 2014). Similarly, an odontologist from Mexico published his patent for hydration of entire bodies, to include the hands, using an ammonium hydroxide and sodium bicarbonate solution. These solutions, when properly applied, permit full rehydration, allowing fully rolled impressions to be obtained from once unusable friction ridge skin.

7.6.2.3.1 Sodium Hydroxide Reconditioning

A solution of 3–5% sodium hydroxide dissolved in water can be used to rehydrate the hands and/or digits of mummified remains. This process generally works within 4–24 hours; however, frequent monitoring is advised after 8–12 hours as the tissue may start to disintegrate, rendering the skin unprintable. The epidermis will dissolve quickly, but the resulting rehydrated dermal layer can be photographed or dried for one to two days in a towel and printed. The skin may also be dried with acetone and then printed (Figure 7.6).

7.6.2.3.2 Ammonium Hydroxide Reconditioning

A solution of 2% ammonium hydroxide and 25 g/L sodium hydroxide in distilled water will take longer to rehydrate than when using sodium hydroxide. This solution does not damage the epidermis, however, and will not dissolve the skin if left soaking for a longer period of time (accidentally or intentionally) (Cardenas 2010). A hand can take up to 36 hours, whereas a disarticulated finger may be rehydrated within a day. The skin can usually be rinsed and printed or

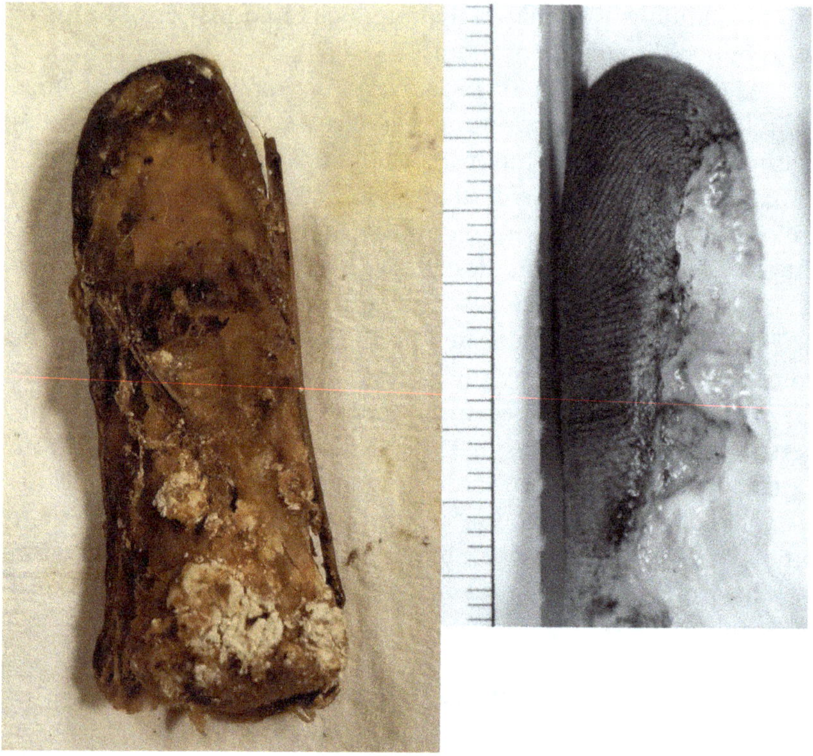

Figure 7.6 Before and after images of a mummified, dissociated finger rehydrated through sodium hydroxide reconditioning.

enhanced even further with a very brief dip (3–5 seconds) in boiling water to clean it before printing.

7.6.2.3.3 Detergent Soaking Reconditioning

It is necessary to note that water and detergent rehydration is common practice. Though this method is not specifically useful for DVI due to how long it may take, it is the safest method. Soaking the fingers in the Lexol® leather conditioner or Palmolive® dishwashing liquid can be used to rehydrate desiccated skin over time. The rehydration of the fingers may take days or even months in some cases, depending on the extent of desiccation. Even after hydration, the skin may not fully swell to the original shape and size as it does with the hydroxide methods. After soaking, tissue injection or massaging and stretching the skin flat to remove any creases may be necessary to obtain a higher-quality print without wrinkles. There is little to no risk of dissolving the skin with this method over any amount of time. The main concern with its usage is whether it will be effective enough to achieve printable skin.

7.6.3 Collecting PM Prints

As research advances, the focus will shift toward first employing new technology to expedite identifications, then using analog methods as backup methodologies. Undeniably, the most important part of the DVI fingerprinting process is capturing the prints, as this directly leads to identifications. There are several ways to capture the prints, ranging from high-tech scanners to the traditional ink and paper method. It is inappropriate to say that any available method is entirely sufficient, as each technique has benefits and limitations associated with it. Obtaining high-quality fingerprints should always be the ultimate priority, not just the expediency of print capture. Decomposition and skin trauma at DVI scenes often lead to the epidermis quickly deteriorating in a manner that makes traditional ink and paper or digital capture less viable as printing options. While most living records are recorded with either ink and paper or live scan, the friction ridge skin of deceased persons often will not reproduce adequate quality and clarity by these methods once decomposition begins. An effective alternative method is to use adhesive lifters and black fingerprint powder, resulting in a much higher resolution capture. Recognizing these subtle differences in print capture can make a drastic difference when examining difficult prints in the comparison phase of the identification process. The procedure listed below is in order of "best practices" generally speaking, with the understanding that there is no ultimate "right" way.

7.6.3.1 Digital Capture

Digital fingerprint technologies were originally designed and built for printing live persons at booking stations. The technology has greatly improved over the past decade and continues to do so; it no longer requires a giant capture block to be attached to a desktop computer or ruggedized laptop. There are simple, accessible platforms that operate on Android and iOS devices so that work can be done on location and utilized for deceased printing. This mobile advancement has rendered the digital collection of postmortem prints both feasible and the most logical first option. Assuming the conditions of the remains allow for it, the fastest and most efficient method of fingerprint capture is the use of a biometric scanner (Figure 7.7). Biometric scanners come in a variety of shapes, sizes, and types of technologies. They can also vary in the quality, or resolution, of the images they produce (Johnson and Riemen 2019). Some scanner technologies necessitate that the subject being printed is alive. This renders this genre of scanner useless for a DVI setting. If properly utilized, many setups have the ability to directly search the collected biometrics on scene and cascade them against multiple local, state, and federal databases in real-time. It is important to understand the limitations and capabilities of the devices available for use prior to deploying them during a DVI event. It is also imperative that end users have training in advance with the chosen setup. For the searching functionality to work, most databases require five or more high-quality finger recordings for high accuracy, which may be an issue in a highly fragmented DVI event. Searches of the Department of Defense (DOD) biometric database, for instance, will error out if less than two unique finger recordings are submitted, regardless of the quality of capture. If the situation allows for biometric capture with a scanner, a device should be chosen that can be manipulated against the deceased. Most live scan systems are designed so that a live person can be manipulated against the device setup on a table. This is challenging in DVI because decedents cannot always be moved in the way required. Now, many mobile sensor platforms factor this into their designs and can easily be moved around the station as needed. As is the case with all recordings, it is imperative that fingers be recorded in order, as one finger out of order can yield a false-negative result.

7.6.3.2 Powder and Adhesive Lifters

If the aforementioned resources are unavailable or the ability to digitally capture prints is not possible, the next best strategy for recording postmortem fingerprint impressions from deceased individuals

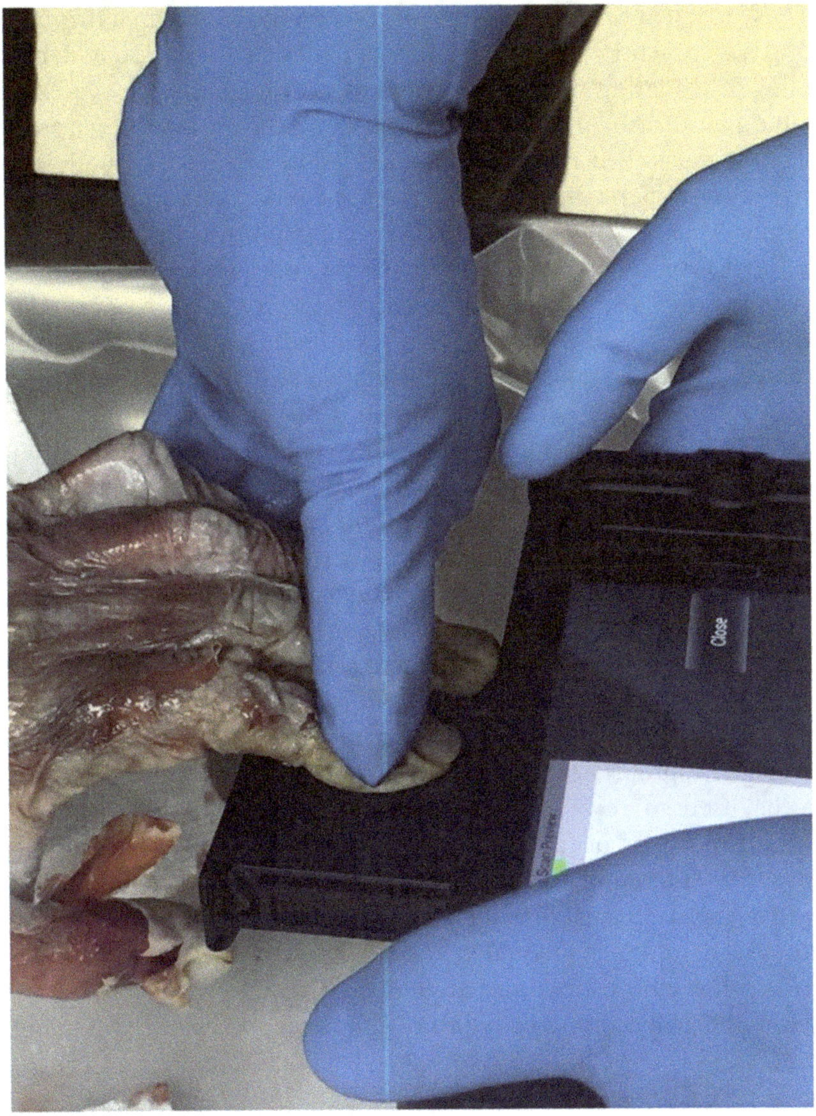

Figure 7.7 Use of a digital scanning platform to quickly print PM remains.

involves using black powder and white adhesive lifters applied to acetate sheets. This technique can be useful for daily morgue cases but can be cost-prohibitive in smaller municipalities. This method is quick and easy to use, producing clearer prints than those obtained through inking. The practitioner simply applies a light coat of black powder to the fingers, covering the entire pattern area, using a sponge-type disposable paintbrush or traditional camel or squirrel hair fingerprint brush. Fiberglass brushes used to detect latent prints are not advised as they do not perform well once they encounter any moisture. An adhesive lifter (such as Handiprint®, Quickprint®, or an address label) that is pre-cut to the approximate size of the finger blocks on a fingerprint card is then placed on each finger or surface of friction ridge skin. For best results on fingers, the lifter is placed on the side of the finger of the first joint and then wrapped around the finger, nail to nail, to record the impression. If debris or skin from the finger is being lifted along with the powder and obscures ridge detail, a lifter with weaker adhesive such as an address label should be used, or subsequent lifts may be tried. If too much powder is applied, lifting again without applying more powder will likely result in a better impression than trying to cleanse the finger and starting the process over. Once a satisfactory lift has been created, the recorded impression is next affixed to the back of an acetate fingerprint card. This type of clear plastic card can be produced by photocopying a standard fingerprint card onto transparency sheets or freeform cards can be created and labeled appropriately on the front of the card. This same procedure may be used to record palm prints, footprints, and fragments of unknown portions of friction ridge skin. The resultant adhesive lifts from the powdered digits will be of higher resolution and can easily record even fine dermal ridge detail, in situations where ink and paper methods are often inadequate. The resultant prints are already in correct color and position and are easily searched in biometric databases or manually compared without additional processing after being scanned.

7.6.3.3 Ink and Paper

Traditional methods of fingerprinting using ink and paper still exist as they remain affordable, accessible, and most people in the industry have experience with this approach. This technique has been utilized almost as long as friction ridge impressions themselves have been used for identification. The format of the fingerprint card has not changed dramatically since its inception, and it functions well for high throughput. The main reason the ink and paper method does not surpass other recording techniques is the lack of ridge quality in the recordings compared to some digital scanners and powder/lift setups. It is, however, still a viable option in some DVI settings. For cases with minimal postmortem degradation, such as a mass shooting or a transportation incident without extensive trauma to the remains, ink and paper is a cheap and efficient means of print capture. Caution should be taken, however, when the remains begin to exhibit postmortem degradation and the conditions are no longer standard for ink printing. If attempting to utilize ink for macerated or thermally degraded remains, the resultant quality may be so poor that it inhibits searching and comparing the prints. When setting up a mortuary station in a mass fatality event based off the preliminary information, it is imperative to consider the limitations of this technique.

The ink and paper method is, for the most part, straightforward. First, there is the application of a thin layer of black printer's ink to the fingers and then a recording of the friction ridge impressions onto a fingerprint card or piece of paper. When printing a live individual, the person's finger or palm is manipulated against a plate with ink rolled onto it or onto an ink pad, and then it is rolled again, nail to nail onto a card. While this works well with live individuals who have such mobility, deceased persons will be placed supine on a gurney when intact, and likely be in some stage of rigor mortis. This position, in combination with rigidity, prevents the practitioner from being able to manipulate the body against the ink medium, and requires the medium to be manipulated against the remains. An ink pad, roller, or spatula can assist with applying the ink, although over-inking is a common issue when utilizing these devices. Once the skin has an even layer of light printer's ink applied, paper or a fingerprint card (commonly cut into strips) can be rolled against it. The use of a postmortem spoon, a curved device used to hold the paper while applying the digits, can greatly assist in obtaining both clean and clear prints using the paper strips. The recorded card is filled out similarly as it would be when used to print the living, and then must be scanned at a minimum of 500 ppi to digitize it for automated searches. Because the identity is not yet known, the biographical descriptor fields on the card should be used to track the ME/C number or barcode assigned to the remains. It is important to *always* record all available fingers, as this greatly increases the chances of a quick identification through a ten-print search. Ten extra minutes spent to record more than just one or two fingers can equate to days saved on the searching and comparing end of the work.

7.6.3.4 Casting

One of the least time-consuming methods available for capturing difficult, mummified, or hardened remains is casting. Although less frequently used than photography in the daily work of morgues, casting can achieve reproduction of the ridges that photography may not resolve within a single shot. Casts can still be scanned or photographed and searched. Using high-resolution casting material such as AccuTrans®, Mikrosil™, or other similar two-part epoxy silicon casting materials enables even a wrinkled, hardened digit to be physically printed. This method is faster than rehydrating the fingers, as it dries and is usable within minutes versus the hours that rehydration requires. Casting may also be performed after rehydration has been attempted if the skin is not capable of being fully dried for other recording techniques. Ideally, the practitioner lightly covers the friction ridge skin with black fingerprint powder and subsequently applies a thin but consistent layer of white casting material onto the same area, having already mixed it to the manufacturer's specification. After the casting material has dried, the cast can be gently peeled off and scanned or photographed for retention. While other colors of casting materials such as transparent, red/brown, purple, and black may exist, the black powder on a white cast provides ideal contrast, results in an image that does not require digital tonal reversal before use, and is much easier to quickly capture. Casts may also be powdered after being lifted for additional contrast, as long as the cast has fully cured. This can be an expedient method to cast multiple hardened digits or fragments and keep the remains moving in the assembly line without waiting on lengthy rehydration. Recovered castings will be in correct position and color (if black powder is used on a white cast) when compared to AM records. It should be noted that these castings, while durable, are not permanent and, if left in a full filing cabinet or placed in a stack of records, they may lose their shape and eventually flatten out beyond use.

7.6.3.5 Photography

DVI events resulting in thermal damage, high trauma, or advanced decomposition may prevent the collection of physical recordings from the skin. Remains are almost always photographed during intake for documentation purposes, but the use of photography for fingerprinting is often overlooked. It is important to re-state that photographs of fingers in most cases cannot be directly searched for identification in the most prevalent AFIS ten-print databases, even if digitally processed and added to a digital fingerprint template. Instead, each of the photographs would require searching the image as latent prints for identification as the latent searching software's accuracy is optimized for individual print searching. When photographing fingers, the goal is to capture focused, detailed imagery of the friction ridges. It takes a photographer who is properly trained with the right equipment to obtain the necessary images. There is widely accessible technology, including cellphone cameras, that possess the requisite imaging resolution. The most integral part, however, is knowing how to frame and focus the pictures.

Ideally, photography should involve the appropriate use of direct, reflected, oblique, or transmitted lighting to create optimal contrast in the ridges to be captured by the image. Friction ridges on a clean dry hand are visible, but not easily photographed directly. Instead, a small amount of fingerprint powder or ink can be applied first to the skin, to create contrast even on wet and slippery skin. A proper amount of oblique side lighting may accomplish the same contrast, but care should be taken to illuminate the whole finger without having hot spots as this can cause issues later on when the prints are compared. It is also essential to capture 1 : 1 images of the friction ridge skin using a macro lens because the prints will be subsequently compared with AM impressions of natural size. If this cannot be accomplished, a scale or object of a known size should be included in the photograph so that image dimensions can be corrected and calibrated. The images should be of high enough resolution to be later calibrated to minimally 500 ppi. Images in excess of 1000 ppi when calibrated are ideal.

If using variable lenses or agency-approved cell phone cameras, they should be set to macro mode and images should be taken as closely as the device will allow for focus to ensure highest resolution. A hand or finger documented from 12 to 24 inches away will likely have insufficient resolution or detail once zoomed in to view the ridges for comparison. If possible, for fragmented remains, a copy stand should be used to allow for stable, close-up images. When the hand is still associated with the body or a large remains portion, a tripod allows for a clear shot in close proximity. Most cameras cannot capture a full palm with attached fingers at proper resolution; therefore, individual fingers should be captured. It is also important to label the finger, if the finger number is known. This can be done on the included scale, or by denoting it on a card or post-it within the image. The images will be in reverse position, and possibly reverse color depending on the layer of skin that is being photographed. Images can later be digitally rotated horizontally and processed to grayscale to make the ridges black and the furrows appear white. The resultant photos for fingers should follow the same guidance previously discussed for recorded prints on fingerprint cards, where the image is centered on the pattern area of the finger, fully capturing the appropriate core and deltas when present. Photographs of the sides or tips of the fingers may not permit identification, as traditional AM records may not have this corresponding area recorded. These areas should be photographed only if the core part of the fingerprint is compromised or missing.

7.7 Searching/AM Records

The AAFS Standards Board (ASB) published an American National Standard (ANS), titled "ANSI/ASB Best Practice Recommendation 007, Postmortem Impression Submission Strategy for Comprehensive Searches of Essential Automated Fingerprint Identification System Databases" (ASB 2018). This standard was finalized through ASB's DVI Consensus Body and accredited by the American National Standards Institute (ANSI). The document details information needed to effectively search postmortem fingerprints in DVI operations and is a great resource for understanding the complexities of biometric databases in the United States.

7.7.1 Database Searches

It is essential to understand what to do with PM fingerprint records once they have been obtained from the remains. Fingerprint databases in the United States are admittedly confusing and complex when attempting to get a "comprehensive" search of all recordings. The FBI, DHS, and DOD each run very large, independent, federal fingerprint databases (Mulawka 2014; Stokes 2019). In addition, most states have a centralized fingerprint repository, and many large cities or counties also maintain their own databases. While there is continued progress toward interoperability among the systems, sharing prints does not occur efficiently or automatically. These systems do not always reciprocate in data sharing, even federally, and many systems cannot "talk" to one another without special requests from one agency to the next. This dialogue may involve litigation due to the civil rights considerations associated with such information sharing. In an open-population DVI event, this lapse in communication among systems is incredibly straining, as it is not logical or even feasible to be able to provide all PM records to every database in the United States for searching. Some databases are not searchable, such as the DMV fingerprint records in states that record prints (ex: CA, CO, HI, and TX). If there is a tentative identity for someone, a manual comparison to that record can be conducted by the proper authorities, but no searching can be done with a true unknown within these population databases. Additional sources of AM fingerprint records may come from the employer of the missing person. Employers are more frequently requiring fingerprints for background checks prior to hiring an applicant. These records may remain in the employee's file for future checks, but the prints often do not permanently reside in any government database. The same logic applies for schools as well, as many schools retain recorded fingerprints of their students to use for biometric entry into the facilities or as a mean of paying for school lunch, etc.

It is common for multiple nationalities to be involved in a DVI event, especially in tourist destinations or in transportation incidents. The majority of mass fatalities occur on transportation vessels, such as planes, boats, busses, or trains. These are utilized by tourists visiting the country and, as such, can create an international event without occurring in an international location. In general, almost all foreign persons over the age of 14 entering the United States are fingerprinted at border entry sites. The US Department of Homeland Security maintains this database, and it can be crucial for obtaining AM records for any foreign persons involved. The DHS database has also been very useful for foreign police cooperation in that persons may not have been fingerprinted in their own country, but these records are retained by the United States and under certain circumstances can be provided for use in DVI events elsewhere (Box 7.2) (DHS 2017).

In a twenty-first-century approach, it is expected that most entities will have live-scan/dead-scan capabilities and real-time searching in a DVI scenario as part of their mass fatality plan. Typically, these agencies already use digital capture and searching within their daily operations. Others may not have the capability but may already have an agreement with larger agencies to deploy this type of technology in the event of a disaster. By and large, the majority of the systems rely on NIST file systems, in the electronic fingerprint file formats (i.e., EBTS, EFT, EFTS, WSQ, and NIST). By doing so, they are seamlessly shareable among agency databases both within the United States and the rest of the world as needed (Mangold 2016). It is the responsibility of each agency covering a particular region of the United States to know their capabilities and understand who they can call on to request rapid assistance if they do not possess the required technologies.

7.7.2 AM Purported Knowns

In the hours or even days following an incident, a properly run mass fatality recovery effort should have a version of a Family Assistance Center and a Victim Identification Center. These entities allow those who believe their loved one may be involved in a disaster, to come forward and provide as much detail and AM information as possible. Through a series of vetting efforts, the true list of missing persons is eventually assembled. Using this information, the investigators can begin to fill in the gaps in AM data, looking for fingerprints, taking familial DNA samples, and requesting AM dental records. In the absence of AM fingerprint records, in accordance with local law enforcement, the houses or hotel rooms of the missing persons can be processed as though it were a crime scene, to collect DNA and fingerprints from items that individual may have come into contact with. These items will likely need to be processed by a local crime lab to detect purported latent prints and can delay the identification process, but still may be the only viable primary identifier to establish the identity of the deceased. This AM data research should be done concurrently with the processing of the victims at the morgue to expedite the DVI operation as much as possible. Because the fingerprints are collected from uncontrolled items, and the ground truth source of the prints cannot be verified, they can be used as purported knowns for identification. Caution should be taken when excluding a victim from being the source if no match is made. Likewise, if a match to purported knowns is made, it should always be followed up with further analysis of other primary identifiers, such as DNA and dental exams when possible.

7.7.3 Palm Prints and Footprints

One of the most overlooked areas in DVI is the use of palm prints and footprints as means for identification. Palm prints are being increasingly collected by local law enforcement, especially in larger cities that have the capability in their standard booking stations. It is uncommon for police to take footprints, unless a specific investigation warrants it. Additionally, the prints of a newborn taken at the hospital may possibly be used for a short period based on the comparable wrinkles, but the friction ridges are not yet strong enough to be printed with most recording means currently being used. These newborn records, however, almost never equate to a usable AM record for comparison to an adult victim. Unfortunately, fingers often do not fair well in catastrophic events because they are one of the first things placed between a person and the trauma source. In a mass shooting type of incident, the use of fingerprints can be expected. In a transportation incident such as a large plane crash, however, it is not uncommon for there to be in excess of 10,000 fragmented remains as was seen in the ET302 crash. The fingers are often sheared off in a crash, or damaged in a way that they cannot be printed. The palms and feet, however, have more muscle and skin than the fingers and more often remain intact in a crash. Feet are typically covered by shoes, so they have an added layer of protection during a traumatic event. It is worth reiterating that all friction ridge skin found in a highly fragmented mass fatality should be printed, as it is never known what the AM sample may contain or if any of the fingers will ever be recovered. Footprint identification is just as effective as fingerprint identification, provided that AM footprints can be located. Many AFIS systems already have a palm print searching and comparison tool or component, and it is plausible that the same technology could be used to develop a footprint database in the future. Palm print algorithms may also currently be used to inter-compare populations of footprints recovered from scenes and the morgue. While footprints may not be used in most forensic casework, they are a very valuable tool for identification. It is not uncommon for a person to attempt to refrain from giving their fingerprints while they are living, for fear of self-incrimination in any future offenses. The collection of footprints would, however, be much less incriminating. A database of known footprints solely for identification purposes could be established to allow the deceased to be identified more easily, regardless of how they died. While this is not current practice, it should be considered for the future of biometric advancement. Scientific modalities (friction ridge prints, DNA, dental, etc.) are heavily depended on for identification purposes, and the reason deceased persons go unidentified is due to lack of viable AM data that is searchable.

7.8 Conclusion

The terms "Disaster Victim Identification," "Mass Fatality Incident," and "Mass Disaster" all imply the need for victims to be identified in a timely and scientifically accurate manner. Regardless of the jurisdiction, coroner or medical system distinction, or the geographic region, there will inevitably be a family waiting to learn the fate of their loved one and begin the closure process. It is imperative to ensure that whoever is handling the overall operation considers logical, realistic timeframes and the capabilities of those doing the work. At the same time, it is up to the practitioners to make sure they are prepared to efficiently do their best work in an expeditious manner. This chapter outlined each step of the process and provided the tools and guidance to achieve a high-quality work product, but such methods work only if practiced in advance, and followed when the event occurs. It is essential that all agencies have a proper and detailed mass fatality plan and know in advance how to implement it when the time comes. Sadly, it is inevitably a "when," not an "if," that such a plan will be needed.

References

ASB (2018). *Postmortem Impression Submission Strategy for Comprehensive Searches of Essential Automated Fingerprint Identification System Databases*. ANSI/AAFS.

Ashbaugh, D.R. (1999). *Quantitative-qualitative Friction Ridge Analysis: An Introduction to Basic and Advanced Ridgeology*. Boca Raton: CRC Press.

Johnson, B.T. and Riemen, J.A.J.M. (2019). Digital capture of fingerprints in a disaster victim identification setting: a review and case study. *Forensic Sciences Research* 4 (4): 293–302. 10.1080/20961790.2018.1521327.

Caplova, Z., Obertova, Z., Gibelli, D.M., Mazzarelli, D., Fracasso, T., Vanezis, P., Sforza, C. and Cattaneo, C. (2017). The reliability of facial recognition of deceased persons on photographs. *Journal of Forensic Sciences* 62: 1286–1291. 10.1111/1556-4029.13396.

Cardenas, A.H.R. (2010). *Rehydration and Preservation of Soft Tissues in Mummified Corpses, with the Forensic Purpose of Identifying and Diagnosing the Cause of Death*. Mexico Patent of Invention. MX20100011682. 24 October 2010.

DHS (2017). Biometrics [online]. Available at: https://www.dhs.gov/biometrics (Accessed 14 September 2020).

Dutch Police (2016). Jaarverslagen dactyloscopie en HAVANK [online]. Available at: https://www.politie.nl/binaries/content/assets/politie/algemeen/onderwerpteksten/algemeen/2017-jaarverslagen-2014-2015-dactyloscopie-en-havank.pdf (Accessed 14 September 2020).

FBI (1977). *The Science of Fingerprints: Classification and Uses*. Washington, D.C.: Department of Justice.

Hernandez, G. and Hess, G.L. (2014). Rehydrating mummified hands: The pima county experience. 2014. *Academic Forensic Pathology* 4 (1): 114–117.

Hickman, M.J., Hughes, K.A., Strom, K.J. and Ropero-Miller, J.D. (2007). *Medical Examiners and Coroners' Offices, 2004. Bureau of Justice Statistics Special Report*. Washington, D.C.: Department of Justice, Office of Justice Programs.

Holder, E.H., Robinson, L.O. and Laub, J.H. (2011). *The Fingerprint Sourcebook*. Washington, DC: U.S. Dept. of Justice, Office of Justice Programs.

INTERPOL (2014). *INTERPOL Disaster Victim Identification (DVI) Guide*. Lyon: The International Criminal Police Organization.

Mangold, K.C. (2016). *Data Format for the Interchange of Fingerprint, Facial and Other Biometric Information ANSI/NIST-ITL 1-2011 NIST Special Publication*

500-290 Edition 3. Gaithersburg, MD: National Institute of Standards and Technology.

Mulawka, M. (2014). *\postmortem Fingerprinting and Unidentified Human Remains*. Philadelphia: Routledge.

NRC (2009). *Strengthening Forensic Science in the United States: A Path Forward*. Washington D.C.: The National Academies Press.

Scanlon, J. (2008). Identifying the tsunami dead in Thailand and Sri Lanka: Multi-national emergent organizations. *International Journal of Mass Emergencies and Disasters* 26 (1): 1–18.

Siwek, D. and Reinecke, G.W. (2014). Relaxation of clenched digits in cadaveric hands to facilitate the recovery of postmortem friction ridge impressions. *Journal of Forensic Identification* 64 (1): 13–17.

Stokes, J. (2019). Technical note: next generation identification – A powerful tool in cold case investigations. *Forensic Science International* 299: 10.1016/j.forsciint.2019.03.033.

Uhle, A.J. (2010). Fingerprints and human identification. In: *Forensic Dentistry, Second Edition* (ed. D. Senn and P. Stimson), 79–101. Boca Raton: CRC Press.

Uhle, A.J. and Leas, R.L. (2007). The boiling technique: A method for obtaining quality postmortem impressions from deteriorating friction ridge skin. *Journal of Forensic Identification* 57 (3): 358–369.

CHAPTER 8

DNA Technology and the Future of Disaster Victim Identification

Taylor M. Dickerson III

SNA International, contractor at the Armed Forces Medical Examiner System (AFMES) Armed Forces DNA Identification Laboratory (AFDIL), Dover, DE, USA

8.1 Introduction

Forensic DNA testing is one of the many modalities of identification used to identify victims of a mass fatality event. Historically, DNA testing has proven to be effective and reliable as the sole means to identify individuals. It has also been used to complement other modalities and confirm an identification, or re-associate fragmented remains when other modalities are not possible. Many notable mass fatality events worldwide have utilized DNA testing for these purposes.

One of the earliest efforts to use DNA testing was for the burn victims in the Branch Davidian Compound in Waco, Texas, in 1993. The Armed Forces DNA Identification Laboratory (AFDIL) and the United Kingdom's Forensic Science Service were able to use polymerase chain reaction (PCR) methods to develop DNA profiles from short tandem repeat (STR) locations within the nuclear DNA of the severely burned human remains [1]. The crash of Swissair Flight 111 in 1998 off the coast of Nova Scotia required the use of DNA testing to identify all 229 victims and demonstrated the success of DNA testing of human remains exposed to sea water. The Royal Canadian Mounted Police utilized PCR for STR testing and provided a model for DNA-led

Disaster Victim Identification in the 21st Century: A US Perspective, First Edition.
Edited by John A Williams and Victor W Weedn.

identifications in a closed population incident where a variety of DNA reference samples were needed for comparisons [2,3].

The terroristic events of September 11, 2001 (9/11) in New York City (NYC), Pennsylvania, and Washington, D.C., brought the world's attention to large-scale disaster victim identification (DVI) efforts. Even though all modalities of identification were used at each incident site, DNA testing was particularly useful to identify the large number of fragmented remains, especially in NYC. The collapse of the twin towers at the World Trade Center (WTC) site reduced the 2,753 decedents to more than 21,000 separate remains and posed serious challenges for the DNA testing efforts. STR testing worked on a small percentage of samples in the initial phases of testing. Exposure of the remains to chemicals, building materials, and fire, along with the normal course of biological degradation, warranted the use of DNA methods not traditionally employed with mass fatality identification. NYC's Office of Chief Medical Examiner led the DNA identification effort, but partnered with other laboratories to help with the testing of reference samples and remains; and to develop procedures to utilize mitochondrial DNA, single nucleotide polymorphisms (SNPs), and mini-STRs [3–7]. Never had such a combination of DNA technologies been used before in a DVI effort. Improvements in DNA extraction techniques, sensitivities in typing platforms and STR amplification kits, and the expansion of the number of locations tested with STR amplification kits have ushered new phases of DNA testing that continue for the remains recovered from the WTC [8].

Natural disasters like the Southeast Asia tsunami in 2004 and Hurricane Katrina in 2005 required multi-agency, and even international, response due to the large number of deceased. Human remains were exposed to warmer climates and large volumes of water over a longer period of time, leading to rapid decomposition. Both disasters reminded scientists of the difficulties associated with DNA testing of degraded human remains [9–15]. Mitochondrial DNA was necessary to help identify victims from both disasters when STR testing did not work [10,14]. It was also difficult to obtain suitable reference samples for the victims in Southeast Asia and Louisiana. Many personal items used as direct reference samples were destroyed by flood waters. The Swedish government was able to use blood cards collected for newborn babies as direct references for some of its citizens who died in the tsunami [12]. For Hurricane Katrina, volunteer genetic counselors and DNA analysts worked at the Louisiana Family Assistance Center to assist in finding family members, who were dispersed all over the country, to use as DNA references for kinship analysis [15]. Both approaches to find DNA references proved beneficial for the DNA identifications and provided a model for their use in future DVI efforts.

All of the mass fatality events mentioned so far, and many not mentioned here, have spurred discussion and debate in the DVI and forensic DNA communities on how to proceed with DNA testing in a mass fatality event. These discussions resulted in the publication of recommendations and guidelines to be used by anyone involved in any step of the DNA identification process – from sample collection through issuing a DNA report [16–21]. One of the more recent documents, "Best Practice Recommendations for DNA Analysis for Human Identification in Mass Fatality Incidents," was published by the American Academy of Forensic Sciences (AAFS) Standards Board (ASB) in 2019. It is a culmination of best practice recommendations set forth by the Disaster Victim Identification subcommittee within the Organization of Scientific Area Committees (OSAC) for Forensic Science after originating from the disbanded Scientific Working Group on Disaster Victim Identification [22]. While these best practices provide a framework for DNA identification, they do not discuss the different technologies in use for DNA testing. The aim of this chapter is to provide an overview of the different DNA testing technologies, their applicability in a DVI effort, and some of the advances made which may lead to future applications.

8.2 STRs and Mini-STRs

Forensic DNA testing is widely used in publicly and privately funded laboratories all over the world. It not uncommon for those laboratories with the technology and experience using it to be involved with a DVI effort. Most, if not all, of those laboratories use STR-based testing from commercially available PCR amplification kits. The kits are designed to test from 9 to 25 different locations (loci) found within human chromosomes. These loci were selected by the forensic DNA community because of their distance from one another and their location in non-coding regions – areas of DNA that are not responsible for physical traits or potential diseases. These loci are well conserved from generation to generation, making them useful for kinship related comparisons. A person inherits their DNA from both mother and father. A decedent's DNA profile generated with STRs will have alleles in common with both parents. This allows for comparison of an unidentified remain to a set of family references tested with the same STR loci. Most often, parents, children, and/or siblings are asked to donate a reference sample, but in some cases more distantly related family members may be used as well. A kinship report is usually generated providing the likelihood of the unidentified remain belonging to that family [3,23].

As long as laboratories test the same STR loci, their DNA profile results will be compatible. This is critical for any effort to construct a DNA database, where DNA profiles need to be searched against each other and reference samples to find potential matches. Most forensic DNA databases are designed to handle direct matches and kinship comparisons. A direct match is usually made when an unidentified remain matches a direct reference sample that contains the decedent's DNA (i.e., toothbrush, hairbrush, razor, etc.). This type of match also occurs when fragmented remains have the same DNA profile and are believed to be from the same decedent. A statistical calculation is then performed and provided for all matches to ensure confidence before making an official identification [24–27].

STR testing improved over the years as changes were made to the amplification kits commonly used by laboratories. One major improvement included an increase in the number of loci tested per kit. As that number increased, the discriminatory power also increased and provided more assurance that a DNA profile was unique to an individual. The sensitivity of testing increased with the adjustment or addition of components in the amplification kits. Depending on the location and circumstances surrounding the death, a variety of chemical and environmental contaminants could be present on human remains. Some of these contaminants may inhibit DNA testing, which often results in a partial profile or no DNA profile.

Sometimes a dilution of the sample's DNA extract prior to amplification will overcome the effects of inhibition. Use of an amplification kit designed to overcome inhibition will also increase a laboratory's success in obtaining a DNA profile. Using a kit with these improvements could minimize the amount of troubleshooting needed and may shorten the overall time to complete DNA testing. Laboratories will often perform comparison studies to evaluate the sensitivities of different amplification kits on the same types of samples. This allows the laboratory to select an amplification kit that works best for the samples they most commonly encounter. A laboratory may find the amplification kit they use for crime scene samples works just as well with samples from human remains. They may simply need to make adjustments to the volume of DNA amplified or amount of DNA injected into the capillary electrophoresis system to increase their success with samples that have low yields of DNA or may be degraded [3,28–30].

A laboratory may choose to implement an amplification kit with mini-STRs to overcome issues with sample degradation. A mini-STR is the same location as a regular STR with the same name but reduced in size to allow for amplification of that location in a smaller format, where no result was obtained in its regular format. As long as DNA degradation is not too extreme, mini-STRs may provide a DNA profile when amplification with a regular STR kit fails. Mini-STRs may also be used to supplement a partial profile that exhibits degradation at the larger loci within a regular STR kit. If those larger loci are present in the mini-STR format, and a result is obtained, the results can be combined with the original partial profile to give a more complete DNA profile for the sample [31,32].

8.3 Lineage Markers

Mitochondrial DNA testing is performed by sequencing the bases found within two hypervariable regions (HV1 and HV2) of the mitochondrial DNA genome. These regions are not responsible for any visible traits or potential diseases, which is attractive for forensic purposes just like the STR loci chosen for testing. PCR amplification is used to generate separate sections of HV1 and HV2. Those sections are then sequenced with Sanger-based methods in both forward and reverse directions along the DNA. This process is repeated, with the sections pieced together until a full DNA sequence is obtained at each region. The resulting DNA sequence is then compared to a reference sequence, referred to as Anderson or revised Cambridge, to determine if there are any differences at each base position. The differences, or polymorphisms, are considered the forensic profile for the mitochondrial DNA sample, which can be compared to references or other human remains samples for identification or re-association, respectively. The mitochondrial DNA testing process is more labor-intensive and expensive compared to STR-based testing. Additional equipment, reagents, and training on interpretation are all needed and handled separately from traditional STR testing. For these reasons, mitochondrial DNA is often not tested by forensic DNA laboratories. However, mitochondrial DNA testing has its utility when STR testing fails. Mitochondria are found in greater numbers, than the single nucleus, within a human cell and have a circular genome, which makes it less susceptible to damage. Samples that exhibit DNA degradation through failed or poor quality STR results may produce a result with mitochondrial DNA testing [3,23].

Y-STR testing is performed in a similar fashion as STR testing, making it easier for laboratories to implement. Y-STRs are found on the Y chromosome, which is male-specific. Simply put, if a Y-STR result is obtained from a human remains sample, that sample is expected to be male. As with STRs, the Y-STR loci were chosen for testing by the forensic DNA community and are tested via commercially available amplification kits. The resulting DNA profile shows one or two alleles at each location tested and can be compared to references or additional human remains samples.

The regions tested within mitochondrial DNA and Y chromosomal DNA are commonly referred to as lineage markers due to their inheritance from an individual's parents. Mitochondrial DNA is inherited from an individual's mother and found to be in common with their maternal line of relatives. Since the Y chromosome is found only in male individuals, it is inherited from the individual's father and found to be in common with their paternal line of relatives. Family reference samples collected for DVI purposes are usually designated as being from maternal or paternal relatives, just in case testing for lineage markers is needed. Since mitochondrial DNA sequences and Y-STR profiles are expected to be in common with relatives, these results are not as discriminatory as STRs. A mitochondrial DNA match indicates the sample may be from the unidentified individual or a maternal relative. A Y-STR match indicates the sample may be from the unidentified individual or a paternal relative. The laboratory reporting these results will also provide a statistic to indicate how common the profiles are within specific population groups [3,23].

Improvements made to mitochondrial DNA testing have also come about to address issues with degradation and inhibition. Laboratories may change the volumes of reagents or DNA within an amplification reaction to affect a better downstream result. Some laboratories may employ mini-primers for mitochondrial DNA. Mini-primers have a function similar to mini-STRs by providing the same testable regions, but in smaller formats, to overcome issues with DNA degradation [33]. A laboratory may use different size primer sets based on the perceived quality of the human remains sample. Choosing the appropriate primer set initially may save time and prevent the need for troubleshooting.

A mitochondrial DNA sequence may be used to determine its haplogroup, or ancestry information. If the victims of the mass fatality have different ancestries, this information may be useful in differentiating the remains [34].

Y-STR amplification kits have seen the same improvements over the years as STR kits. The kits are more sensitive and able to overcome inhibition. Additional Y-STR locations have also been incorporated, providing more loci for comparison. Some of these locations are referred to as rapidly mutating Y-STRs due to their higher mutation rates between generations. A different result, or allele, may be seen at one or more of these locations when comparing a sample to its reference, indicating a mutational event occurred during inheritance. A laboratory testing these locations will need to take this into consideration and determine if the mutational event is the likely cause for the mismatch, or if the sample is from a different individual altogether [35,36].

8.4 Next Generation Sequencing

The Forensic DNA community has adopted a DNA sequencing technology referred to as next generation sequencing (NGS), or massively parallel sequencing (MPS). This technology is widely used in clinical settings to study and diagnose genetic disorders and has been adapted for forensic use with targeted regions of interest within nuclear and mitochondrial DNA. The sequencing method employed will vary depending on the commercially available reagents and instrumentation chosen by the laboratory, but the workflow of NGS has common features. First, a library of targeted DNA regions is constructed and pooled together. Clusters of DNA are then created for each DNA fragment to serve as the sequencing reaction. Finally, millions of data points are read and interpreted by customized software. The method is considered "massively parallel" since multiple regions can be tested in a single reaction and analyzed together. For example, where traditional Sanger sequencing of mitochondrial DNA relied on piece-by-piece construction of the HV1 and HV2 regions, NGS can produce the whole mitochondrial genome in one shot. Having more data available for analysis could be useful in certain situations. If unrelated individuals have a common mitochondrial sequence in the HV1 and HV2 regions, discovering differences in other parts of the genome would allow discrimination between those individuals. NGS of STR and Y-STR loci provides the ability to test more loci than are present in existing amplification kits. Additional information may be obtained about the alleles for those loci since the sequence of the alleles is developed rather than an allele number. DNA technologies that are not widely used, such as single nucleotide polymorphisms (SNPs) and X chromosomal testing, are more attainable with an NGS platform already validated for STRs, Y-STRs, and/or mitochondrial DNA. SNP and X-STR regions are tested to identify an individual by comparison to reference samples just as STRs and lineage markers. Different SNP regions can also provide information about an individual's ancestry and phenotypic traits, such as eye, hair, and skin color, thereby aiding the identification by comparison to their biological profile [37–39].

All of these features of NGS can be advantageous in a DVI effort. The ability to streamline testing and have more data available after the initial round of testing may save time and add more information to the DNA identification process. An ideal scenario would show a human remain that is associated to family reference samples via STRs, Y-STRs, and mitochondrial DNA, while also matching the missing individual's biological profile via SNPs. All of this information taken together would strengthen the DNA identification. While that is certainly an attainable goal for NGS, there are some difficulties with this technology that must be taken into consideration. Most laboratories will not purchase an NGS method just for the possibility of a DVI event. The added expense of having another method online is not always feasible for a laboratory, especially when it requires additional instrumentation, training, and competency of its scientists. A laboratory is more likely to use NGS in a DVI effort if they have already incorporated the method into their normal casework procedures. Before it becomes more commonly used in the forensic DNA community, naming conventions for STR loci have to be agreed upon to ensure compatibility with existing DNA databases [40]. Most NGS procedures take multiple days to complete, so improvements made to the turnaround time would make it more attractive for widespread use. There is also concern that samples with extreme degradation may not yield the necessary results with every NGS method. Laboratories that encounter degraded specimens may need to validate methods that are more sensitive and able to overcome these issues. AFDIL has developed such a method to aid in the identification of soldiers recovered from past US military conflicts [41,42]. A laboratory may have to resort to such a method if traditional testing does not yield results.

8.5 Rapid DNA

Having the ability to perform DNA testing in a quicker manner and outside of a traditional laboratory has been discussed for many years. Even though many laboratories have made improvements to their workflows to speed up testing, the time spent waiting for sample incubation or an instrument to finish is a limiting step in decreasing the turnaround time from sample preparation to profile generation. The use of microfluidics to develop a "lab on a microchip" has always been a reasonable solution, but difficult to implement [43,44]. With the recent development of rapid DNA instruments, which may be purchased commercially, this notion of a quicker turnaround time for DNA testing is more realistic.

All steps in the nuclear DNA testing process from extraction through separation and detection of STRs are included in one instrument run which can be completed within two to three hours. Data analysis can also be automated and presented with a pass/fail "flag" for the user [45]. Rapid DNA instruments can be used outside of a laboratory and have already been deployed by numerous law enforcement agencies. Police stations can develop DNA profiles of those arrested and search them in CODIS to determine if that individual is linked to another crime. The FBI in conjunction with the Scientific Working Group on DNA Analysis Methods developed standards for the use of rapid DNA in police booking stations [46]. However, the use of rapid DNA to develop a DNA profile from criminal evidence and perform subsequent searches in CODIS is not approved by the FBI [47]. Despite this ruling, some laboratories are using this technology for different sample types, and specifically for cases that will not need CODIS entry and searching. Use of rapid DNA for a DVI effort falls into this category.

The technology has already been used in some jurisdictions with success for quicker identification of human remains [48,49]. It is feasible to set up and run a rapid DNA instrument in a mobile morgue, family assistance center, or other DVI setting to develop DNA profiles from both remains and reference samples in real-time [50]. A jurisdiction hoping to utilize rapid DNA in this way will need to consider a number of factors. They must determine the logistics of deploying the instruments; whether they are purchased for the DVI effort or borrowed from laboratories that already use them. The staff using the instruments will need training on all aspects of the procedure, to include sample collection and how the data is used and interpreted at the end of a run. A consideration needs to be made about the validation of the instrument and the STR loci-tested, so a forensic DNA laboratory's involvement with data interpretation, searching of DNA profiles, and report writing are addressed for the medicolegal authority making the official identification of remains. Many of the requirements and standards that an accredited forensic DNA laboratory follows may be applicable to the use of rapid DNA and have to be followed. While studies suggest a great success rate of DNA profile generation for high-quality samples, some have seen lower success rates for poor quality, degraded DNA samples [51–54]. If the manufacturer provides a more sensitive cartridge for samples with expected low yields of DNA, that may be useful for these samples [55–57]. If some or all samples do not work with rapid DNA or require additional technologies (i.e., Y-STR or mitochondrial DNA), there needs to be a DNA laboratory in place to handle that additional work.

8.6 Conclusion

All of the DNA technologies discussed here will continue to improve with ongoing research and contributions from forensic professionals. As the technologies progress, decisions have to be made whether to adopt them for laboratory use and if they will be applicable to help identify victims of a mass fatality event. Some situations will warrant the use of one technology over another or even the combination of technologies to complement one another. A change in DNA technology will be beneficial only if it provides accurate and timely results to aid the identification of remains in a DVI effort. Medicolegal authorities and forensic DNA specialists should work together to make these decisions and ensure continued success.

References

1. Clayton, T.M., Whitaker, J.P., and Maguire, C.N. (1995, Nov 30). Identification of bodies from the scene of a mass disaster using DNA amplification of short tandem repeat (STR) loci. *Forensic Science International* 76 (1): 7–15.
2. Leclair, B., Fregeau, C.J., Bowen, K.L., and Fourney, R.M. (2004, Sep). Enhanced kinship analysis and STR-based DNA typing for human identification in mass fatality incidents: The Swissair Flight 111 disaster. *Journal of Forensic Science* 49 (5): 1–15.
3. Butler, J.M. (2012). *Advanced Topics in Forensic DNA Testing: Methodology*. San Diego, CA: Elsevier Academic Press.

4. Budimlija, Z.M., Prinz, M.K., Zelson-Mundorff, A., Wiersema, J., Bartelink, E., MacKinnon, G., Nazzaruolo, B.L., Estacio, S.M., Hennessey, M.J., and Shaler, R.C. (2003). World Trade Center human identification project: Experiences with individual body identification cases. *Croatian Medical Journal* 44 (3): 259–263.
5. Holland, M.M., Cave, C.A., Holland, C.A., and Bille, T.W. (2003). Development of a quality, high throughput DNA analysis procedure for skeletal samples to assist with the identification of victims from the World Trade Center attacks. *Croatian Med Journal* 44 (3): 264–272.
6. Biesecker, L.G., Bailey-Wilson, J.E., Ballantyne, J., Baum, H., Bieber, F.R., Brenner, C., Budowle, B., Butler, J.M., Carmody, G., Conneally, P.M., Duceman, B., Eisenberg, A., Forman, L., Kidd, K.K., Leclair, B., Niezgoda, S., Parsons, T.J., Pugh, E., Shaler, R., Sherry, S.T., Sozer, A., and Walsh, A. (2005). DNA identifications after the 9/11 World Trade Center attack. *Science* 310: 1122–1123.
7. Shaler, R.C. (2005). *Who They Were. Inside the World Trade Center DNA Story: The Unprecedented Effort to Identify the Missing*. New York, NY: Free Press.
8. Gill, J.R., Desire, M., Dickerson, T., and Adams, B.J. (2011). The 9/11 attacks: The medicolegal investigation of the World Trade Center fatalities. In: *Forensic Pathology Reviews* (Editor(s) E. Turk), 6. New York,NY: Humana Press.
9. Ladika, S. (2005). DNA helps identify missing in the Tsunami zone. *Science* 307 (5709): 504.
10. Deng, Y.J., Li, Y.Z., Yu, X.G., Li, L., Wu, D.Y., Zhou, J., Man, T.Y., Yang, G., Yan, J.W., Cai, D.Q., Wang, J., Yang, H.M., Li, S.B., and Preliminary, Y.J. (2005). DNA identification for the tsunami victims in Thailand. *Genomics, Proteomics & Bioinformatics* 3 (3): 143–157.
11. Lessig, R., Thiele, K., and Edelmann, J. (2006). Tsunami 2004 – Experiences, challenges and strategies. *International Congress Series* 1288: 747–749.
12. Holmlund, G., Lodestad, I., Nilsson, H., and Lindblom, B. (2006). Experiences from DNA analysis in Sweden for the identification of tsunami victims. *International Congress Series* 1288: 744–746.
13. Wright, K., Mundorff, A., Chaseling, J., Maguire, C., and Crane, D.I. (2015). An evaluation of the Thai tsunami victim identification DNA operation. *Forensic Science Policy & Management: An International Journal* 6 (3-4): 69–78.
14. Donkervoort, S., Dolan, S.M., Beckwith, M., Northrup, T.P., and Sozer, A. (2008). Enhancing accurate data collection in mass fatality kinship identifications: Lessons learned from Hurricane Katrina. *Forensic Science International: Genetics* 2: 354–362.
15. Dolan, S., Saraiya, D., Donkervoort, S. et al. (2009). The emerging role of genetics professionals in forensic kinship DNA identification after a mass

fatality: Lessons learned from Hurricane Katrina volunteers. *Genetics in Medicine* 11: 414–417.

16. U.S. Department of Justice, National Institute of Justice (2005). Mass fatality incidents: A guide for human forensic identification. June. NCJ 199758.

17. U.S. Department of Justice, Office of Justice Program, President's DNA Initiative (2006). Lessons Learned from 9/11: DNA Identification in Mass Fatality Incidents.

18. Prinz, M., Carracedo, A., Mayr, W.R. et al. (2007). DNA Commission of the International Society for Forensic Genetics (ISFG): Recommendations regarding the role of forensic genetics for disaster victim identification (DVI). *Forensic Science International: Genetics* 1: 3–12.

19. International Committee of the Red Cross (2009). Missing people, DNA analysis and identification of human remains: A guide to best practice in armed conflicts and other situations of armed violence.

20. American Association of Blood Banks (2010). Guidelines for mass fatality DNA identification operations.

21. International Criminal Police Organization (2014). Interpol disaster victim identification guide.

22. ANSI/ASB (2019). Best practice recommendations for DNA analysis for human identification in mass fatality incidents. 1.

23. Sozer, A.C. (2014). *DNA Analysis for Missing Person Identification in Mass Fatalities*. Boca Raton, FL.: CRC Press.

24. Cash, H.D., Hoyle, J.W., and Sutton, A.J. (2003). Development under extreme conditions: Forensic bioinformatics in the wake of the World Trade Center disaster. In: *Biocomputing Pacific Symposium on Biocomputing*. (Editor(s) R.B. Altman, A.K. Dunker, L. Hunter, T.A. Jung, T.E. Klein). 638–653. River Edge, NJ: World Scientific.

25. Alonso, A., Martin, P., Albarran, C., Garcia, P., De Simon, L.F., Iturralde, M.J., Fernandez-Rodriguez, A., Atienza, I., Capilla, J., Garcia-Hirschfeld, J., Martinez, P., Vallejo, G., Garcia, O., Garcia, E., Real, P., Alvarez, D., Leon, A., and Sancho, M. (2005). Challenges of DNA profiling in mass disaster investigations. *Croatian Medical Journal* 46: 540–548.

26. Bradford, L., Heal, J., Anderson, J., Faragher, N., Duval, K., and Lalonde, S. (August, 2011). Disaster victim investigation recommendations from two simulated mass disaster scenarios utilized for user acceptance testing CODIS 6.0. *Forensic Science International: Genetics* 5 (4): 291–296.

27. Osborn-Gustavson, A.E., McMahon, T., Josserand, M., and Spamer, B.J. (2018). Chapter 12 – The utilization of databases for the identification of human remains. In: *New Perspectives in Forensic Human Skeletal Identification* (Editor(s) K.E. Latham, E.J. Bartelink and M. Finnegan), 129–139. San Diego, CA: Academic Press.

28. Butler, J.M. (2006). Genetics and genomics of core short tandem repeat loci used in human identity testing. *Journal of Forensic Sciences* 51: 253–265.
29. Irwin, J.A., Lene, Y., MD, Loreille, O., Barritt, S.M., Christensen, A.F., Holland, T.D., Smith, B.C., and Parsons, T.J. (2007). Application of low copy number STR typing to the identification of aged, degraded skeletal remains. *Journal of Forensic Sciences* 52: 1322–1327.
30. Hill, C.R., Butler, J.M., and Vallone, P.M. (2009). A 26plex autosomal STR assay to aid human identity testing. *Journal of Forensic Sciences* 54: 1008–1015.
31. Opel, K.L., Chung, D.T., Drábek, J., Tatarek, N.E., Jantz, L.M., and McCord, B.R. (2006). The application of miniplex primer sets in the analysis of degraded DNA from human skeletal remains. *Journal of Forensic Sciences* 51: 351–356.
32. Hill, C.R., Kline, M.C., Coble, M.D., and Butler, J.M. (2008). Characterization of 26 miniSTR loci for improved analysis of degraded DNA samples. *Journal of Forensic Sciences* 53: 73–80.
33. Gabriel, M.N., Huffine, E.F., Ryan, J.H., Holland, M.M., and Parsons, T.J. (2001). Improved MtDNA sequence analysis of forensic remains using a mini-primer set amplification strategy. *Journal of Forensic Science* 46: 247–253.
34. Marshall, C., Taylor, R., Sturk-Andreaggi, K., Barritt-Ross, S., Berg, G.E., and McMahon, T.P. (2020). Mitochondrial DNA haplogrouping to assist with the identification of unknown service members from the World War II Battle of Tarawa. *Forensic Science International: Genetics* 47: 102291.
35. Ballantyne, K.N., Keerl, V., Wollstein, A., Choi, Y., Zuniga, S.B., Ralf, A., Vermeulen, M., De Knijff, P., and Kayser, M. (2012). A new future of forensic Y-chromosome analysis: Rapidly mutating Y-STRs for differentiating male relatives and paternal lineages. *Forensic Science International: Genetics* 6 (2): 208–218.
36. Boattini, A., Sarno, S., Bini, C., Pesci, V., Barbieri, C., De Fanti, S., Quagliariello, A., Pagani, L., Ayub, Q., Ferri, G., Pettener, D., Luiselli, D., and Pelotti, S. (2016). Mutation rates and discriminating power for 13 rapidly-mutating Y-STRs between related and unrelated individuals. *PLoS One* 11 (11): e0165678.
37. Yang, Y., Xie, B., and Yan, J. (2014). Application of next-generation sequencing technology in forensic science. *Genomics, Proteomics & Bioinformatics* 12 (5): 190–197.
38. Børsting, C. and Morling, N. (2015). Next generation sequencing and its applications in forensic genetics. *Forensic Science International: Genetics* 18: 78–89.

39. Bruijns, B., Tiggelaar, R., and Gardeniers, H. (2018, Nov). Massively parallel sequencing techniques for forensics: A review. *Electrophoresis* 39 (21): 2642–2654.

40. Gettings, K., Kiesler, K.M., Faith, S.A., Montano, E., Baker, C.H., Young, B.A., Guerrieri, R.A., and Vallone, P.M. (2016). Sequence variation of 22 autosomal STR loci detected by next generation sequencing. *Forensic Science International: Genetics* 21: 15–21.

41. Loreille, O., Koshinsky, H., Fofanov, V.Y., and Irwin, J.A. (2011). Application of next generation sequencing technologies to the identification of highly degraded unknown soldiers' remains. *Forensic Science International: Genetics Supplemental Series* 3: 540–541.

42. Marshall, C., Sturk-Andreaggi, K., Daniels-Higginbotham, J., Oliver, R.S., Barritt-Ross, S., and McMahon, T.P. (2017). Performance evaluation of a mitogenome capture and Illumina sequencing protocol using non-probative, case-type skeletal samples: Implications for the use of a positive control in a next-generation sequencing procedure. *Forensic Science International: Genetics* 31: 198–206.

43. Horsman, K.M., Bienvenue, J.M., Blasier, K.R., and Landers, J.P. (2007). Forensic DNA analysis on microfluidic devices: A review. *Journal of Forensic Science* 52: 784–799.

44. Bruijns, B., Van Asten, A., Tiggelaar, R., and Gardeniers, H. (2016). Microfluidic devices for forensic DNA Analysis: A review. *Biosensors (Basel)* 6 (3): 41.

45. Butler, J.M. (2015). The future of forensic DNA analysis. *Philosophical Transactions of the Royal Society B* 370: 20140252.

46. FBI (September, 2020). Standards for the operation of rapid DNA booking systems by law enforcement booking agencies.

47. Hares, D.R., Kneppers, A., Onorato, A.J., and Kahn, S. (2020). Rapid DNA for crime scene use: Enhancements and data needed to consider use on forensic evidence for State and National DNA Databasing – An agreed position statement by ENFSI, SWGDAM and the Rapid DNA Crime Scene Technology Advancement Task Group. *Forensic Science International: Genetics* 48: 102349.

48. Gin, K., Tovar, J., Bartelink, E.J., Kendell, A., Milligan, C., Willey, P., Wood, J., Tan, E., Turingan, R.S., and Selden, R.F. (2020). The 2018 California wildfires: Integration of rapid DNA to dramatically accelerate victim identification. *Journal of Forensic Science* 65: 791–799.

49. Turingan, R.S., Brown, J., Kaplun, L. et al. (2020). Identification of human remains using rapid DNA analysis. *International Journal of Legal Medicine* 134: 863–872.

50. Sozer, A. (Summer, 2019). Rapid DNA & mass fatality incidents. *Evidence Technology Magazine* 17 (2).

51. Hennessy, L.K., Mehendale, N., Chear, K., Jovanovich, S., Williams, S., Park, C., and Gangano, S. (2014). Developmental validation of the GlobalFiler express kit, a 24-marker STR assay, on the RapidHIT system. *Forensic Science International: Genetics* 13: 247–258.

52. Romsos, E.L., French, J.L., Smith, M., Figarelli, V., Harran, F., Vandegrift, G., Moreno, L.I., Callaghan, T.F., Brocato, J., Vaidyanathan, J., Pedroso, J.C., Amy, A., Stoiloff, S., Morillo, V.H., Czetyrko, K., Johnson, E.D., de Tagyos, J., Murray, A., and Vallone, P.M. (2020). Results of the 2018 rapid DNA maturity assessment. *Journal of Forensic Science* 65: 953–959.

53. Turingan, R.S., Tan, E., Jiang, H., Brown, J., Estari, Y., Krautz-Peterson, G., and Selden, R.F. (2020). Developmental validation of the ANDE 6C system for rapid DNA analysis of forensic casework and DVI samples. *Journal of Forensic Science* 65: 1056–1071.

54. Kitayama, T., Fukagawa, T., Watahiki, H., Mita, Y., Fujii, K., Unuma, K., Sakurada, K., Uemura, K., Sekiguchi, K., and Mizuno, N. (2020, Sep). Evaluation of rapid DNA system for buccal swab and disaster victim identification samples. *Legal Medicine (Tokyo)* 46: 101713.

55. Buscaino, J., Barican, A., Farrales, L., Goldman, B., Klevenberg, J., Kuhn, M., Lin, F., Nguyen, P., Salceda, S., Schueren, R., Smith, C., Troup, C., Tsou, D., Vangbo, M., and King, D. (2018). Evaluation of a rapid DNA process with the RapidHIT ID system using a specialized cartridge for extracted and quantified human DNA. *Forensic Science International: Genetics* 34: 116–127.

56. Turingan, R.S., Vasantgadkar, S., Palombo, L., Hogan, C., Jiang, H., Tan, E., and Selden, R.F. (2016). Rapid DNA analysis for automated processing and interpretation of low DNA content samples. *Investigative Genetics* 7: 2.

57. Cihlar, J.C., Kapema, K.B., and Budowle, B. (2021). Validation of the Applied Biosystems RapidHIT ID instrument and ACE Globalfiler Express sample cartridge. *International Journal of Legal Medicine* https://doi.org/10.1007/s00414-021-02722-9.

CHAPTER 9
The Victim Information Center and Data Collection

Its Evolving Role in DVI

Jason H. Byrd

Department of Pathology, Immunology and Laboratory Medicine, University of Florida, Gainesville, FL, USA

9.1 Introduction

When considering a mass fatality event, one must first consider the spectrum of victims impacted by the event. Many individuals may be involved in an event that causes fatalities but may remain unaffected and not requiring supplemental aid or assistance. Within the group of individuals who are affected or impacted by the event, there are those who may be injured as a result of the incident, and there are also fatalities. Mass fatality incidents are generally divided into two main groups – natural incidents and man-made incidents. Natural incidents include tornados, wildfires, hurricanes, floods, winter storms/blizzards, mudslides, and wildfires. Man-made incidents include transportation incidents, mass shootings, fires, building/structure collapse, asphyxiation, and stampedes. Across all categories of mass fatality events, the vast majority (approximately 89%) of incidents have fatalities ranging from 10 to 50 individuals. Approximately 9% of mass fatalities involve 51–300 individuals, leaving only very few incidents that involve more than 300 individuals (Carroll et al. 2017).

Disaster Victim Identification in the 21st Century: A US Perspective, First Edition.
Edited by John A Williams and Victor W Weedn.

This raises the question, what constitutes a mass fatality event in terms of number of affected individuals? Strictly speaking, there is no singular number of individuals that must be affected for an event or incident to be classified as a mass fatality. Rather, the number of fatalities must be high enough that it overwhelms the capacity of local resources. In some smaller, rural areas that do not have abundant resources, as few as 10 deaths from a single incident may overwhelm their resources. In larger, more urban areas with vast resources, as many as 50 deaths from a single incident may be well within their capacity to handle without necessitating a designation of a mass fatality event or otherwise requesting the aid of outside resources.

9.1.1 History of the Family Assistance Center

The models in use for Family Assistance Centers (FACs) today evolved from response models developed for aviation disasters. They were created because families often expressed concern about the lack of timely and official information provided to them. The concept of the FAC was then established to provide support services to families near the disaster location while waiting on the identification and release of the deceased. It also served to provide family support services in a private venue away from the media and the general public. One of the first FACs was known as the "Compassion Center" and was established after the bombing of the Murrah Federal Building in Oklahoma City in 1995. Families gathered privately and drew support from one another while waiting to receive updates on the recovery of remains and the identification efforts. They were also given access to the various service providers that were located at the compassion center which included mental health counseling, religious services, and access to funeral directors and organizations such as the Red Cross and Salvation Army. Since 1995, this model has been used repeatedly and further refined to address various types of incidents.

One aspect of the refinement of this model was the identification of the role of obtaining antemortem information from decedent family members. This function, the required associated tasks, and the space in which to conduct this operation have become known as the Victim Information Center (VIC), which is one aspect of the larger, more encompassing, role of the FAC, which provides victim services under a large scope of activities other than the required need for antemortem data collection. The roles of the VIC and FAC were further defined by the Aviation Disaster Family Assistance Act of 1996 (ADFAA) (449 USC § 1136, 41313 and 41113) that created the framework and defined responsibilities for the FAC. This legislation required a task force led by the National Transportation Safety Board (NTSB) to develop a Federal Family Assistance Plan for aviation disasters. The Aviation Disaster Family Assistance Act of 1996 required a process for providing information to and coordinating service provision for family members of those killed and survivors of major aviation accidents within the United States. Specific responsibilities were assigned to the NTSB, the air carrier(s), and agencies designated to provide mental health counseling and other services (Schroeder 2002). The Rail Passenger Disaster Family Assistance Act of 2008 assigned similar responsibilities to the NTSB, the American Red Cross, and interstate passenger rail operators following an accident resulting in major loss of life.

9.2 Overall Function of the Victim Information Center

According to the Federal Emergency Management Agency (FEMA), the Victim Information Center "collects and manages information about missing persons and coordinates antemortem investigation, information gathering, and recording, under the authority of the presiding law enforcement and medico-legal agencies" as it relates to fatality management (FEMA 2018). The purpose of the VIC is to help family members in the aftermath of a mass fatality incident. While primarily designed to assist family members of those who perished in the incident, the VIC model can be modified to also assist families of those injured or otherwise impacted by the event. The general VIC model provides direct access to medical examiner/coroner services, grief counseling, funeral service options, and information on the investigation from the relevant law enforcement and jurisdictional authorities, but services may vary based on the specific needs of those affected by the incident. The VIC also provides a controlled facility where family members can receive specific information about the event and ensuing investigations while ensuring their privacy remains protected. This allows investigators and Medical Examiners/Coroners access to family members to more effectively collect antemortem information for victim identification.

The VIC model was developed to provide a venue for responding agencies within the local jurisdiction to provide information to victims, ensure access to support services, and allow for the collection of information from families that may be required for victim identification. Even though an incident may involve or affect individuals from multiple jurisdictions, only one VIC should be established to meet these needs (see Chapter 9.5). The VIC should be staffed for the interviewing of family members and friends of the incident victims to provide an opportunity to obtain vital information that may lead to a positive identification of the victim. It also provides for identification consultation with forensically trained specialists.

9.2.1 Incident Operations

The Victim Information Center should be a basic and standard component of the local mass fatality plan as it is a critical component of family support. The local jurisdiction's decision to establish a VIC should be based on factors including the number of injuries, fatalities, and overall community impact. Factors affecting the operation and function of the VIC will vary between incidents, but the VIC should operate – at a minimum – for the duration of the period of victim recovery and identification. Local jurisdictions should develop plans to provide continuing assistance to families once they depart the VIC.

The VIC model within a local mass fatality management plan should be scalable and focused such that it most effectively and appropriately meets the needs of the victims' families and the impacted community. According to FEMA, there are specific guidelines that a VIC team should meet and follow when responding to a mass fatality incident. The suggested minimum number of personnel needed to fully staff a VIC team is 27 and should be composed of the following members (Box 9.1). Due to the scalable nature of the VIC, additional call takers and interviewers may be utilized based on the size and scope of the incident (FEMA 2018).

Box 9.1 Victim Identification Center Staffing Roles. The number of individuals (suggested in parentheses) to staff roles will vary with the scope of the MFI.

Team Leader (1)
Information Collection Coordinator (1)
Call Taker Specialist (5)
Interview Specialist (7)
Volunteer Training Specialist (2)
Behavioral Health Chaplaincy Specialist or other Behavioral Health Specialist (1)
Data and Records Coordinator (1)
Dental and Medical Records Acquisition Specialist (1)
Data Entry Specialist (5)
Records Management Specialist (2)
Documentation Specialist (1)

9.2.2 Meeting the Needs of Families and Survivors

Every mass fatality incident differs in the impacts it has on those affected. Although there is no singular model that will account for all potential needs of those affected, there are common needs among the families of those known or presumed to have been killed, as well as injured victims and their families. Family needs will likely change over time based on individual reactions, overall incident response, victim identification process, and the requirements of the overall incident investigation. Support and service organizations within the VIC must ensure their efforts are tailored to best meet the needs of both the families and survivors, particularly as they relate to identifying victims, returning personal effects, ongoing investigations, and any potential future prosecution of criminal acts.

In the wake of a mass fatality incident, family members of those affected will often quickly gather near the incident site or nearby hospitals seeking information about victims. This will likely occur prior to the official opening of the VIC. To assist in the overall management of initial information gathering, a call center should be designated, and a temporary reception center should be established to provide information on the opening of a full-scale VIC.

9.2.3 Briefings and Communication

Communication and proper flow of information are critical when working with families of victims and those affected by a mass fatality incident. Family briefings should be conducted on a set schedule so that family members feel they are receiving consistent and timely information regarding the ongoing investigation and identification process. Family members should be briefed before the media; it is paramount to avoid family members finding out information about their loved ones from the media before hearing it directly from investigators. VIC staff should ensure family members are given appropriate notice of the briefings and that the tone they use is suitable for the gravity of the incident, ensuring they operate with sensitivity to diversity. Within these briefings, VIC staff should inform families about the status of identifications, the process for the return of personal effects, and an explanation of time requirements. Each briefing should also include a summary of any key points and status of the incident operations, any remaining "housekeeping" items (such as food service, transportation, and lodging issues), and the time of the next briefing. Be open about the procedures and steps used in the identification process and be realistic about the time it may take to identify remains.

While it is, of course, essential to ensure that the family briefings contain appropriately substantive information, it is equally important to ensure that the method of communication used to impart the information is appropriate. Perception of communication is critical during these briefings as 55% of the perception of communication is non-verbal, including eye contact and body language. Vocal communication including volume and tone account for 38% of perception, and only 7% of communication perception is verbal – that is, the actual words being said (Mehrabian 1981).

9.3 Components of the Victim Information Center

9.3.1 Temporary Reception Center

A temporary reception center should be established as quickly as possible after the incident to provide family members and victims with information and immediate attention. The number of staff and type of services should be limited at the temporary reception center. Instead, the primary focus should be on establishing the VIC for full-scale operation. Staff at the temporary reception center should focus their efforts on making family members aware of the impending creation of the VIC including its location and available services. The temporary reception center also serves as a point of initial information gathering in order to more effectively determine what services should be offered at the VIC to better meet the needs of the families.

9.3.2 Call Centers

Call centers are a critical component of the VIC in that they are the mechanism for gathering information about potential missing persons. Importantly, the call center within the VIC is the official source for families to use to report missing individuals. When establishing and opening a call center within the Victim Information Center, there are several standard protocols that should be followed as well as others that may change based on the nature of the incident. The call center should be opened as soon as reasonably possible and the numbers for the call center should be published immediately after the incident. When opening a call center, one must consider how the call center information will be publicized, what the target capacity of the call center might be, and how long the call center will likely remain open. A standard protocol for information collection should be established such that all call center staff are obtaining the same information regarding potential victims of the mass fatality event. Considerations must be made for how the collected information will be quality-controlled to determine what may or may not be useful for victim identification. Information that is collected at the call center must then be transmitted to the organizations who will use the data for identification purposes, and the security and protection of the data must be ensured.

9.3.2.1 Missing Persons Call Center

The most common type of call center within the VIC is the Missing Persons Call Center (MPCC). The MPCC should be established immediately after the incident to start gathering victim information. By quickly opening the MPCC after an incident, it can help to reduce the volume of calls going to 911 and other *11 dispatch centers. For incidents that occur within multiple jurisdictions, there initially may be multiple incident-related call centers, but these should all be consolidated into one unified MPCC as quickly as possible. The goal of the MPCC is to receive calls and collect information from members of the public wishing to report someone missing. Staff of the MPCC should gather information on who is being reported missing, who is reporting the missing individual (relationship to the missing individual), and information on the likelihood of the potentially missing individual's involvement in the incident. They should also provide information on the Victim Identification Center in general. It is important to note that the determination of which agency manages the MPCC, how the call-in numbers are publicized, what specific information is collected, and access to collected data is made by the local jurisdiction within the incident. Once victim accounting has been completed, the MPCC may be deactivated at the discretion of the local jurisdiction or it may be converted into a services call center to provide information on behavioral health support, crisis counseling, and legal services for those affected by the incident.

9.3.2.2 Air Carrier Call Center

The Aviation Disaster Family Assistance Act of 1996 requires the establishment of a specific type of call center for aviation disasters – the Air Carrier Call Center (ACCC). The ACCC will be responsible for making notifications of involvement based on the information from the passenger manifest (Schroeder 2002). Similarly, rail disasters are also federally mandated to aid victims and their families. Both air and rail carriers need to know the location of the victim's families so that assistance can be provided, thus similar information must be collected by the ACCC as would be collected by the MPCC. It is a determination of the local jurisdiction on utilization of a separate MPCC as an additional call center.

9.4 Accounting for the Victims

A primary goal of the Victim Information Center's team is to successfully facilitate matching a victim from the incident to a missing person's report. In order to do so, the VIC team is tasked with the collection and organization of critical data. This includes antemortem data such as fingerprints, dental X-rays, medical records, photographs, and DNA which may be useful in the process of victim identification. By providing subject matter expertise in mass fatality management and victim information procurement, the VIC team will also serve as a liaison to the victim's families to better facilitate the matching and identification process. They are responsible for training partners working with the VIC to appropriately gather the information required for victim identification from the family interview process. The VIC team is also responsible for managing the missing persons list, updating the victim database, and – eventually – coordinating the release of remains.

An important component of matching an incident victim to a missing person's report is using DNA. Family reference samples and personal effects of the victim containing biological material may provide the only method by which processed victim remains can be identified. DNA specialists should be incorporated into or consulted on the VIC interview process to ensure proper DNA collection procedures, prevent cross contamination, and ensure that the best possible specimens are collected for subsequent testing.

Often, victim data will be compiled from multiple sources beyond just the MPCC data. Law enforcement reports, passenger manifests, and patient tracking information from hospitals and ERs will also be used to compile a victim information database. The compiled victim data associated with missing person's reports will then be matched with decedent information which will result in overall victim accounting (Figure 9.1). Victim accounting is the responsibility of the local jurisdiction in which the incident occurred.

9.4.1 Victim Information Program

As a component of efforts to match incident victims to collected missing person's reports, a Victim Information Program (VIP)

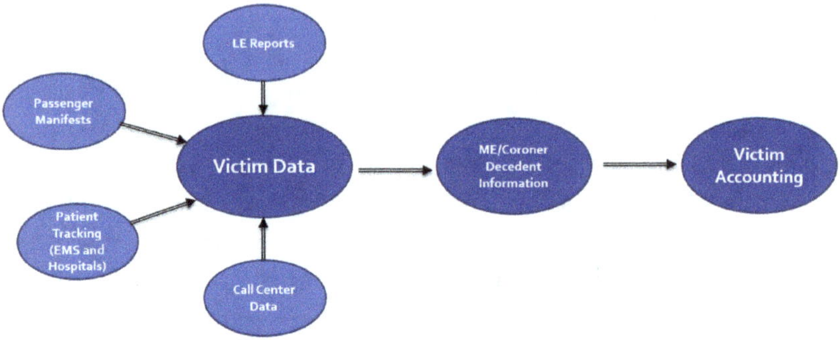

Figure 9.1 Victim accounting is accomplished by matching victim data – compiled from multiple sources – to decedent information.

database should be established. This helps to streamline the collection of data related to missing persons information and antemortem records with collected postmortem data from the incident victims. The antemortem menu component should contain information regarding missing persons such as the interview form as collected from the MPCC, including demographics of the missing individual, physical descriptions, medical history, clothing/jewelry/personal effects descriptions, family history, and any other relevant background information. Within the antemortem menu, there should be forensic reports that allow antemortem data to be searched by age, gender, height, weight, and other potentially identifying information such as fingerprints, dental records, or other medical information (Figure 9.2). General reports should also be included in the antemortem page to include general missing person lists, informant lists, funeral home lists, and other information. Finally, the antemortem menu should contain administrative reports including daily stats, positive identifications, family notifications, and others.

Likewise, the postmortem menu component should contain information regarding incident victims such as the postmortem exam forms, including victim site recovery, radiology, pathology, clothing/jewelry/personal effects inventory, fingerprint, DNA sample, and other relevant postmortem exam information (Figure 9.3). It should also contain both general and forensic reports including a victim list,

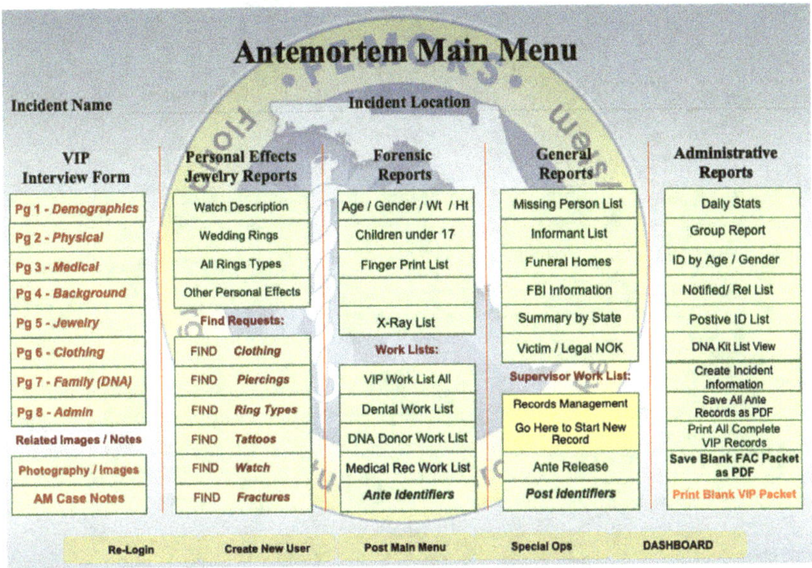

Figure 9.2 An example of the antemortem main menu of the victim information program database.

identification reports, morgue reports, tracking forms, remains management, and other case notes as appropriate.

9.5 Considerations for the Victim Information Center

9.5.1 Equipment and Personnel

When considering staffing, interviewers should be limited to personnel specially trained in dealing with grieving individuals such as funeral directors, medicolegal investigators, social workers, or law enforcement personnel. Technical specialists should also be available for the collection of physical evidence such as family reference and other antemortem DNA samples. The staff of the VIC should be easily and readily identifiable to be distinguished from other visitors.

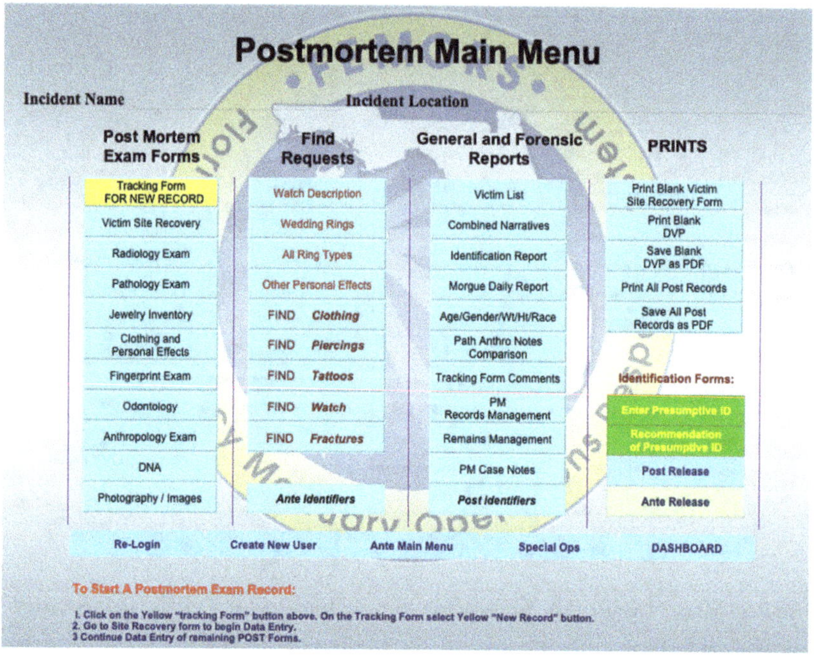

Figure 9.3 An example of the postmortem main menu of the victim information program database.

Likewise, family members should be issued badges in an unobtrusive manner to ensure they are appropriately distinguished from onlookers and media.

In some instances, the VIC may need to provide 24/7 assistance which would require additional staffing beyond the recommended minimums. Considerations should be made for special needs family and visitors as well as the possibility of providing child-care services. Medical treatment and general first aid should also be available on-site. Although numerous family members of victims will likely choose to travel to the incident location and to the VIC, many will not. Considerations must be made for the support of family members who choose not to, or are unable to, travel to the incident location such as the use of a "virtual" VIC. This would likely involve additional equipment, technology, and staffing needs and must be considered in the planning stages of establishing the VIC.

The FEMA has published guidelines for the minimum equipment needs to staff a VIC which include considerations for information technology (IT) equipment, personal protective equipment (PPE), and communication equipment. IT requirements include 26 laptop computers and software necessary to run the Victim Information Program Database, 19 scanners, 3 printers, and 19 bar code or QR readers for use in records tracking. PPE requirements include respirators, eye protection, gloves, and protective footwear – although it is important to consider that PPE requirements are incident-specific and may vary greatly based on the nature of the incident. Communication requirements include 14 short-range, two-way portable radios, 28 cell phones, and 1 satellite phone (FEMA 2018). As the VIC is meant to be scalable from the minimum operational team of 27 members to as large as the incident necessitates, all equipment considerations must be made on a case-by-case basis. Other general equipment needs may include basic office supplies, a reliable internet connection, equipment for making and issuing identification and credential badges, and televisions for local and national news feeds.

9.5.2 Function and Location

The Victim Information Center may be part of a Joint Family Assistance Center, a Reunification Center, or a Joint Family Support Operations Center (in the case of transportation incidents for the latter). Usually, the VIC is established under a unified incident command system (ICS). The designated facility management support organization should have experience and operating procedures for the establishment of a VIC, and the efforts of personnel at the VIC should be coordinated with the involved law enforcement agency/agencies' missing persons investigators. The VIC differs from a disaster services center in that its functions address the unique needs of family members of those who were injured and killed in the incident, rather than those who may have been affected or impacted by the incident but did not suffer an injury or fatality.

When choosing a location to establish and operate a VIC, consideration must be given to factors including incident proximity, privacy, security, functional space, and access. A good rule of thumb when allocating space is to plan on 10–15 family members at the VIC per incident victim. Functional areas must be considered to include family-only entrances and exists as well as staff-only entrances and exits. Check-in and check-out procedures should be established to ensure information confidentiality and overall security of the VIC by requiring identification and verifying credentials at these checkpoints. Other functional areas within the VIC may include: administrative offices, family briefing area, family interview area, family communication center, quiet rooms for reflection and counseling, child-care area, forensic specialist area, individual rooms for next-of-kin notifications, medical and first-aid area, food area, and transport staging. Because each of these areas must be discrete and separate from others, not all locations are readily suitable for use as a VIC but must be considered when choosing the location of the VIC.

9.5.3 Closing the Victim Information Center

Before making the determination to close the VIC, there are several essential points of consideration that must be evaluated. The most critical component to consider is the probability that all remains will be recovered, identified, and returned to their family members within a reasonable period of time. Once the initial surge of remains identification has been completed, the process may slow down dramatically, and the remaining identifications may take months or even years to complete. In such instances, it is not practical to continue operating the VIC indefinitely; rather, staff should communicate long-term plans to the family members and inform them of the plans to close the VIC and how they would still be able obtain information regarding the ongoing identification process. This should consider the geographic location of the surviving family members and should also include a method of obtaining contact information for the family members.

Box 9.2 Mass Fatality Management Resources

National Transportation Safety Board (NTSB)
National Disaster Medical System (NDMS)
Disaster Operational Response Teams (DMORT)
Disaster Portable Morgue Unit (DPMU)
Victim Information Center (VIC)
National Guard Fatality Search and Recovery Teams (FSRT)
Family Assistance Plan for Aviation Disasters

Box 9.3 General Disaster Resources

American Red Cross
Department of State
Department of Health and Human Services
Department of Justice Agencies
Federal Bureau of Investigation (FBI)
Department of Homeland Security
Federal Emergency Management Agency (FEMA)
Department of Defense

9.6 Available Resources

There are numerous federal and state resources available to assist in mass fatality management, specifically the establishment and operation of a Victim Information Center. Some of these more specialized resources, such as the National Disaster Medical System (NDMS), have infrastructure already in place to establish a VIC as needed. Others, such as the Family Assistance Plan for Aviation Disasters, assign airline and federal responsibilities and describe the parameters for each. (Box 9.2). Other available resources are more general in nature but still may be useful based on the specific situation (Box 9.3).

References

Carroll, E., Johnson, A., Depaolo, F., Adams, B.J., Mazone, D. and Sampson, B. (2017). Trends in United States mass fatality incidents and recommendations for medical examiners and coroners. *Academic Forensic Pathology* 7 (3): 318–329.

Federal Emergency Management Agency (2018). *Fatality management victim information center team. Resource typing definition for fatality management services – medical and public health* [online]. Available at: https://rtlt.preptoolkit.fema.gov/Public/Resource/View/12-508-1249?p=8 (Accessed 30 August 2020).

Mehrabian, A. (1981). *Silent Messages: Implicit Communication of Emotions and Attitudes*. Belmont, CA: Wadsworth Pub. Co.

Schroeder, K.B. (2002). Failing to prevent the tragedy, but facing the trauma: The Aviation Disaster Family Assistance Act of 1996 and the Air Transportation Safety and System Stabilization Act of 2001. *Journal of Air Law and Commerce* 67(1): 189–232.

CHAPTER 10

Ethical and Legal Considerations

Victor W. Weedn

George Washington University, Dept. of Forensic Sciences, Washington, D.C., USA
Office of the Maryland Chief Medical Examiner, Baltimore, MD, USA

10.1 Introduction

The specialty of disaster law is not widely studied, and there are few books on the subject [1–5]. These texts do not discuss mass fatality management or disaster victim identification as a topic area. No specific journal articles cover legal issues of DVI, but there is a chapter on the subject in one book [6].

10.2 State Authority for Fatality Management

The US Constitution is the supreme law of the United States of America. It represents a grant of power by the states to the union – the federal government. The Tenth Amendment declares that the federal government is limited to enumerated powers delegated to it and other residual powers are reserved to the states. Among the traditional powers left to the States are the so-called police powers (here a constitutional term and is not referring merely to local law enforcement), defined as the "power inherent in the state to prescribe within the limits of the federal and state constitutions reasonable regulations necessary to preserve the public order, health, safety, or morals" [7]. These police powers are quite broad and encompass public safety and public health, as well as fatality management and the disposition of

Disaster Victim Identification in the 21st Century: A US Perspective, First Edition.
Edited by John A Williams and Victor W Weedn.

remains. It can also be argued that the primacy of state and local disaster response is a legacy of policy arising at a time when the federal government was quite limited.

In the United States, medical examiner and coroner offices are legally responsible for the bodies and human remains falling under their jurisdiction by state statutes, and thus they have the primary responsibility for mass fatality management and disaster victim identification. There are approximately 2,000 county coroner systems in the United States and approximately 400 medical examiner systems headed by forensic pathologists and may be state-, regional-, county-, or city-based [8]. Most mass fatality incidents are not declared disasters and are thus governed only as other non-natural deaths by medical examiner and coroner legislation [9]. In general, small medical examiner and coroner offices are not well prepared for large mass fatality incidents [10].

State and local medicolegal death authorities are governed by state statutes [11]. Although coroners were inherited as part of the common law of England, both medical examiners and coroners are now universally authorized by and operate according to state statutes. These statutes vary widely and are often poorly written and in need of updating as they do not generally receive much attention in state legislatures [12,13].

While law enforcement is responsible for evidence at death scenes, the body is the province of the medical examiner or coroner – even though the body is itself considered to be evidence. This duality can be confusing; see *People v. Roehler*, 167 Cal.App.3d 353 (1985). Furthermore, law enforcement is in charge of missing persons, but medical examiners and coroners are responsible for unidentified remains – they are not missing; they are merely unidentified. Missing persons and identification missions impinge on each other, but they are distinct roles, even if sometimes confused.

State mortuary laws and health codes will regulate the disposition of remains [14]. In cases of *hazardous human remains*, some laws may require cremation or allow the public health authorities to commandeer the remains.

10.3 Federal Medicolegal Death Investigations

The only federal medical examiner office is the Armed Forces Medical Examiner System (AFMES), headquartered in Dover, DE [15]. The AFMES was established in 1988, but not statutorily authorized until 1999 [16]. The AFMES has jurisdiction over deaths of military members overseas according to Status of Forces Agreements and of deaths occurring on exclusive federal jurisdiction properties (10 USC. §1471) [17]. The military has an elaborate structure and sophisticated plans to deal with its own past and present war dead [18,19]. State and local medical examiners and coroners may waive jurisdiction and permit the AFMES to investigate deaths of military members and military bases without exclusive federal jurisdiction on a case-by-case basis. The AFMES may assist the Department of State, the NTSB, or the FBI, as well as state and local medicolegal death authorities when requested.

10.3.1 Assassination of the President or Other Federal Officials

When President John F. Kennedy (JFK) was assassinated in late 1963, it was not a federal crime to kill the president of the United States. This prompted Congress in 1965 to make it a federal crime to kill the president, president-elect, vice president, or other person in succession (18 USC. §1751) [20]. After JFK's brother, Senator Robert F. Kennedy (RFK) was assassinated in 1968, Congress in 1971 and several later amendments extended the federal reach to the deaths of congressional, cabinet, and Supreme Court justices, as well as major presidential and vice-presidential candidates (18 USC. §351) [21]. The legislation places the FBI in charge of the investigations. Although not explicitly stated, it is anticipated that the Armed Forces Medical Examiner will conduct the autopsy.

10.4 Legislatively Mandated Scientific Identification

On April 26, 2006, a university van carrying nine students and staff members collided with a tractor-trailer in Indiana [22]. Five people died at the crash scene, including a young blonde woman identified as

Whitney Cerak by the coroner. "Whitney" was interred in a marked grave at a funeral with 1,400 people in attendance. Meanwhile, a similar looking young blonde woman who survived the accident but was unable to communicate was identified as Laura van Ryn. For several weeks, the van Ryn family kept a bedside vigil over the patient they believed to be their daughter. Five weeks passed before suspicion about their identity arose. This incident prompted Indiana and Michigan to enact legislation requiring scientific identification of unknowns.

10.5 Missing Persons Acts and Presumptive Deaths

Most states allow for a legal declaration of death despite the absence of direct proof of the person's death – so-called *presumptive deaths*, whether by statute or by judicial recognition of the common law rule [23–25]. At common law, if a person is missing for seven years then the person may be presumed dead. At least eleven states have passed missing persons acts and sometimes reduce the time for the presumption to four or five years.

Missing persons statutes explicitly authorize law enforcement to collect certain personal information as well as prescribe certain data to be collected or steps to be taken during such investigations.

The National Institute of Justice sponsors the NamUS program that is useful for linking unidentified remains and missing persons at a national level [26]. Nine of the state missing persons acts require use of NamUS (NY, TN, IL, MI, OK, AR, WV, NM, NC) [27]. Billy's Law was introduced three times at the national level to mandate entry of missing persons and unidentified information, but ultimately failed to pass [28,29]. The laws range regarding timeframe for entry (e.g. immediately or 60 days) and whether there is a required entry of biometrics (DNA, dental and fingerprints) or not. A version, NamUS *for* Critical Incidents (NamUS-CI), has recently been launched specifically for use in mass fatality incidents [30].

Specific peril statutes will allow issuance of a death certificate based upon a presumption of death earlier than otherwise if the deceased is thought to have died from a certain circumstance [31]. Many of these statutes are temporary and specific to a given incident, such as Hurricane Katrina. An alternative to such statutes was used in response to the 9/11 World Trade Center mass fatality incident, where a declaratory judgment allowed the NYC medical examiner's office to conclude that a missing person had died in the 9/11 attacks [32]. An international perspective of presumption of death is discussed below.

10.6 Rights of the Dead

At common law, the rights of the deceased are extinguished at death; the primary exception is the testamentary power of individuals to allocate distribution of their estates after death in wills. However, increasingly rights have been given to individuals that persist after death [33]. Perhaps most significantly here, the Uniform Anatomical Gift Act (UAGA), initially promulgated in 1968 and revised since, creates the right of individuals to donate their organs, tissues, and body parts after death [34]. Some courts have enforced various stated desires of deceased individuals, but other courts have upheld different outcomes desired by the survivors [35].

10.7 Rights of Others in the Dead

Centuries ago, in England, judges determined that bodies, as the sacred remnants of living human beings, should not be thought of as *property* [36,37]. Families have a sepulchral right to dispose of the body, but they cannot own the body. The unintended consequence of families lacking a property interest in the bodies is that they could not sue grave robbers! England passed Anatomical Acts to give families the ability to bring lawsuits for the mutilation or abuse of corpses or other tortious disturbance of the dead. The *no property rule* was inherited into American jurisprudence, but instead of passing legislation, American judges determined that the bodies were *quasi-property* with sufficient property-like interests that families could sue [38].

Medical examiners and coroners must release bodies to the next-of-kin for disposition after completing their examination of the body, although they may retain tissues and specimens for their own purposes. Where the remains have not been identified, at least in the case of the World Trade Center disaster, courts have held that family claims to burial were untenable [39].

10.8 Constitutional Considerations in Responding to Disasters

The Constitution does not provide an explicit provision for federal assistance of states, localities, or individuals in times of need, but the enumerated powers do provide a basis for permitting federal disaster mitigation and response. Seemingly the most obvious reference would be the *Preamble* that declares that "We the People of the United States, in Order to form a more perfect Union, establish Justice, insure domestic Tranquility, provide for the common defense, promote the general Welfare, and secure the Blessings of Liberty," but the Preamble has never been given legal force [41]. The *General Welfare Clause* (Art. I, Sec. 8, Clause 1) gives Congress near-plenary power to tax and spend in support of the general welfare of the nation [41]. The Fourth Congress did not believe it had the authority to provide financial relief for Savannah's Great Fire of 1796, which destroyed two thirds of the city, because it would be for the special welfare of the city and not the general welfare of the nation's taxpayers [42,43]. Arguably more important is the *Commerce Clause* (Art. I, Sec. 8, Clause 3) that gives Congress the power to "regulate commerce with foreign nations, and among the several states, and with the Indian tribes" [44]. Both the General Welfare Clause 12 and the Commerce Clause have been expansively interpreted over the last century to allow near-unfettered congressional power to act. Furthermore, the *Necessary and Proper Clause* (Art. I, Sec. 8) grants Congress power to make laws necessary to effect the duties of the federal government and the Sec. 5 *Enforcement Power* of the Fourteenth Amendment grants Congress the power to enforce by appropriate legislation equal protection and due process of law [45].

Article II of the Constitution vests the president with "executive power" to "take Care that the Laws are be faithfully executed." The Stafford Act, discussed below, incorporates a massive congressional delegation of power to the president to commit federal resources immediately to respond to save lives and property.

10.9 Emergency Powers

Emergencies generally do not create exceptions to the law and thus disasters are addressed within the ordinary legal scheme; this is becoming even more true as planning and statutes evolve to anticipate disasters [46]. So-called emergency powers are suspect (*Youngstown Sheet & Tube Co. v Sawyer*, 343 US 579, 1959).

Whether or not the executive power of the president has an inherent authority in emergency situations to respond without congressional authorization or even over their legislated proscriptions is debated within legal scholarship. The arguments are usually cast in terms of wartime powers, but presumably would also apply to domestic crises [47–51].

So-called martial law has no specific meaning within the law, but generally refers to the use of the military actions taken during wars or emergencies [52,53]. Article I of the Constitution grants militia powers to the federal government which permits the federal government to federalize state militias (i.e., National Guard units) to respond to disasters – but this should not be construed as a state of martial law.

10.10 Stafford Act

The primary statutory scheme governing federal disaster relief in the United States is the Robert T. Stafford Disaster Relief and Emergency Assistance Act (Stafford Act), 42 USC. §§5121-5207 [54,55]. This scheme envisions the federal government to step in to assist state and local efforts when the incident is of sufficient magnitude and severity that it overwhelms state and local capacity to respond. Congress funds a Disaster Relief Fund (DRF) to pay for this [56,57], although the federal government may or may not demand repayment from the state. Short of federal assistance, states can also receive assistance from neighboring states through preexisting Emergency Management

Assistance Compacts (EMACs) – interstate mutual aid agreements overseen by FEMA.

The president may declare an *emergency* or *major disaster* at the request of a governor or on her own [58]. They are defined (§102) as:

(1) "Emergency" means any occasion or instance for which, in the determination of the President, Federal assistance is needed to supplement State and local efforts and capabilities to save lives and to protect property and public health and safety, or to lessen or avert the threat of a catastrophe in any part of the United States.

(2) "Major Disaster" means any natural catastrophe (including any hurricane, tornado, storm, high water, winddriven water, tidal wave, tsunami, earthquake, volcanic eruption, landslide, mudslide, snowstorm, or drought), or, regardless of cause, any fire, flood, or explosion, in any part of the United States, which in the determination of the President causes damage of sufficient severity and magnitude to warrant major disaster assistance under this Act to supplement efforts and available resources of States, local governments, and disaster relief organizations in alleviating the damage, loss, hardship, or suffering caused thereby.

If an incident does not constitute a major disaster, then the incident might qualify as an emergency, although the aid to states, localities, and individuals is more limited. The definitions of both "emergency" and "major disaster" include some "non-natural" events. "Emergency" is defined broadly in terms of the scope of the damage, rather than the cause, which may be "any occasion or instance." "Catastrophe" is not defined, but clearly encompasses both emergencies and major disasters. Historically, FEMA has interpreted biologic disasters as falling outside the Stafford Act, but the Homeland Security Counsel included influenza pandemic planning in declarations of emergency or major disasters. Congress has since unsuccessfully attempted to explicitly include infectious disease outbreaks in the statutory definition of major disaster.

Under this statutory regime, a state governor or Indian tribal chief may request a presidential declaration of a major disaster (§401) or an emergency (§501), which triggers financial, technical, and other assistance through the Federal Emergency Management Agency (FEMA). The request must be based upon a finding that the disaster is of such severity and magnitude that effective response is beyond the capabilities of the state and local governments and that federal assistance is necessary. The state must have executed its own emergency plan and expended its own resources. Furthermore, the state must agree to comply with the cost-sharing requirements of the Act.

The Preliminary Damage Assessment (PDA) process is a mechanism used to determine the impact and magnitude of damage and resulting needs of individuals, businesses, public sector, and community as a whole [59]. PDAs are posted to FEMA's website: https://www.fema.gov/preliminary-damage-assessment-reports. The PDA will be a basis for the governor's request and the president's response. After criticisms that the declaration process was too political in the wake of Superstorm Sandy, Congress directed FEMA to provide more objective criteria and give more consideration to the trauma suffered by the affected community. This resulted in the codification of factors considered to determine whether assistance is warranted in FEMA's regulations (44 CFR §206.48).

The president has ultimate discretion and decision-making authority to declare major disasters and emergencies under the Stafford Act. A denial of a request may be appealed for reconsideration. *Kansas v. United States,* 748 F. Supp. 797 (D. Kan., 1990) held that the presidential decision was not subject to judicial review.

Under Section 501(b) of the Stafford Act (42 USC. §5191(b)), the president may provide federal emergency assistance without a declaration, "when he determines that an emergency exists for which the primary responsibility for response rests with the United States because the emergency involves a subject area for which, under the Constitution or laws of the United States, the United States exercises exclusive or preeminent responsibility and authority." Although the section provides that the president should consult with the governor if practicable, the president may proceed without the governor's consent.

After Hurricane Katrina, Congress amended Section 402 (42 USC. §5170a(6)) to permit the president to provide "accelerated" federal assistance and support without a request, when necessary to save lives, prevent human suffering, or mitigate severe damage. This provision allows FEMA to lean forward and push to take proactive steps, rather than merely react in a traditional pull system.

Major disaster assistance may include: (1) response and recovery aid to states and localities, (2) hazard mitigation assistance, and (3) individual assistance. General federal assistance may include the directing of any federal agency with or without reimbursement, coordination of disaster relief assistance, and assistance in distributing resources. Essential assistance may include use of federal resources; medicine, food, or consumables; work and services, or contributions. Furthermore, the federal government may provide grants or community disaster loans.

The Act establishes penalties for misuse of funds and other violations of the Act and permits the Attorney General to bring a civil action for relief. Section 308 provides that disaster relief "shall be accomplished in an equitable and impartial manner, without discrimination on the grounds of race, color, religion, nationality, sex, age, disability, English proficiency, or economic status." Special populations, such as low-income, the elderly, or the unemployed, may indicate a greater need for assistance (44 C.F.R. §206.48(b)(3)). By law, federal disaster assistance cannot duplicate insurance coverage (42 USC. §5155 and 44 C.F.R. §206.48(b)(5)).

The Act provides protection from civil lawsuits for discretionary functions of federal employees. In *Freeman v. United States*, 556 F.3d 326 (5th Cir., 2009) the court held that discretionary decisions to provide Katrina survivors was statutorily immune from civil liability (FTCA 28 USC. §2680(a); Stafford Act Sec. 305, 42 USC. §5148). However, *Graham v. FEMA*, 149 F. Supp. 997 (9th Cir., 1998) and *McWaters v. FEMA*, 436 F. Supp. 2nd 802 (E.D. La., 2006) held the non-discretionary mandates could be a basis for civil liability.

Numerous other laws address specific areas of disaster response outside the Stafford Act, such as for flood insurance, earthquakes, and nuclear accidents.

10.11 Federal Executive Administration

The Homeland Security Council (HSC) is an entity within the White House and Chaired by the president. It is the counterpart to the National Security Council (NSC). The Homeland Security Advisor and the Secretary of Homeland Security are members along with other executive officials, agency heads, and military and intelligence leaders.

The Department of Homeland Security (DHS) is responsible for domestic public safety, similar to departments of interior and home ministries of other countries. Authorizing legislation explicitly includes anti-terrorism, border security, immigration and customs, cyber security, and disaster prevention and response. The department has an operating budget of approximately $50B and a quarter million employees, making it the third largest cabinet department – behind DOD and the VA.

The Federal Emergency Management Agency (FEMA) is an agency within DHS responsible for disaster prevention and response [60]. The budget is approximately $18 billion, much of which is redistributed to the states according to the relief needed. There are 10 FEMA regions. A National Response Coordination Center (NRCC) coordinates response efforts.

The National Response Frameworks (NRFs) guide the national response to declared disasters and emergencies; it outlines roles and responsibilities. There are national response frameworks for prevention, protection, mitigation, response, and recovery. The National Response Framework (NRF) [61] includes the National Incident Management System (NIMS) [62] which provides operational guidance. NIMS includes the Incident Command System (ICS) [63] as a structure for managing incident response. The NRF has 23 supporting annexes that include Emergency Support Function (ESF) annexes.

Within the ICS, the DVI/fatality management operations are typically a "branch" under the Operations Section. The NIMS ICS structure has traditionally placed mass fatality management as a branch of the Operations Section, but a 2017 NIMS update introduces an Intelligence/Investigations Function that would place mass fatality management under a forensic section in certain cases such as criminal, terrorist, or epidemic incidents [64].

Under ESF #8, the Department of Health and Human Services (HHS) has primary responsibility for coordinating the federal public health and medical assistance to supplement state, tribal, territorial, and local (STTL) disaster efforts [65]. These efforts include providing shelter for the displaced, medical rescue, patient movement, medical care of the injured, and disposition of human remains. Attention and resources for the living will always be prioritized above those of dead and accordingly DVI planning and resourcing have not been well supported.

The HHS Office of the Assistant Secretary for Preparedness and Response (ASPR) [66] is responsible for implementing this tasking. The National Disaster Medical System (NDMS) [67] is a federally coordinated program that augments local medical needs through dispatch of small teams, including the Disaster Medical Assistance Teams (DMATs), Trauma and Critical Care Teams, National Veterinary Response Team (NVRT), Disaster Mortuary Response Teams (DMORTs), and a Victim Information Center Team. DMORTs are the primary mechanism for assistance to medical examiner and coroner offices in mass fatality incidents [68].

10.12 State and Local Executive Administration

State, tribal, territorial, and local (STTL) governments have their own emergency management agencies that will take charge of the disaster/emergency operations. All STTLs have Emergency Operating Plans (EOPs) and Emergency Operations Centers (EOCs) or Emergency Operations Integrations Centers (EOICs) which support a Unified Command to respond to incidents.

The federal government established a Target Capabilities List (TCL) as guidance to STTL [69]. Fatality management is a Recover Mission Capability and is intended to be used by STTL to assist their own mass fatality planning efforts. State emergency managers may assess the mass fatality plans of medical examiners and coroners against this document.

10.13 Military Assistance

The military, as a significant source of manpower and resources, is often called upon for federal relief and participates in homeland security [70,71]. The Department of Defense (DOD) is a federal agency that the president may call upon in a declared major disaster to provide general federal assistance or essential assistance. Moreover, the Stafford Act singles out the DOD as the agency the president may call "in the immediate aftermath of an incident, which may ultimately qualify" as a major disaster or emergency, but before the declaration has been made. The DOD may, in advance of a declaration, be requested by a governor "for the purpose of performing on public and private lands any emergency work which is made necessary by the incident and which is essential for the preservation of life and property" for a period of up to ten days (Sec. 403; 42 USC. §5170b(c)).

In 1876, President Ulysses S. Grant sent federal troops to polling places in the Deep South to enforce the voting rights of Blacks, which resulted in the presidential election of the Republican Rutherford B. Hayes over Samuel Tilden by one electoral vote. In reaction to this, Congress in 1878 passed the Posse Comitatus Act (18 USC. § 1385) that prohibits the direct use of federal troops in law enforcement activities; *United States v. Red Feather*, 392 F. Supp 916 (D.S.D., 1975), *United States v Casper*, 541 F. 2nd 1275 (8th Cir., 1976) [72,73]. This prohibition does not apply to supplies, materiel, or equipment. It also does not apply to state National Guard troops unless they have been federalized (Title 10 status). The Act also does not apply where other laws have expressly authorized the use of federal troops, the most prominent of which is the Insurrection Act (10 USC. §§331-335), originally promulgated in 1807, that specifically permits use of the military to suppress lawlessness and restore public order [74].

During the 1906 San Francisco earthquake, Major General Adolphus Greely, Commander of the US Army's Pacific Division, unilaterally ordered 4,000 federal troops to patrol the streets, stop looting, fight fires, and protect buildings, including the US Mint, post office, and county jail. Mayor Schmitz issued a proclamation that the police and federal troops were authorized to shoot-to-kill persons engaged in looting other crimes. The mayor appointed Captain Edward Ord to be a Special Police Officer. Although most soldiers served the community well, some soldiers themselves engaged in looting. The army also sheltered, fed, and clothed tens of thousands of displaced residents. Soldiers commandeered civilians for work details. Civilian authorities assumed these responsibilities after a couple of months and the army withdrew from the city [75].

In 2005, after Hurricane Katrina, President Bush considered, but did not order, federal troops into New Orleans to stop looting, citing the Posse Comitatus Act. Congress in response to President Bush's request for greater authority to use the military in disaster responses passed legislation amending the act, but it was repealed the following year over objections of all 50 state governors for the ability of the president to federalize the National Guard without the consent of the affected governor [76].

The military expects and plans for civil-military integration through Defense Support of Civil Authorities (DSCA) in overwhelming disasters. The US Northern Command (USNORTHCOM), created in 2002, is responsible for homeland defense (HLD) and homeland security (HLS). USNORTHCOM supports states and locals in HLS disaster response and will not take the lead unless the event occurs on a military base [77]. The National Guard (NG) is also an important component of both HLS and HLD. NG units are state assets (Title 14 status), unless they are *federalized* (Title 10 status); thus they may be first responders on behalf of the Governor or serve later as part of the federal support. The Army National Guard (ARNG) maintains Weapons of Mass Destruction Civil Support Teams (WMD-CSTs). The Air National Guard (ANG) maintains Fatality Search and Recovery Teams (FSRTs) to assist recovery of bodies when requested.

10.14 Transportation Incidents

Congress consolidated all transportation agencies into the Department of Transportation (DOT) in 1967. Responsibility for investigations of domestic civil transportation incidents was given to the National Transportation Safety Board (NTSB). In 1974, the NTSB was made an independent agency, administratively supported by the DOT (49 USC. Chapter 11) [78]. The statutory scheme grants the NTSB the ability to order an autopsy performed, unless local law protects observance of religious beliefs and is consistent with the needs of the investigation (49 USC. §1134(f)) [79]. The Aviation Disaster Family Assistance Act of 1996 (49 USC. §1136) gives the NTSB the additional role of managing the federal response to aviation disaster victims and their families [80]. NTSB family assistance was extended to foreign air carriers in 1997 (49 USC. §41313) [81] and to railroad accidents in 2008 (49 USC. §1139) [82].

10.15 Terrorist Incidents

Through various statutes, presidential directives, and Attorney General Authorities, the FBI has jurisdiction to investigate terrorist incidents and can supersede state and local investigations. The FBI is the lead agency for crisis management, as opposed to consequence management, activities in assessing and responding to potential or credible threats of terrorism within the United States. The Terrorism Incident Law Enforcement and Investigation Annex establishes policy in FEMA's National Response Plan [83]. The Domestic Emergency Support Team (DEST) [84] is a rapid deployment team, staffed by the FBI, DOD, DOE, DHHS, EPA, and FEMA, to provide guidance to the FBI Special Agent in Charge (SAC) concerning weapons of mass destruction (WMD) actual incidents and threats. The FBI asserts its authority aggressively and specifically has asserted their authority over the bodies of victims, but it is unclear that its authority extends this far – as medical examiners and coroners claim jurisdiction over bodies despite law enforcement's authority over criminal investigations.

10.16 Infectious Epidemics

As a generality, response to bioterrorist and natural infectious disease outbreaks are a shared responsibility between emergency services and public health. This results in some confusion and less well-developed plans and responses. Privacy issues and government authority loom as large issues in public health law [85,86]. Furthermore, the role of medical examiner and coroners is often neglected, although deaths from natural disease may be seen as falling outside their jurisdictions.

There is a reluctance to invoke the Stafford act in response to infectious disease outbreaks [87]. The 2009 H1N1 influenza pandemic tested the system [88,89]. Nonetheless, the current COVID-19 pandemic has exposed problems with the existing system and may result in changes [90–94]. There is a call for greater federal leadership, rather than merely offering state assistance. Furthermore, it is not clear who is in charge – FEMA, ASPR, CDC, HHS Asst. Secretary for Health, the White House Task Force? Nonetheless, responsibilities are divided generally as follows:

- WH – overall coordination, funding, messaging
- FEMA – distribute supplies, release national stockpiles
- ASPR – ESF #8 responsibilities, informative resources for STTL [95]
- CDC – oversee laboratory testing, surveillance, oversee public health response
- FDA – emergency use authorizations for commercial PPE, tests, medications, and vaccines
- CMS – medical licensure waivers (allows healthcare workers to work where needed)
- EPA – decontamination
- OSHA – workplace safety

At the state level, public health emergencies may trigger significant empowerments of public health officials [96–98]. In 2001, legal experts at Georgetown and Johns Hopkins drafted the Model State Emergency Powers Health Act which addresses planning, surveillance, and responding to public health emergencies [99]. It grants mandatory quarantine powers. It limits liability to "gross negligence or willful misconduct." A more comprehensive Turning Point Model State Public Health Act (MSPHA) was drafted by a diverse group representing governments and public health agencies [100]. More than half of the states have adopted one or the other of these two model laws.

10.17 National Emergency Family Registry and Locator System/National Call Center

The Post-Katrina Emergency Management Reform Act of 2006 mandated the creation of a National Emergency Child Locator Center (6 USC. §774) and National Emergency Family Registry and Locator System (6 USC. §775) [101]. These capabilities were designed to assist reunification of families, but have not been activated in recent times.

The author discussed with DHS officials the possibility of the inclusion of deceased family members, but there was no interest in this. The National Forensic Science Commission has recommended the establishment of a National Call Center to be activated in times of need for families inquiring of their loved ones, but advocacy on this point has yet to be successful [102].

10.18 International Legal Considerations in DVI

The ease and extent of mobility today ensures that most mass fatality incidents will involve international victims. In a NTSB study of 16 aviation accidents from 1996 to 2009 involving 20 to 265 victims, there were 3 to 33 nationalities involved, with an average of 4 on US domestic flights and 12 on international flights.

10.18.1 The US Department of State

The US Department of State (DOS) has primary authority for repatriation of recovered remains of those dying or recovered in other countries. The DOS will also assist other countries repatriate the remains of their citizens who die within the United States.

Moreover, the DOS may assist the disaster response of other countries [103]. Embassies have Disaster Assistance Authority for immediate provision of small sums or supplies. The DOS US Agency for International Development (USAID) maintains an Office of Foreign Disaster Assistance (OFDA) [104] and an International Disaster Response Subcommittee [105]. OFDA may activate a Response Management Team (RMT) in Washington D.C. and deploy a Disaster Assistance Response Team (DART) or other emergency teams. The response will transition to other USAID offices for longer-term mitigation and prevention efforts, although OFDA supports disaster risk reduction efforts.

10.18.2 Nation-specific Laws

Disaster victim identification operations must function under the "rule of law" of the jurisdiction which controls the site where the remains are found, presumably also the site of the incident or action that resulted in the deaths. Interpol DVI Guidelines recognizes this when they state:

> Every DVI operation should be subject to the laws and rules of the country in which the disaster occurs. This premise is fundamental to ensuring that the legal framework in which the Lead Authority operates within is supported both legally and constitutionally.
>
> Furthermore, adherence to the laws of the nation where the DVI response occurs enables national, regional and local authorities to activate their rules and procedures in accordance with approved and agreed arrangements. A departure from this well established principle could not only undermine the legal processes operating in a particular region, but hinder the overall operation of the DVI process.
>
> Agreements regarding the integration of international DVI teams operating in foreign countries are therefore highly beneficial, as points of legal and procedural conflict can be resolved before teams are deployed. In order to progress such agreements, it is desirable for nominated representatives to develop protocols with their counterparts from other nations. [106]

Laws governing mass fatality management vary significantly between countries [107–112]. Generally, in the United States and commonwealth countries medicolegal death investigation is a function outside law enforcement, but for others it is a law enforcement function. Regardless, missing persons investigations is always a law enforcement function. The identification of unidentified human remains and DVI in particular may be a law enforcement function even where routine medicolegal death investigation are independent. Thus, other than the United States, DVI is generally a police operation. Outside of this broad categorization, the laws of individual nations vary substantially in their specifics. For instance, health regulations may require that remains be ruled not hazardous prior to transport across borders.

10.18.3 Obligation to Identify Victims

The notion of a right to be identified and the right of families to have the remains of their loved ones returned, imposing an obligation on states to identify remains and repatriate them, has been advanced [113] and is probably required under international humanitarian and human rights laws (see below). Regardless of any national or international legal mandate or not, countries will customarily recognize the needs of other countries to have the remains of their citizens recovered, identified, and repatriation through the legal notion of "comity," which is a legal notion of reciprocity – we will respectfully treat the remains of your citizens, if you respectfully treat the remains of our citizens. Moreover, as the capability to do so has improved, individual identification of remains is an increasing worldwide expectation of the public and the media, due to the increasing technological capability to do so. This expectation acts as a powerful moral imperative and motivation for governments to do so.

10.18.4 International Disaster Response Law

There is a growing area of International Disaster Response Law (IDRL), but there are as yet relatively few sources on the topic [114–117], although there are annual conferences on the subject [118] and a database maintained of global disasters [119]. There is no overarching international convention that governs disaster response [120], although the International Federation of Red Cross and Red Crescent's (IFRC) International Disaster Response Law (IDRL) Guidelines are highly influential [121]. Nor is there a single international standard definition of *disaster*. The IFRC's International Disaster Response Guidelines defines "disaster" as:

> serious disruption of the functioning of society, which poses a significant, widespread threat to human life, health, property or the environment, whether arising from accident, nature or human activity, whether developing suddenly or as a result of long-term processes, but excluding armed conflict. [122]

The United Nations International Strategy for Disaster Reduction (UNISDR) defines "disaster" as:

> serious disruption of a community or a society causing widespread human, material, economic or environmental losses which exceed the ability of the affected community or society to cope using its own resources. [123]

International human rights law and humanitarian law (IHRL and IHL described below), such as non-discrimination and respect for diversity, are the legal underpinning of IDRL. Of course, there is a political dimension to this as well [124].

The UN Inter-Agency Standing Committee (IASC) is the primary mechanism for coordination of international humanitarian assistance. The IASC is the longest-standing and highest-level humanitarian coordination forum of the UN system and is chaired by the Emergency Relief Coordinator (ERC) [125]. The IASC has promulgated operational guidelines [126] and field manual [127] for itself. These documents are based upon the Universal Declaration of Human Rights (UDHR) [128], and other relevant human rights instruments. While they are primarily devoted to the living survivors of disasters and armed conflicts, the operational guidelines do address fatalities (see Box 10.1).

10.18.5 International Treaties

Customs, norms, and comity (the doctrine of mutual respect) have traditionally dominated international law and was particularly shaped by diplomacy and maritime trade. However, it has increasingly been codified by international treaties. Furthermore, international organizations (IOs) have become important actors on the world stage.

The US Constitution gives international treaties supremacy over other laws (Art. VI), however, such treaties must be signed by the president and ratified by the Senate. The treaty clause (Art. II, Sec. 2, Clause 2) empowers the president to propose and negotiate treaties with other countries upon the advice and consent of a two-thirds supermajority of the Senate. The United States is a signatory to the Geneva Convention and the Universal Declaration of Human Rights, but many treaties have been left unsigned, unratified, or signed and then withdrawn.

As mentioned above, there is not yet a stand-alone international legally binding convention or treaty specifically governing disasters, but there is guidance and numerous international treaties that impinge on international aspects of fatality management.

Box 10.1 Key IASC Operational Guidelines

D.3.5 Appropriate measures should be taken to collect and identify the mortal remains of those deceased, to prevent their despoliation or mutilation, and to facilitate the return of the remains to the next of kin. If remains cannot be returned—for example, when the next of kin cannot be identified or contacted—they must be disposed of respectfully and in a manner which will help their future recovery and identification.

D.3.6 Cremation of unidentified bodies should be avoided. Instead, they should be stored or buried temporarily, pending future identification and return to families.

D.3.9 Family members should be fully informed about the location of gravesites, and have full access to them. They should be given the opportunity to erect memorials and conduct religious ceremonies as needed.

D.3.10 Family members should have the opportunity to recover the remains of their dead for further forensic investigations and to dispose of them according to their own religious and cultural beliefs and practices [129].and …

- Ensure that a comprehensive census or registration exercise is conducted to determine the number, age and gender of people who have died in the disaster.
- Ensure that the bodies are numbered and photographed and details of the deceased are identified or recorded before mass burials or other forms of disposal. In addition to photographs, personal effects and documents of the deceased, methods of forensic human identification are based on matching antemortem data (AMD) of the missing with post-mortem data (PMD) obtained from the remains (e.g. fingerprints, dental records, unique medical traits, general physical characteristics, DNA, etc.). Careful and adequate recovery of the remains and associated evidence will facilitate the identification process. If mass graves are used, commingling of bodies should be avoided and the position of each body within the grave should be noted, marked and mapped.

- Ensure that the proper collection and management of antemortem data (AMD) is incorporated into the identification process, since AMD of the missing is essential for identifying the dead.
- In the aftermath of a disaster, ensure that public statements are made to dispel unfounded beliefs that cadavers spread diseases in order to avoid the hasty disposal of the dead. Ensure that any official responsible for handling or disposing of the dead know and understand that cadavers should not be hastily buried for this reason [130].

10.18.6 International Humanitarian Law

International Humanitarian Law (IHL) pertains to the protection of life, health, and dignity during war and other armed conflicts. The first international legal guidance on victim identification was advanced in the 1949 Geneva Conventions and their Additional Protocols, which embody IHL [131,132]. The Geneva Conventions and Protocols are maintained by the World Medical Congress. The United States is a signatory and is bound by its provisions. The Geneva Conventions and its Additional Protocols specifically address the handling of the war dead. Unlike the IASC operational guidelines, these should be considered legal requirements. They require that the dead are searched for, collected, documented, identified, and disposed of in a dignified manner, ideally by returning the remains to bereaved families. Specifically, they declare that parties to armed conflict shall facilitate inquiries about individuals missing as a result of hostilities and search for the combatants and civilians who have been reported by the adverse party to be missing or dead; prevent the bodies from being despoiled; identify, if possible, the bodies of combatants, including a medical examination; gather identifying information and materials and convey them to an Information Bureau; facilitate correspondence with and the reunion of dispersed families; and honorably inter the combatant dead and otherwise honor family rights, religious convictions and practices, and manners and customs without prejudice of

Table 10.1 Provisions of the Geneva Conventions and Additional Protocols referring to the War Dead [133].

GC III, Art. 17(3) requirement for military ID card
GC I, Art. 15(1); GC II, Art. 18(1); GC IV, Art. 16(2); CIHL, Rule 112 requirement to search and evacuate dead bodies
AP I, Art. 33(4) search recovery teams must be protected
GC I, Art. 16; GC II, Art. 19; AP I, Art. 33(2); CIHL, Rule 116 Requirement to collect identifying information
GC I, Art. 16(2) and GC II, Art. 19(2) information exchange through National Information Bureau of ICRC' Central Tracing Agency
GC I, Art. 16(3); GC II, Art. 19(3); GC IV, Art. 129; CIHL, Rule 114 must forward personal property of deceased
GC I, Art. 15; GC II, Art. 18; GC IV, Art. 16; AP I, Art. 34(1); CIHL, Rule 113 requirement that remains are respected and not mutilated
GC I, Art. 17; GC II, Art. 20; GC III, Art. 120(3)-(5); GC IV, Art. 130(1) and (2); CIHL, Rule 115 remains may not be cremated except for hygiene or religious reasons
GC I, Art. 17; GC III, Art. 120(6); GC IV, Art. 130(3); AP I, Art. 34(1); CIHL, Rule 116 belligerents must establish a graves registration service
AP I, Art. 34(2)(c); CIHL, Rule 114 states must facilitate repatriation
AP I, Art. 34(2)(a) must conclude agreements for access to graves by families and graves registration personnel
440 AP I, Art. 34(3) must maintain graves of adversaries
441 AP I, Art. 34(4) exhumations not allowed except for repatriation and home country must be notified

health, age, status, race, religion, or political conviction. However, these IHL provisions provide no legal guarantees for families, but instead simply stipulate obligations of the parties to a conflict toward each other (see Table 10.1).

10.18.7 International Human Rights Law

International Human Rights Law (IHRL), which is distinct from complementary to IHL, is concerned with the protection of life, health, and dignity at all times – both war and peace; it encompasses modern conceptions of universal rights. IHRL does not explicitly call for victim identification, but its positive entitlements may be construed to imply such, particularly in regard to enforced disappeared and other human abuses [134,135]. Such human rights include the right to recognition everywhere as a person before the law, right to justice, and the right to truth. The most prominent IHRL, but not universally adopted, is embodied in the International Bill of Human Rights [136]. The United Nations Human Rights Council (UNHRC) has stated that the international community must "endeavor to recognize the right of victims of gross violations of human rights, and their families, and society as a whole to know the truth to the fullest extent practicable" [137]. The European Court of Human Rights (ECtHR) has ruled that a state's failure to conduct an effective investigation into a missing persons case constitutes a violation of the state's procedural obligation to protect the right to life under Article 2 and a violation of the rights of families of the missing under Article 3 (the prohibition of torture); an effective investigation must be official, transparent, independent, impartial, and capable of establishing the circumstances of the case to meet the human rights standard [138].

10.18.8 Missing and Disappeared Treaties

Beyond the fundamental IHL and IHRL treaties, there is a network of treaties and conventions among many countries that creates obligations of countries to assist death investigations of the disappeared and missing. These include: the International Convention for the Protection of All Persons from Enforced Disappearance [139] approved by the UN General Assembly in 2006; the Inter-American Convention on Forced Disappearance of Persons [140]; and the Declaration on the Role of the State in Addressing the Issue of Persons Missing as a consequence of Armed Conflict and Human Rights Abuses [141].

10.18.9 International Resources

Interpol: The International Criminal Police Organization (Interpol) is an intergovernmental agency formed to facilitate information sharing by law enforcement agencies across borders [142]. Membership includes 190 countries. It does not function as a law enforcement agency with its own police force, but instead is a networking intermediary to facilitate law enforcement and security officials to make contact and exchange information. Interpol maintains databases of fingerprints and DNA profiles that are useful to DVI operations which can be accessed through specified agents within National Central Bureaus of each of the member countries. When requested by a member state, Interpol will coordinate or otherwise assist victim identification efforts from natural disasters and terror attacks. Interpol may send Incident Response Teams (IRTs) from member nations that function similarly to DMORT teams. Interpol has a DVI subcommittee that oversees the Disaster Victim Identification Guide [143] and DVI software (DVI System International from Denmark-based Plass Data) [144].

International Commission on Missing Persons: The International Commission on Missing Persons (ICMP) was originally formed at the behest of President Clinton to perform identifications of victims of the former Yugoslavian conflicts [145]. It developed a significant DNA identification capability. It is now a treaty-based international organization recognized by the UN, headquartered in The Hague, the Netherlands, that addresses missing persons and performs disaster victim identification on a global basis.

International Red Cross, International Federation for Red Cross and Red Crescent Societies: The International Red Cross (ICRC) and the International Federation for Red Cross and Red Crescent Societies (IFRC) are global humanitarian organizations that coordinate, direct, and provide international assistance following natural and man-made disasters in non-conflict situations [146]. The IFRC has published Guidelines for the Domestic Facilitation and Regulation of International Disaster Relief and Initial Recovery Assistance [147].

United Nations Office for the Coordination of Humanitarian Affairs: The United Nations Office for the Coordination of Humanitarian Affairs (OCHA) was established by the United Nations General Assembly Resolutions 46/182 of 1991, calling for the strengthening of the coordination of humanitarian and disaster relief assistance [148]. OCHA has a Central Emergency Relief Fund

(CERF) which it has used to disburse billions of dollars in emergencies and crises from natural disasters and violent conflicts.

Pan American Health Organization and World Health Organization: The Pan American Health Organization (PAHO) and the World Health Organization (WHO) are active in mass casualty management efforts [149]. Among other things, they have published guidelines on mass fatality management [150].

Association of Southeast Asian Nations (ASEAN): The Association of Southeast Asian Nations (ASEAN) is a regional coalition that has published an Agreement on Disaster Management and Emergency Response [151].

10.18.10 Aviation and Maritime Deaths

Jurisdiction is generally determined by where a death occurs; however, when a death occurs in international waters or international air space, then the jurisdiction is determined by the final port-of-call or destination airport. Warships are an exception, in that they, like embassies, they are considered sovereign territory of their home country. In cases of deaths at sea (international waters), a medicolegal death investigation authority should assert their jurisdiction if there is a suspicion of foul play, investigate the death, and issue a death certificate. However, if the death is not suspicious, then prior to the *disembarkment* of the body, perhaps after a brief scene investigation and on-board body inspection, the office may wish to decline jurisdiction to avoid the family having to bear the enormous expense of repatriating the body. As a practical matter, medicolegal death investigation authorities might list the place and time of death corresponding to the disembarkment to avoid jurisdictional disputes.

Maritime incidents are governed by the Convention on Facilitation of International Maritime Traffic maintained by the International Maritime Organization (IMO) [152].

Aviation incidents are governed by the Convention on International Civil Aviation (Chicago Convention), which was originally signed in 1944 [153]. Annex 9 pertains to the facilitation of landside formalities for clearance of aircraft and passengers, goods and mail, with respect to the requirements of customs, immigration, public health and agriculture authorities [154]. Annex 13 pertains to aircraft accident and incident investigation [155]. Section 5.1 declares: "The State of Occurrence shall institute an investigation into the circumstances of the accident,... shall use every means to facilitate the investigation." Sections 5.2 and 5.3 describe circumstances where the site is in a non-signatory, and Section 5.18 *et. seq.* describes participation by others. Section 5.9 specifically describes autopsy examinations:

> The State conducting the investigation into a fatal accident shall arrange for complete examination of fatally injured flight crew and, subject to the particular circumstances, of fatally injured passengers and cabin attendants, by a pathologist, preferably experienced in accident investigation. These examinations shall be expeditious and complete. Note.—Guidance material related to autopsies is provided in detail in the Manual of Civil Aviation Medicine (Doc8984) and the Manual of Aircraft Accident Investigation (Doc 6920), the former containing detailed guidance on toxicological testing.

The National Transportation Safety Board (NTSB) will investigate overseas incidents involving US-registered marine vessels and aircraft, in collaboration with local investigative authorities, especially when there is significant loss of American lives, or when the involved ship or aircraft is American-built.

10.18.11 Presumed Deaths

Missing persons, presumed to be dead, is a significant issue to the international community [156–158]. An international mechanism for issuing presumed death certificates when a person was missing but death was certain was agreed to at the Athens Convention in 1966. The 2004 Indian Ocean tsunami agreement exposed two main flaws in the Athens Convention: (1) it was primarily concerned with maritime and flight mishaps, and (2) it spoke only to instances of certain deaths. The European Council adopted the *Recommendations on Principles Concerning Missing Persons and the Presumption of Death* on December 9, 2009, which allow for an immediate declaration of death when death is certain, a one-year waiting period when death is probable, and a five-year waiting period when death is uncertain [159].

10.18.12 Customs

Moving bodies through customs and immigration is governed by The International Convention on the Simplification and Harmonization of Customs Procedures (Kyoto Convention) (1974; revised 1999) [160].

10.18.13 Telecommunications

Telecommunications during a disaster response is governed by The Tampere Convention on the Provision of Telecommunication Resources for Disaster Mitigation and Relief Operations (1998) [161].

10.18.14 International Framework for Risk Reduction

Confronted with a constant stream of global disasters, the international community has sought measures to mitigate and prevent the impact of those disasters. Efforts produced the Yokohama Strategy for a Safer World: Guidelines for Natural Disaster Prevention, Preparedness, and Mitigation and its Plan of Action in 1994 and the Paris Declaration, Conclusions and Recommendations of the Conference on Natural Disasters Prevention, Land-Use Planning and Sustainable Development in 1999. In January of 2005, the World Conference on Disaster Reduction met in Kobe, Japan, by coincidence days after a tsunami killed more than 225,000 in 11 countries. All members of the United Nations agreed to reduce disaster loss by strengthening the resilience of nations and communities at risk. One result was a plan to establish an international early warning system to identify storms and tsunamis to allow for evacuations as possible. Moreover, 168 countries adopted The Hyogo Framework for Action (HFA), named after the prefecture in which Kobe resides, a 10-year plan to make the world a safer place from natural hazards through risk reduction and disaster mitigation [162]. It sought to substantially lower the loss of lives, economic damages, and environmental impact. The HFA expired in 2015 and was succeeded by the 15-year Sendai Framework for Disaster Risk Reduction [163]. The four priorities of the plan are: (1) understanding the risk, (2) strengthening disaster governance, (3) investing in disaster reduction for resilience, and (4) enhancing disaster preparedness. The UN Office for Disaster Risk Reduction (UNDRR) is the UN agency charged with overseeing the implementation of the Framework [164]. The associated Global Facility for Disaster Reduction and

Recovery (GFDRR) is an entity of the World Bank that provides a grant funding mechanism [165]. Mass fatality management is not discussed.

10.19 Ethical Considerations in DVI

"Show me the manner in which a nation cares for its dead, and I will measure with mathematical exactness, the tender mercies of its people, their loyalty to high ideals, and their regard for the laws of the land."

Attributed to William Gladstone, Prime Minister of England (1868–1874) [166]

There are few sources on the ethics of mass fatality management. There are several books on ethics and disasters [167–171] and on ethics and anthropology [171,172], but they are generally focused on other issues. Occasional articles touch on the subject of fatality management and DVI [174,175], but a report of a conference on the subject at the Carnegie Mellon University speaks squarely to the ethics of DVI operations [176].

Ethical obligations extend beyond legal obligations. In fact, legal duties traditionally cease upon death.

Modern concern regarding the ethics of research involving human subjects developed as the result of the Nazi regime's atrocities during World War II. Then in response to public outcry over a series of domestic public health studies, Congress passed the 1974 National Research Act which created a National Commission for the Protection of Human Subjects of Biomedical and Behavioral Research. The National Commission published its report, Ethical Principles and Guidelines for the Protection of Human Subjects of Research (commonly referred to as the *Belmont Report*) in 1979 [177]. The Belmont Report remains the foundation for ethical considerations of the US Department of Health and Human Services. It concluded that the basic ethical principles to guide behaviors are respect for persons, beneficence, and justice. Later, Beauchamp and Childress in the leading textbook on biomedical ethics declared there are four basic principles: autonomy, beneficence, non-maleficence, and justice [178].

The World Medical Association (WMA) promulgated a Statement on Medical Ethics in the Event of Disasters in 2017 [179]. However, this statement refers exclusively to the clinical medical response. Its recommendations include that physicians be trained in disaster medicine, that triage of patients be appropriate and the safety of physicians and other responders be recognized as essential. In the aftermath of a disaster, the needs of survivors and families should be considered and treated with dignity, and their customs, rites, and religions are respected. The four principles of humanitarian action include humanity, impartiality, neutrality, and independence have been applied to disaster response, but again with the living in mind [180].

The overarching ethical principle for mass fatality management and disaster victim identification operations is *respect for persons*. This universal ethical principle applies to all aspects of DVI operations and should be built into the planning documents for such.

Respect for persons embodies the Golden Rule – that we should treat others as we would want others to treat us. Here we recognize that this principle extends into death. The principle also incorporates the ethical notions of human dignity and autonomy:

- *Human Dignity* incorporates a reverence for the sanctity of life and the understanding that every human being has an innate and inalienable right to be valued and treated equally as a human person.
- *Autonomy* is the notion that individuals have a fundamental natural right to self-determinism, particularly as it relates to their own body, and therefore governments do not have the moral authority to intrude on the personhood and body without specific and proportional cause. Every person should be treated as an autonomous individual who has desires, make choices, and hold beliefs while living their life that should not be dismissed, disregarded, or denigrated, but rather should be respected and heeded as possible and appropriate.

In a 2011 report summarizing a conference at Carnegie Mellon University on the ethics of the recovery and identification of disaster victims, the authors wrote:

> All people have a special moral worth, or dignity, that comes from each individual's equal value as a human being. Because of their moral worth, there is a duty to respect the dignity of all living individuals. This duty commands a minimum standard of consideration for survivors of natural disasters. ... Unlike the living, the dead have only one element of individuality: identity. Having an identity gives the dead an enduring individuality. [181]

It is instructive that the 2016 WHO DVI Manual declares that the first two of the five responses for managing the dead in a disaster are: (1) consideration for the dignity of the dead and (2) respect for the bereaved [182].

10.19.1 Community Resilience

The Carnegie Mellon report makes clear that respect for the dead during DVI operations is important to the living and ultimately the resilience of the community:

> When a survivor is uncertain as to the fate of a loved one, his suffering can be exceptionally debilitating. However, relief efforts can help alleviate the misery of the living and ease further anguish. The wrongful treatment of remains affects the dignity of the living by prolonging their suffering, depriving them of the opportunity to acknowledge and mourn their losses, and limiting their abilities to envision the future. If societies meet the minimum standards of treatment of the dead, the surviving communities will have a better chance to rebuild their lives after the disaster. [183]

Human remains deserve respect and should be treated with dignity at all times precisely due to the fact that human remains are the residual posthumous manifestations of the living person and because the needs and welfare of families and loved ones can be deeply affected by the way they are treated. Thus, laws in the United States and elsewhere recognize the right of the dead to be free from abuse and desecration and to rest undisturbed and unmolested.

Furthermore, DVI provides closure from ambiguous loss for families and the community. Successful DVI efforts when done well enhance trust in government. It is a crucial aspect of community resilience.

10.19.2 Equal Treatment

Human remains should be treated equally as all humans are equally entitled to respect and dignity. Favoritism for certain nationalities or the wealthy or politically connected should not be condoned. The objectives of DVI operations should focus on the identification of the dead and return of remains to families and loved ones and should not succumb to political interests.

10.19.3 Respectful Treatment of the Remains

The DVI operations, including the practices and resources utilized, should demonstrate proper dignity and respect, i.e., trampling upon remains at recovery scenes should be avoided. Bodies and remains should also be secured from public view and white sheets placed over the remains. Additionally, visible markings relating to the operations should be appropriate (i.e., refrigerated storage vans should not display advertising on their sides, or they should be covered).

10.19.4 Respect for the Beliefs of the Deceased

Respect for the persons includes respect for their autonomy, personal decisions, and choice of lifestyle. Religious beliefs and cultural norms of the deceased are bound up in the appropriate dignity and respect accorded to the remains. Race, ethnicity, ancestry, and sexual orientation are components of the identity of the deceased. These various considerations may dictate practices that should be determined in consultation with families and community leaders.

10.19.5 Respect for Loved Ones

Respecting the families and friends of the deceased victims is a particularly important aspect of respecting the dead. Engagement of the families and friends for antemortem information and DNA specimens will be important to the DVI operation, as well as for the disposition of the remains and funerary arrangements. This engagement is voluntary and thus good relations with the families and friends of the deceased victims are not only a moral imperative but also a practical need. Their religious customs and beliefs should be honored to the extent possible.

In New Zealand, where the Maori believe that the spirit of the deceased is not released until burial and thus should be treated as alive, forensic pathologists might introduce themselves or even ask permission to perform the autopsy of the dead body before proceeding.

However, sometimes the customs and beliefs of the deceased and their loved ones are in conflict with DVI operations. For example, religious objections to autopsy might arise. An autopsy might be performed before someone is identified and found to be associated with a family of a certain faith. Where there is putative knowledge of identity, then discussions with the family would seem appropriate and may overcome the objection. The DVI team would have to balance the need to perform an autopsy to achieve their objectives against the interests of the objecting parties, before proceeding over family objections.

10.19.6 Respectful Communications

Communications should be appropriate, respectful, reverent, and truthful, both in personal communications and in public announcements. This is true for public discussions as well as with family members and loved ones. Effective and honest communication of information should be provided to permit families to make informed decisions regarding their participation in the DVI process, including information on expectations of outcome. Publication of the names of the deceased should not precede notification of families, to the extent possible. Genetic and medical information should be kept confidential.

There is a tension between the public's right to know and the privacy of families. Publication of the list of the dead at the close of the DVI operations may satisfy the public need.

The Navaho and Apache of the Southwest United States and the aborigines of Australia have belief systems in which speaking the name of the dead is forbidden and must be considered as these cases arise.

10.19.7 Haitian Example [184–186]

The 7.0-magnitude earthquake that struck Haiti on January 12, 2010, collapsed 100,000 structures, killed more than 316,000 people, injured 300,000 others, and displaced more than 1 million people. The Haitian government was virtually decapitated and the surviving government officials made an urgent request for US assistance. President Barack Obama directed a "whole-of-government" response led by the US

Agency for International Development (USAID) Office of US Foreign Disaster Assistance (OFDA) with significant support from the US Department of Defense (DoD) through US Southern Command (SOUTHCOM). OFDA deployed a Disaster Assistance Response Team (DART) to Haiti within 24 hours. Within two days, SOUTHCOM established Joint Task Force–Haiti (JTF-Haiti) to provide US military support to the international response and relief effort through Operation Unified Response, primarily composed of US Army forces. Operation Unified Response rendered the stricken nation humanitarian assistance (HA) and disaster relief (DR) until June 1, 2010, when JTF-Haiti stood down and all remaining US forces were withdrawn except for a small coordination cell.

The US Department of State demanded the return of the "American" bodies. Of course, the Haitians consider themselves "Americans" as well. Moreover, the determination of which bodies were US citizens would have to await DVI operations. Many Haitian bodies were piled into dump trucks and bulldozed into mass graves, making surviving families feel frustrated and resentful toward the recovery teams. Reacting to the Haitian government's inefficiency, the United States, the UN, other international actors, and NGOs stepped in. However, the foreign DVI teams tended to privilege their own nationals over Haitian victims in their relief efforts. By tossing Haitian bodies aside in the search for remains, the DVI teams did not respect universal equal human value but instead placed a higher value on their own nationals. The lack of cooperation among aid groups resulted from the disorganization and chaos of the disaster and exacerbated an already ineffective treatment of the living and dead.

10.20 Conclusion

The United States, as well as other countries, has established policies and infrastructure to respond to disasters, but less so for DVI operations – this is not surprising given a priority of the living over the dead. The need for DVI is recognized universally and is considered a human right. The ethical and legal concerns specific to DVI *per se* centers on the notion of respect for persons.

References

1. Farber, D.A., Chen, J.M., Verchick, R.R.M., and Sun, L.G. (2015). *Disaster Law and Policy*, 3rd ed. 574. NY, NY: Wolters Kluwer. pages; ISBN-13: 978-1454869252.
2. Hunter, N.D. (2018). *The Law of Emergencies: Public Health and Disaster Management*, 2nd ed. 434. Butterworth-Heinermann, Oxford, UK: pages; ISBN-13: 978-0128042755.
3. (2014). *The International Law of Disaster Relief* (ed. by D.D. Caron, M.J. Kelly and A. Telesetsky), 412. NY, NY: Cambridge Univ Press. pages; ISBN-13: 978-1107061316.
4. (2017). *Law and the Management of Disasters: The Challenge of Resilience* (ed. by A. Herwig and M. Simoncini), 292. NY, NY: Routledge. pages; ISBN-13: 978-1138193529.
5. Miller, R.A. (2009). *Law in Crisis: The Ecstatic Subject of Natural Disaster*. 247. Redwood City, CA: Stanford Law Books. pages. ISBN-13: 978-0804762564.
6. Greenberger, M., Henson, T., Kates, S., and Major, A. (2012). Chapt. 9. Legal issues in mass fatality events. In: *Death in Large Numbers: The Science, Policy, and Management of Mass Fatality Events* (ed. by E.A. Gursky and M.F. Fierro), 491. Chicago, IL: American Medical Association. pages; ISBN-13: 978-1603596299.
7. *Tighe v. Osborne*, 131 A. 801, 803 (MD Ct of App, 1925).
8. Medical Examiners and Coroners' Offices, 2004, Bureau of Justice Statistics, NCJ 216756. (2007). https://www.bjs.gov/content/pub/pdf/meco04.pdf.
9. Carroll, E., Johnson, A., DePaolo, F., Adams, B.J., Mazone, D., and Sampson, B. (2017). Trends in United States mass fatality incidents and recommendations for medical examiners and coroners. *Acad For Path* 7 (3): 318–329. 10.23907/2017.029.
10. Gershon, R.R.M., Orr, M.G., Zhi, Q., Merrill, J.A., Chen, D.Y., Riley, H.E.M., and Sherman, M.F. (2014). Mass fatality preparedness among medical examiners/coroners in the United States: A cross-sectional study. *BMC Public Health* 14 (1275): 1–15. http://www.biomedcentral.com/1471-2458/14/1275.
11. Coroner/Medical Examiner Laws, by State, CDC Public Health Law website; https://www.cdc.gov/phlp/publications/topic/coroner.html.
12. National Commission on Forensic Science, Model Legislation For Medicolegal Death Investigation Systems (Jan 9, 2017). DOJ archive; https://www.justice.gov/archives/ncfs/page/file/934406/download.
13. Weedn, V.W. (2015). Model medical examiner legislation. *Acad For Path* 5 (4): 614–627. 10.23907/2015.065.
14. Gilligan, T.S. and Steve, T.F.H. *Mortuary Law*, 10th ed. 132. Cincinnati, OH: Cincinnati Foundation for Mortuary Education. pages; ISBN-13: 978-1883031022.

15. Armed Forces Medical Examiner System, military health system website; https://health.mil/afmes.
16. Weedn, V.W. (2020). Origins of the Armed Forces Medical Examiner System. *Acad For Path* DOI.
17. 10 U.S.C. Section §1471 Forensic Pathology Investigations (from Cornell Legal Information Institute); http://www.law.cornell.edu/uscode/text/10/1471.
18. Mortuary Affairs, Joint Publication 4-06, DOD. (Oct 12, 2011). https://fas.org/irp/doddir/dod/jp4_06.pdf.
19. The Capstone Document Mass Fatality Management for Incidents Involving Weapons of Mass Destruction, US ARDEC (2005). https://www.hsdl.org/?abstract&did=460809.
20. 18 U.S. Code §1751, Presidential and Presidential staff assassination, kidnapping, and assault; penalties, Legal Information Institute, Cornell Law School https://www.law.cornell.edu/uscode/text/18/1751.
21. 18 U.S. Code §351, Congressional, Cabinet, and Supreme Court assassination, kidnapping, and assault; penalties, Legal Information Institute, Cornell Law School https://www.law.cornell.edu/uscode/text/18/351.
22. Van Ryn, D., Van Ryn, S., Colleen, N., and Cerak, W. (2009). *Mistaken Identification: Two Families, One Survivor, Unwavering Hope*. 278. NY, NY: Howard Books. pages; ISBN-13: 978-1439153550.
23. Cornelius, N. (Mar 28, 2019). Life insurance claims for a missing persons. *Quotacy*, https://www.quotacy.com/life-insurance-claims-for-a-missing-person.
24. Carriere, J.L. (1990). The rights of the living dead: Absent persons in the civil law. *La L Rev* 50: 901–972.
25. Sentell, C.E. (2004). The missing insured and the life insurance death claim. *FDCC Quart* 54 (2): 197–210. https://search.proquest.com/docview/201095367?pq-origsite=gscholar&fromopenview=true.
26. NamUs website; https://www.namus.gov.
27. Billy's Law, H.R. 3695 (111th): Billy's Law (2010). https://www.govtrack.us/congress/bills/111/hr3695/summary.
28. Casolino, P. (Oct 5, 2015). *Bill Inspired by Billy Smolinski to Aid Families of Missing Sees New Hope*. New Haven Register. https://www.nhregister.com/connecticut/article/Bill-inspired-by-Billy-Smolinski-to-aid-families-11349919.php.
29. Illinois Missing Persons Identification Act 50 ILCS 722/1. https://www.ilga.gov/legislation/ilcs/ilcs3.asp?ActID=2911&ChapterID=11.
30. NamUs for Critical Incidents, YouTube (Dec 10, 2019). https://www.youtube.com/watch?v=IfuSCK8szBU.
31. Henson, T. (2012). Before next time: The continued evolution of statutory responses to mass fatalities. *The Journal of Contemporary Health*

Law and Policy 29: 7–35. https://heinonline.org/HOL/Page?collection=journals&handle=hein.journals/jchlp29&id=41&men_tab=srchresults.

32. Gill, J.R. (2006). 9/11 and the New York City office of the chief medical examiner. *Forensic Science, Medicine, and Pathology* 2 (1): 29–32. https://link.springer.com/article/10.1385/FSMP:2:1:29.

33. Madoff, R.D. (2011). *Immortality and the Law: The Rising Power of the American Dead*. 191. New Haven, CT: Yale Univ Press. pages; ISBN-13: 978-0300171402.

34. Verheijde, J.L., Rady, M.Y., and McGregor, J.L. The United States Revised Uniform Anatomical Gift Act (2006) (2007). New challenges to balancing patient rights and physician responsibilities. *Philosophy, Ethics, and Humanities in Medicine* 2 (19): 1–8. 10.1186/1747-5341-2-19.

35. Cantor, N.L. (2011). *After We Die: The Life and Times of the Human Cadaver*. 284. Washington, DC: Georgetown Univ Press. pages; ISBN-13: 978-1589016958.

36. Kuzenski, W.F. (1924). Property in dead bodies. *Marq L Rev* 9 (1): 17–24. https://scholarship.law.marquette.edu/cgi/viewcontent.cgi?article=4512&context=mulr.

37. *Boorman v. Nevada Memorial Cremation Society*, 236 P.3d 4 (Nev. 2010).

38. Marsh, T. (2015). *The Law of Human Remains*. 528. Tucson, AZ: Lawyers & Judges Pub. pages; ISBN-13: 978-1936360291.

39. *World Trade Center for Proper Burial, Inc. v. City of New York*, 567 F.Supp.2d 529 (2d Cir. N.Y. 2009); 359 Fed.Appx. 177 (2nd Cir. 2009); 583 F.3d 785 (cert. denied).

40. Chemerinsky E, Paulsen MS, The Preamble, Interactive Constitution (2020). https://constitutioncenter.org/interactive-constitution/interpretation/preamble-ic/interps/37.

41. Spending for the General Welfare, Legal Information Institute, Cornell Law School website; https://www.law.cornell.edu/constitution-conan/article-1/section-8/clause-1/spending-for-the-general-welfare.

42. Eastman, J.C. (2001). Restoring the "general" to the general welfare. *Clause, Chapman L Rev* 4 (1): 63,65,79. http://digitalcommons.chapman.edu/chapman-law-review/vol4/iss1/2.

43. (28 Dec, 1796). Document 23, house of representatives, relief to savannah. *Annals* 6: 1712,1717–26. https://press-pubs.uchicago.edu/founders/documents/a1_8_1s23.html.

44. Commerce Clause, Legal Information Institute, Cornell Law School website; https://www.law.cornell.edu/wex/commerce_clause.

45. Lawson, G. and Siegel, N.S. (2020). Necessary and proper clause, interactive constitution. https://constitutioncenter.org/interactive-constitution/interpretation/article-i/clauses/754.

46. Farber, *op. cit.*, p.90.

47. Hunter, *op. cit.*, pp. 19-38.

48. Healy, G. (2008). *The Cult of the Presidency: America's Dangerous Devotion to Executive Power*. 264. Washington, DC: Cato Institute. pages; ISBN-13: 978-1933995151.
49. Barron, D.J. and Lederman, M.S. (2008). The commander in chief at the lowest ebb – A constitutional history. *Harvard L Rev* 121 (4): 941–1111. https://cdn.harvardlawreview.org/wp-content/uploads/pdfs/barron_lederman2.pdf.
50. Zhong, W., Makridis, C.A., and Diddams, J. (2020). *Emergency Executive Powers: Not Needed Indefinitely*. Mercatus Special Edition Policy Brief. SSRN, 1-6, 2020. 10.2139/ssrn.3590751.
51. Gostin, L.O., Hodge, J.G., and Wiley, L.F. (2020). Presidential powers and response to COVID-19. *JAMA* 323 (16): 1547–1548. 10.1001/jama.2020.4335.
52. Farber, *op. cit.*, p.99.
53. Hunter, *op. cit.*, p.81-82.
54. Stafford, R.T. Disaster relief and emergency assistance act. 42 U.S.C. 5121, *et seq.*; accessible at. https://www.fema.gov/media-library/assets/documents/15271?id=3564.
55. Lindsay, B.R. and Webster, E.M. (June 3, 2020). *Congressional Primer on Responding to and Recovering from Major Disasters and Emergencies*. Congressional Research Service. R41981, updated. https://fas.org/sgp/crs/homesec/R41981.pdf.
56. Painter, W.L. (April 16, 2020). *The Disaster Relief Fund: Overview and Issues*. Congressional Research Service. R45484, updated. https://crsreports.congress.gov/product/pdf/R/R45484.
57. Painter, W.L. (Jul 30, 2019). FY2019 *Disaster Supplemental Appropriations: Overview*. Congressional Research Service. R45844, https://crsreports.congress.gov/product/pdf/R/R45844.
58. Lindsay, B.R. (Nov 12, 2014). *FEMA's Disaster Declaration Process: A Primer*. Congressional Research Service. R43784, updated. https://crsreports.congress.gov/product/pdf/R/R43784.
59. Lindsay, B.R. (Oct 4, 2017). *Preliminary Damage Assessments for Major Disasters: Overview, Analysis, and Policy*. Congressional Research Service. R44977, updated. https://crsreports.congress.gov/product/pdf/R/R44977.
60. FEMA Homepage http://www.fema.gov.
61. FEMA National Response Framework webpage: https://www.fema.gov/media-library/assets/documents/117791.
62. National Incident Management System (2017). 3rd ed., https://www.fema.gov/media-library-data/1508151197225-ced8c60378c3936adb92c1a3ee6f6564/FINAL_NIMS_2017.pdf.
63. FEMA Incident Command System Resources webpage: https://www.fema.gov/national-incident-management-system/incident-command-system-resources.

64. NIMS Intelligence/Investigations Function Guidance and Field Operations Guide, FEMA website, https://www.fema.gov/media-library/assets/documents/84807.
65. Emergency Support Functions, ASPR PHE website: http://www.phe.gov/Preparedness/support/esf8/Pages/default.aspx#8.
66. HHS Office of the Assistant Secretary for Preparedness and Response Organizational Chart: http://www.hhs.gov/about/orgchart/aspr.html; HHS Office of the Assistant Secretary for Preparedness and Response webpage: https://www.phe.gov/about/aspr/Pages/default.aspx.
67. National Disaster Medical System homepage https://www.phe.gov/Preparedness/responders/ndms/Pages/default.aspx.
68. Public Health Emergency Disaster Mortuary Operational Response Teams: https://www.phe.gov/Preparedness/responders/ndms/ndms-teams/Pages/dmort.aspx.
69. Fatality Management (2007). in *Target Capabilities List*, DHS. 519–542. https://www.fema.gov/pdf/government/training/tcl.pdf.
70. Buchalter, A.R. (Feb, 2007). *Military Support to Civil Authorities: The Role of the Department of Defense in Support of Homeland Defense*. Library of Congress. https://www.loc.gov/rr/frd/pdf-files/CNGR_Milit-Support-Civil-Authorities.pdf.
71. Schumacher, L.J. (2011). Dual status command for no-notice events: Integrating the military response to domestic disasters. *Homeland Security Affairs* 7 (4): https://www.hsaj.org/articles/55?utm_source=rss&utm_medium=rss&utm_campaign=dual-status-command-for-no-notice-events-integrating-the-military-response-to-domestic-disasters.
72. Farber, op. cit., pp. 130-149.
73. 18 U.S.C. Section 1385 Use of Army and Air Force as Posse Comitatus (from Cornell Legal Information Institute). http://www.law.cornell.edu/uscode/text/18/1385.
74. Farber, op. cit., pp. 148-149.
75. Gaydos, J.C. and Luz, G.A. (1994). Military participation in emergency humanitarian assistance. *Disasters* 18 (1): 48–57. 10.1111/j.1467-7717.1994.tb00284.x.
76. Farber, op. cit., pp. 146-147.
77. Terbush, J.W., Huckaby, G.C., and Luke, M. (2012). Chapt. 8. Civil-military integration for mass-fatality events. In: *Death in Large Numbers: The Science, Policy, and Management of Mass Fatality Events* (ed. by E.A. Gursky and M.F. Fierro), 491. Chicago, IL: American Medical Association. pages; ISBN-13: 978-1603596299.
78. History of The National Transportation Safety Board, NTSB website: https://www.ntsb.gov/about/history/Pages/default.aspx.
79. 49 CFR Part 831 Accident/Incident Investigation Procedures ("Independent Safety Board Act") (from Cornell Legal Information Institute): http://www.law.cornell.edu/cfr/text/49/part-831.

80. 49 U.S. Code §1136, Assistance to families of passengers involved in aircraft accidents, Legal Information Institute, Cornell Law School; https://www.law.cornell.edu/uscode/text/49/1136.

81. 49 U.S. Code §41313, Plans to address needs of families of passengers involved in foreign air carrier accidents, Legal Information Institute, Cornell Law School; https://www.law.cornell.edu/uscode/text/49/41313.

82. 49 U.S. Code §1139, Assistance to families of passengers involved in rail passenger accidents, Legal Information Institute, Cornell Law School; https://www.law.cornell.edu/uscode/text/49/41313.

83. Terrorism Incident Annex: https://www.fema.gov/media-library-data/20130726-1825-25045-5502/terrorism_incident_law_enforcement___investigation_annex_2004.pdf.

84. FEMA Domestic Emergency Support Team: https://www.fema.gov/media-library-data/1440617086820-f6489d2de59dddeba8bebc9b4d419009/DEST_July_2015.pdf.

85. Hodge, J.G. (2018). *Public Health Law in a Nutshell,* 3d ed. 433. St. Paul, MN: West Academic Publishing. pages; ISBN-13: 978-1634608206.

86. Gostin, L.O. and Wiley, L.F. (2016). *Public Health Law: Power, Duty, Restraint,* 3d ed. 768. Oakland, CA: Univ of Calif Press. pages; ISBN-13: 978-0520282650.

87. Lindsay, B.R. and Lee, E.A. (2020). *Stafford Act Assistance for Public Health Incidents.* IN11229. Congressional Research Service. https://crsreports.congress.gov/product/pdf/IN/IN11229.

88. Lister, S.A. and Redhead, C.S. (Sep 10, 2009). *The 2009 Influenza Pandemic: An Overview.* Congressional Research Service. R40554. https://fas.org/sgp/crs/misc/R40554.pdf.

89. Devlin, S., Gavin, C., Lyle, B., and McGovern, J. (2006). White Paper: Morgue Operations, Identification, and Command and Control of Mass Fatalities resulting from a Pandemic Influenza Event in the United States. https://info.publicintelligence.net/white_paperMFM.pdf.

90. Sekar, K. and Cornell, A.S. (May 13, 2020). Domestic Public Health Response to COVID-19: Current Status. IN11253, updated. https://crsreports.congress.gov/product/pdf/IN/IN11253.

91. Hodge, J.G., Gostin, L.O., Gebbie, K., and Erickson, D.L. (2006). Transforming public health law: The turning point model state public health act. *Journal of Law Medicine & Ethics* 34 (1): 77–84. 10.1111/j.1748-720X.2006.00010.x.

92. Gostin, L.O. and Hodge, J.G. (2020). US emergency legal responses to novel coronavirus balancing public health and civil liberties. *JAMA* 323 (12): 1131–1132. 10.1001/jama.2020.2025.

93. Gostin, L.O. (2020). Governmental public health powers during the COVID-19 pandemic: Stay-at-home orders, business closures, and travel restrictions. *JAMA* 323 (21): 2137–2138. 10.1001/jama.2020.5460.

94. Gostin, L.O., Hodge, J.G., and Wiley, L.F. (2020). Presidential powers and response to COVID-19. *JAMA* 323 (16): 1547–1548. 10.1001/jama.2020.4335.

95. Public Health Emergency homepage: http://www.phe.gov/preparedness/Pages/default.aspx.

96. Gostin, L.O. (2000). Public health law in a new century: Part I: Law as a tool to advance the community's health. *JAMA* 283 (21): 2837–2841. 10.1001/jama.283.21.2837.

97. Gostin, L.O. (31 May, 2000). Public health law in a new century: Part II: Public health powers and limits. *JAMA* 283 (22): 2979–2984. 10.1001/jama.283.22.2979.

98. Gostin, L.O. (2000). Public health law in a new century: Part III: Public health regulation: A systematic evaluation. *JAMA* 283 (23): 3118–3122. 10.1001/jama.283.23.3118.

99. Tharakan, S.M., Salaam-Blyther, T., Gottron, F., and Lawrence, S.V. (June 12, 2020). COVID-19: Global Implications and Responses, IF11421, updated https://crsreports.congress.gov/product/pdf/IF/IF11421.

100. Gostin, L.O., Sapsin, J.W., Teret, S.P., Burris, S., Mair, J.S., Hodge, J.G., and Vernick, J.S. (2002). The model state emergency health powers act: Planning for and response to bioterrorism and naturally occurring infectious diseases. *JAMA* 288 (5): 622–628. 10.1001/jama.288.5.622.

101. Gonzalez, W. and Callahan, M.E. (Aug 27, 2009). National Emergency Family Registry and Locator System (NEFRLS). https://www.dhs.gov/xlibrary/assets/privacy/privacy_pia_fema_nefrls.pdf.

102. National Commission on Forensic Science, National Call Center (Jun 21, 2016). DOJ archive; https://www.justice.gov/archives/ncfs/page/file/880261/download.

103. U.S. Foreign Disaster Fact Sheet DOS website; https://www.usaid.gov/sites/default/files/documents/1866/OFDA_Fact_Sheet.pdf.

104. Office of Foreign Disaster Assistance DOS website: https://www.usaid.gov/who-we-are/organization/bureaus/bureau-democracy-conflict-and-humanitarian-assistance/office-us.

105. International Disaster Response Subcommittee DOS website: https://2009-2017.state.gov/e/eb/adcom/acicip/disasterresponse/index.htm.

106. Interpol Disaster Victim Identification Guide (2014). 7.1 Legal and Jurisdictional Requirements. 19. accessed through: https://www.interpol.int/INTERPOL-expertise/Forensics/DVI-Pages/DVI-guide.

107. Black, S. and Hackman, L. (2009). Disaster victim identification. In: *Wiley Encyclopedia of Forensic Science* (ed. by A. Jamieson and A. Moenssens).

108. Lauta, K.C. (2015). *Disaster Law*. 157. NY, NY: Taylor & Francis. pages; ISBN-13: 978-0415705974.

109. Harper, E. (2009). *International Law and Standards Applicable in Natural Disaster Situations*. International Development Law Organization. ASIN: B003FJ6IL8.

110. Fisher, D. (2007). *Law and Legal Issues in International Disaster Response: A Desk Study, IFRC*. Switzerland: Geneva. https://www.ifrc.org/PageFiles/41194/113600-idrl-deskstudy-en.pdf.

111. Fisher, D. (2007). Chapt. 19, The law of international disaster response: Overview and ramifications for military actors. In: *Global Legal Challenges: Command of the Commons, Strategic Communications, and Natural Disasters* Vol. 83. (ed.by M.D. Carsten), 293–320. Newport, RI: Naval War College. ISBN-13: 978-0160800689. https://digital-commons.usnwc.edu/cgi/viewcontent.cgi?referer=https://www.google.com/&httpsredir=1&article=1175&context=ils.

112. Fischer, H. (2003). Chapt. 2. International disaster response law treaties, trends, patterns and lacunae. In: *International Disaster Response Laws, Principles and Practice: Reflections, Prospects and Challenges* 24–44. IFRC. https://www.ifrc.org/PageFiles/41194/idrl-book-c2.pdf.

113. Disaster Law, IFRC website; https://media.ifrc.org/ifrc/what-we-do/disaster-law.

114. Matsui, S. (2019). *Law and Disaster: Earthquake, Tsunami and Nuclear Meltdown in Japan*. 296. Abingdon, UK: Routledge. pages; ISBN-13: 978-1138481947.

115. (2018). *Disaster Law: Emerging Trends* (ed. by A. Singh), 389. NY, NY: Routledge India. pages; ISBN-13: 978-1138036437.

116. Fisher, D. (Jun 2007). Domestic regulation of international humanitarian relief in disasters and armed conflict: A comparative analysis, IRRC No. 866. https://international-review.icrc.org/articles/domestic-regulation-international-humanitarian-relief-disasters-and-armed-conflict.

117. Model Act for the Facilitation and Regulation of International Disaster Relief and Initial Recovery Assistance (with commentary) (March, 2013). *IFRC/OCHA/Interparliamentary Union*. Switzerland: Geneva. http://archive.ipu.org/PDF/publications/act-en.pdf.

118. 7th International Disaster Law Course brochure (2020). http://iihl.org/wp-content/uploads/2020/03/Sanremo-2020-IDL-programme.pdf.

119. EM-DAT: The International Disaster Database, Centre for Research on the Epidemiology of Disasters (CRED) website; https://www.emdat.be.

120. Fisher, 2007, *op*. cit., pp.

121. International Disaster Response Law (IDRL) Guidelines, IFRC (2011). https://www.ifrc.org/en/what-we-do/idrl/idrl-guidelines.

122. Disaster, Definitions, *ibid.*, p. 14.
123. Disaster, Terms, UNDRR website; https://www.undrr.org/terminology/disaster.
124. Hannigan, J. (2012). *Disasters without Borders: The International Politics of Natural Disasters*. 256. Cambridge, UK: Polity Press. pages; ISBN-13: 978-0745650692.
125. The Inter-Agency Standing Committee, UN website; https://interagencystandingcommittee.org/the-inter-agency-standing-committee.
126. Protecting Persons Affected by Natural Disasters: IASC Operational Guidelines on Human Rights and Natural Disasters (Jan 2011). Washington, DC: Brookings-Bern Project on Internal Displacement. https://www.ohchr.org/Documents/Issues/IDPersons/OperationalGuidelines_IDP.pdf.
127. Human Rights and Natural Disasters: Operational Guidelines and Field Manual on Human Rights Protection in Situations of Natural Disasters, Brookings-Bern Project on Internal Displacement (2008). Washington, DC: https://www.refworld.org/pdfid/49a2b8f72.pdf.
128. Universal Declaration of Human Rights, UN website; https://www.un.org/en/universal-declaration-human-rights.
129. Human Rights and Natural Disasters: Operational Guidelines and Field Manual, *op. cit.*, p. 56.
130. *Ibid.*, pp. 59-60.
131. Geneva Conventions of August 12, 1949 and Their Additional Protocols (2011). *International Committee of the Red Cross*. Switzerland: Geneva. accessed at. https://www.icrc.org/en/war-and-law/treaties-customary-law.
132. Guiding Principles/Model Law on the Missing—Principles for Legislating the Situation of Persons Missing as a Result of Armed Conflict or Internal Violence: Measures to prevent persons from going missing and to protect the rights and interests of the missing and their families, International Committee of the Red Cross, 02/09: https://www.icrc.org/en/document/guiding-principles-model-law-missing-model-law.
133. Geneva Conventions, *op. cit.*
134. United Nations Office of the High Commissioner on Human Rights website, accessed at: http://www.ohchr.org/EN/ProfessionalInterest/Pages/InternationalLaw.aspx.
135. Roht-Arriaza, N. (1990). State responsibility to investigate and prosecute grave human rights violations in international law. *California Law Review* 78 (2): 449–513.

136. United Nations Fact Sheet No. 2 (Rev), The International Bill of Human Rights, http://www.ohchr.org/Documents/Publications/FactSheet2Rev.1en.pdf; The International Bill of Human Rights: http://www.ohchr.org/Documents/Publications/Compilation1.1en.pdf.; The Universal Declaration of Human Rights: http://www.ohchr.org/EN/UDHR/Documents/UDHR_Translations/eng.pdf.

137. United Nations Human Rights Council see: http://www.ohchr.org/EN/HRBodies/HRC/Pages/Home.aspx.

138. Varnava and Others v. Turkey, para. 200; ECtHR, Cyprus v. Turkey (Appl. No. 25781/94), Judgment (10 Mai, 2001). para. 155; Mujkanovic and Others v Bosnia & Herzegovina (Appl. No. 47063/08) http://www.refworld.org/pdfid/50fe93dc2.pdf; http://hudoc.echr.coe.int/sites/eng/pages/search.aspx?i=001-145311#{"itemid":["001-145311"]}.

139. International Convention for the Protection of All Persons from Enforced Disappearance, G.A. res. 61/177, U.N. Doc. A/RES/61/177 (2006), adopted (Dec. 20, 2006). http://www1.umn.edu/humanrts/instree/h4paped.html.

140. The Inter-American Convention on Forced Disappearance of Persons (1994). http://www.oas.org/juridico/english/treaties/a-60.html.

141. The Declaration on the Role of the State in Addressing the Issue of Persons Missing as a consequence of Armed Conflict and Human Rights Abuses (ICMP) https://www.icmp.int/wp-content/uploads/2014/08/signed-declaration-2.pdf.

142. Interpol DVI Website: http://www.interpol.int/INTERPOL-expertise/Forensics/DVI.

143. Interpol Disaster Victim Identification Guide (2014). accessed through. http://www.interpol.int/INTERPOL-expertise/Forensics/DVI.

144. Plass Data English-Language Website: http://www.plassdata.com/products-services/software-products.html#dvi.

145. International Commission on Missing Persons website; https://www.icmp.int.

146. International Federal of Red Cross and Red Crescent Societies website; https://www.ifrc.org/en/who-we-are/the-movement/ifrc.

147. IDRL Guidelines, *op. cit.*

148. Office for the Coordination of Humanitarian Affairs, UN website; https://www.unocha.org.

149. Mass Casualty Management, Fact sheet, WHO website; https://www.who.int/hac/events/drm_fact_sheet_mass_casualty_management.pdf?ua=1.

150. Management of Dead Bodies in Disaster Situations 2d ed., PAHO/WHO/IFRC, (2016). https://www.who.int/hac/techguidance/management-of-dead-bodies/en.

151. Simm, G. (2018). Disaster response in Southeast Asia: The ASEAN agreement on disaster response and emergency management. *Asian Journal of International Law* 8 (1): 116–142. 10.1017/S2044251316000205.

152. Convention on Facilitation of International Maritime Traffic (FAL) (1965). revised 2016, International Maritime Organization. website; http://www.imo.org/en/About/Conventions/ListOfConventions/Pages/Convention-on-Facilitation-of-International-Maritime-Traffic-(FAL).aspx.

153. Convention on Civil Aviation (Chicago Convention), ICAO website; https://www.icao.int/publications/pages/doc7300.aspx.

154. Annex 9 – Facilitation, Border Controls and Procedures, ICAO website; https://www.icao.int/Security/FAL/Pages/Annex9.aspx.

155. Annex 13 – Aircraft Accident and Incident Investigation, ICAO website, https://www.icao.int/safety/airnavigation/AIG/Pages/Documents.aspx.

156. Sarkin, J. (2016). The need to deal with all missing persons including those missing as a result of armed conflict, human trafficking, and human rights violations (including enforced disappearances) in international and domestic law and processes. *Inter-American & European Human Rights Journal* 8: 112–142. https://heinonline.org/HOL/Page?collection=journals&handle=hein.journals/intereur8&id=141&men_tab=srchresults.

157. Legal Frameworks and Rights website, ICMP; https://www.icmp.int/the-missing/legal-frameworks-and-rights.

158. Last Rights: The Dead, the Missing and the Bereaved at Europe's International Borders–Proposal for a Statement of the International legal obligations of States, OHCHR (May, 2017). https://www.ohchr.org/Documents/Issues/Migration/36_42/TheLastRightsProject.pdf.

159. Principles Concerning Missing Persons and the Presumption of Death, Council of Europe (2009). https://rm.coe.int/16807096bd.

160. The International Convention on the Simplification and Harmonization of Customs Procedures (Kyoto Convention) (1974). revised 2006, World Customs Organization website; http://www.wcoomd.org/en/Topics/Facilitation/Instrument%20and%20Tools/Conventions/pf_revised_kyoto_conv/Kyoto_New.

161. Tampere Convention on the Provision of Telecommunication Resources for Disaster Mitigation and Relief Operations, UN website, 1998; https://

treaties.un.org/pages/ViewDetails.aspx?src=TREATY&mtdsg_no=XXV-4&chapter=25.

162. About the Hyogo Framework for Action (2005-2015). UNDRR website; https://www.preventionweb.net/english/hyogo/framework.

163. Sendai Framework for Disaster Risk Reduction, UNDRR website; https://www.preventionweb.net/sendai-framework/sendai-framework-for-drr?pid:22&pil:1.

164. United Nations Office for Disaster Reduction website; https://www.undrr.org.

165. Global Facility for Disaster Reduction and Recovery (GFDRR), GFDRR website; https://www.gfdrr.org/en.

166. Billington, J.H. (2010). entry #363 in *Respectfully Quoted: A Dictionary of Quotations*, Library of Congress, Dover Publications, Mineola, NY,, ISBN-13: 978-0486472881.

167. (2018). *Disasters: Core Concepts and Ethical Theories* (ed. by D.P. O'Mathuna, V. Dranseika and B. Gordijn), 258. NYC, NY: Springer. pages; ISBN: 3030065014.

168. Zack, N. (2010). *Ethics for Disasters*. 164. Rowman & Littlefield Publishers. pages; ASIN: B00292BLUA.

169. (2013). *Disaster Bioethics: Normative Issues When Nothing Is Normal* (ed. by D.P. O'Mathuna, B. Gordjin and M. Clarke), 227. Springer. pages; ISBN-13: 978-9401778459.

170. (2018). *Routledge Handbook of Human Rights and Disasters* (ed. by F.Z. Giustiniani, E. Sommario, F. Casolari and G. Bartolini), 412. NY, NY: Routledge. pages; ISBN-13: 978-1138069916.

171. Saban, L.I.S. (2017). *International Disaster Management Ethics*. 190. Albany, NY: State Univ of New York Press. pages; ISBN-13: 978-1438461700.

172. (2019). *Ethical Approaches to Human Remains* (ed. by K. Squires, D. Errickson and N. Marquez-Grant), 649. Switzerland: Springer. pages; ISBN-13: 978-3030329259.

173. Passalacqua, N.V. and Pilloud, M.A. (2018). *Ethics and Professionalism in Forensic Anthropology*. 146. London, UK: Academic Press. pages; ISBN-13: 978-0128120651.

174. Daley, B. (Aug 28, 2019). Humanitarian forensic scientists trace the missing, identify the dead and comfort the living. *The Conversation*, https://theconversation.com/humanitarian-forensic-scientists-trace-the-missing-identify-the-dead-and-comfort-the-living-115623.

175. Nuzzolese, E. (2012). Missing people, migrants, identification and human rights. *Journal For Odont Stomatol* 30 (2): Supp 1: 47–59. http://www.iofos.eu/Journals/JFOS%20sup1_Nov12/IDEALS%206-96.pdf.

176. Aronson, J.D. and London, A.J. (2011). Recovery and Identification of the Missing after Disaster: Case Studies, Ethical Guidelines and Policy Recommendations, CMU. https://www.cmu.edu/dietrich/ehpp/documents/2011-Recovery-and-Identification-of-the-Missing-after-Disaster.pdf.

177. TheBelmontReport,HHSwebsite;https://www.hhs.gov/ohrp/regulations-and-policy/belmont-report/index.html.

178. Beauchamp, T.L. and Childress, J.F. (2019). *Principles of Biomedical Ethics,* 8th ed. 512. NY, NY: Oxford Univ Press. pages; ISBN-13: 978-0190640873.

179. WMA Statement on Medical Ethics in the Event of Disasters, WMA website. HYPERLINK "https://urldefense.com/v3/__https://www.wma.net/policies-post/wma-statement-on-medical-ethics-in-the-event-of-disasters/__;!!N11eV2iwtfs!uRQWV2Zu6qW0JzQm8tmENxpx58LXZnTaTjedWU3CVL2qEoIA79VdXo6vSGszAfLLtampxItWoGoQ-Wrd08WB$" https://www.wma.net/policies-post/wma-statement-on-medical-ethics-in-the-event-of-disasters/ (accessed 1/14/2022)

180. Humanitarian principles, European Civil Protection and Humanitarian Aid Operations website. HYPERLINK "https://urldefense.com/v3/__https://ec.europa.eu/echo/who/humanitarian-principles_en__;!!N11eV2iwtfs!uRQWV2Zu6qW0JzQm8tmENxpx58LXZnTaTjedWU3CVL2qEoIA79VdXo6vSGszAfLLtampxItWoGoQ-WcRkoVA$" https://ec.europa.eu/echo/who/humanitarian-principles_en (accessed 1/14/2022)

181. CMU, op. cit. p. 48.

182. PAHO/WHO/IFRC Manual, op. cit.

183. CMU, op. cit., p. 20.

184. Cecchine, G., Morgan, F.E., Wermuth, M.A., Jackson, T., Schaefer, A.G., and Stafford, M. (2013). The U.S. Military Response to the 2010 Haiti Earthquake, Rand Corp. ISBN: 978-0-8330-8075-2; https://www.rand.org/content/dam/rand/pubs/research_reports/RR300/RR304/RAND_RR304.pdf.

185. Gupta, K. and Sadiq, A.A. (2010). *Responses to Mass-fatalities in the Aftermath of 2010 Haiti Earthquake, Univ of Colorado Boulder.* Natural Hazards Center. https://hazards.colorado.edu/uploads/quick_report/gupta_2010.pdf.

186. CMU, op. cit., pp. 18-19, 22, 27.

CHAPTER 11
DVI in the Changing Twenty-first Century

Cynthia S. Gavin
Strategic Consultant, Baltimore, MD, USA

11.1 Introduction

"At the time when there is enormous international interest in the future of forensic science … the need for leadership is critical" (Martell 2019)

Change is inevitable. And it can be exciting or terrifying, depending on whether you know where you are going or merely responding to what others propagate. As Rosabeth Moss Kanter said, "Change is disturbing when done to us, exhilarating when done by us" (Kanter 2011). As Medical Examiners and Coroners (ME/C) then, we must consider our future more than our past and begin to ask questions that lead others toward a future Disaster Victim Identification (DVI) vision. Such questions include:

- Based on the future, is there any value in continuing to discuss the differences between Medical Examiner and Coroner Systems, or should our efforts focus on what each system needs to do to meet future challenges?
- Should our identity as ME/Cs continue to be linked with justice, public health, medical, or scientific missions, or do we serve a greater purpose in society?

Disaster Victim Identification in the 21st Century: A US Perspective, First Edition.
Edited by John A Williams and Victor W Weedn.

- In a disaster when there is no crime, and possibly no public health hazard, what is our role?
- Have we developed DVI strategies that will meet the challenges of the changing twenty-first century, or are we merely trying to improve strategies we developed in response to past disaster incidents?
- Have we inadvertently created false obstacles that prevent the forensic community from meeting their needs in the year 2090?

In this chapter, we will answer some of these questions, at least in part, and provide a means our colleagues can employ to create a future vision that will meet the challenges of the twenty-first century. Whereas in the preceding chapters, we reviewed our history and the technical aspects associated with obtaining a decedent identification, in this chapter, we will put the past and these technical aspects in the context of the future and discuss DVI in broader terms. More specifically, we will employ strategic foresight methods to analyze DVI within a future Dynamic Disaster Management System and consider the role ME/Cs offer society, particularly when everyone is experiencing a devastating disaster event. Next, by considering key trends that will impact ME/Cs over the next several decades, we will identify relevant drivers and constrainers of change, as well as areas of uncertainty that will influence our future. With this information, ME/Cs can consider plausible future circumstances and then assess DVI strategies to identify those that provide the greatest value. Following this analysis, more significant issues will become evident when contemplating these findings as DVI strengths, weaknesses, opportunities, or threats. Finally, the discussion will focus on actionable recommendations ME/Cs can put in place today that will help them shape who they are and how they will meet both the known and unknown challenges of the twenty-first century.

11.2 Trend Analysis

In one sense, many might think the preceding chapters of this book identified key trends in DVI. And in a way they did. Authors addressed how ME/Cs and DVI have been historically linked to the King of England when noting the first ME/Cs were called "crowners" (NRC

2009). Other authors brought forward ME/Cs' connection with medicine and science. Still, others identified ME/Cs' work within the criminal justice system and their connection to public health. Yet, most of these analyses focused on the past or what is currently happening. According to Ralston and Wilson (2006), performing future trend analysis, which entails horizon scanning, provides the best means of identifying early signals of change. For ME/Cs, there will be eight predictable megatrends they will experience in the twenty-first century that will shape their perspective about future DVI needs.

11.2.1 Megatrend #1: Population Shift and Megacity Growth

In 2011, the United States (US) Federal Emergency Management Agency (FEMA) reported cities in the next century would experience a population growth between 18 and 30%, and this would affect the surge capacity of the existing disaster response framework (FEMA 2011). Populations will include more ethnically diverse people, and there will be greater than a 6% increase in those over the age of 65. For ME/Cs, this means they will experience a higher annual caseload, a higher disaster caseload, and when gathering antemortem data or revealing postmortem data, they will need to communicate with several types of people groups. Also, while megacity growth itself is not a predictor of crime when other factors such as homelessness, a lack of resources, or perceived injustice exists, civil unrest follows often resulting in mass fatality incidents (MFI) (e.g., shootings, riots), much like we observed with the occurrence of the 1861 Baltimore City Riots (Tkacik 2018; WHP 2020).

11.2.2 Megatrend #2: Change in Disaster Types that Result in MFIs

Not only are disasters no longer novel, but the types of disasters and what we will designate as a disaster will change during the twenty-first century. Disasters likely to impact the ME/Cs and DVI strategies include, but are not limited to, airline-related deaths, terrorism, mass migration, cybercrime, human trafficking, and biological threats.

According to data compiled by the Aviation Safety Network (2020), every year from 1957 to 2006, approximately 1,000 people have lost their lives in airline crashes. The year 1972 was considered the worst year on record when 2,373 people lost their lives in 72 accidents worldwide. Since 2006, however, airline fatalities have significantly dropped, with the lowest number of 59 fatalities occurring in 2017. This statistic is noteworthy, as ME/Cs use a DVI model predicated on airline disasters.

In 2006, Ritter (2006) proffered the criminal justice system will face different social issues by 2040, some of which the US has already experienced in 2018 and 2019 specific to mass migration and border flooding (Dedaj 2018). Although no MFIs have occurred, Latham et al. (2018) more recently reported there had been a growing need to integrate sociopolitical and humanitarian science when identifying migrant deaths. They suggested ME/Cs must become "critical thinkers that go beyond in-house autopsy," and that this type of MFI will prompt transformation within the forensic anthropology community "because such incidents will require leaders to balance social justice and human rights initiatives" (Latham et al. 2018). Future trends will include DVI scenarios involving various adaptations of mass migration to include enemy border invasions.

In addition to reporting an increase in flooding, droughts, and fires, FEMA (2011) identified there would be an increase in domestic and transnational terrorism, which is more likely to result in MFIs. Since 1950, the US has gone from only eight terrorist incidents per decade to 75, and mass fatality shootings have increased from 0 to 26 incidents per decade (Gavin 2019). Furthermore, future DVI circumstances will likely include more:

- Small-scale terrorist incidents.
- Homicide/suicide psychosis resulting from different forms of isolationism.
- Organized riots.
- Terrorist incidents involving chemical (e.g., GB, VX, HD), biological (Ebola, hantavirus, plague, etc.) and radiological agents and materials to include the use of a different category of agents called Non-Traditional Agents (NTAs).
- Terrorist incidents that extend beyond national borders requiring a multination response.

Of course, ME/C may experience an entirely new type of disaster related to cybercrime. Although cybercrimes are not known to result in death, Morgan (2017) reported there will be 6 billion internet users by 2022, and 7.5 billion Internet users by 2030. Cybercrime damages will cost the world $6 trillion annually by 2021, up from $3 trillion in 2015, and global spending on cybersecurity will exceed $1 trillion cumulatively over the next five years (Morgan 2017). Although cybercrime focuses on damage and destruction of data, stolen money, lost productivity, theft of intellectual property, theft of personal and financial data, embezzlement, fraud, and post-attack disruption, healthcare providers have become a "bullseye for hackers" (Morgan 2017). Siwicki (2017) also pointed out medical device failure is on the horizon. Couple the City of Baltimore's recent 2019 Ransom Attack, which resulted in a $18.2 million recovery, with a healthcare attack able to disrupt 226,000 US pacemaker users, and ME/Cs may find themselves needing to institute a very different DVI response model than the one they are currently employing (Duncan 2019; Facty.com 2020).

A more recent type of disaster is related to human trafficking. Lu (2018) reported, "the business of bodies is very lucrative. When Libya lost its government, the first thing the country did was sell people as slaves. When groups needed resources, they used sex as the way to keep up the livelihood of the community" (Lu 2018). Considering there is no governmental structure that effectively punishes human trafficking internationally and the US is only now starting to discuss the issue, ME/C could find themselves engaged in MFIs that involve various human trafficking adaptations including but not limited to sex trafficking and slavery of various age groups, gender, and people groups. All these factors combined will challenge the way ME/Cs implement existing DVI practices.

More recently, the Johns Hopkins Center for Health Security conducted a study in 2018 to reveal naturally occurring microorganisms that could result in a global catastrophic biological risk or a new pandemic. They defined the new pandemic as "biological agents – whether naturally emerging or reemerging, deliberately created and released, or laboratory engineered and escaped – could lead to sudden, extraordinary, widespread disaster beyond the collective capability of national and international governments and the private sector to control" (Adalga et al. 2018). One example of this is RNA viruses, as they are the most likely class of microorganisms that can "evolve or be manipulated" (Adalga et al. 2018). Such biological threats result in loss of life, damage to national governments and international relationships; create societal and economic instability; and create a global security risk. For ME/Cs, a 2008 pandemic influenza analysis revealed they could experience their annual caseload within eight weeks, challenging all DVI approaches even for the largest ME offices in the nation (NYC OCME 2008). Even more interesting to note, in January 2020, the World Health Organization and other authorities started to announce the international spread of the new coronavirus, which started in China, stating it would likely become the next pandemic (Langreth and Cortez 2020).

11.2.3 Megatrend #3: Massive Technological Advancement

Over the next 100 years, ME/Cs will experience massive technological advancement that will impact their DVI strategies both directly and indirectly. ME/Cs will integrate advanced tools that will improve their ability to identify decedents but also need to consider how they will employ transformative networks and smart spaces. For instance, the global digital forensics market is expected to reach $7 billion by 2024, a 12.6% growth between 2016 and 2024 alone (Giiresearch.com 2017). Not only will digital forensic techniques continue to develop, but the associated need to appropriately recover samples and interpret the findings for use in a court of law will also grow. Furthermore, Moore (2019) pointed out there will be a need to develop automated algorithms to explore related DVI hypotheses to look for relevant patterns, which means there will be a need for unique types of forensic data scientists.

The forensic community will also experience other technical tool advancements. For example, medical 3D bioprinters, a technology that combines living cells and other biomaterials to fabricate biomedical tissue-like structures, will become common (Bolwell 2018). The obvious DVI implication is that ME/Cs will start to assess medical device malfunction. An adapted use of this technology, however, is that ME/Cs can use the same technology to construct temporary locations. Such a technical tool can provide ME/Cs an alternative field location to perform DVI work.

So, too, will be tools ME/Cs can use when detecting decedent recovery locations. Ubelaker (2019) reported, "forensic anthropology likely will involve more economical and mobile technology specific to molecular analysis of bone or tooth using solid-phase double-antibody protein radioimmunoassay (pRIA)" (Ubelaker 2019). This type of advancement, along with immersive technologies, will change how users interact with the world (Moore 2019). ME/Cs, for example, can use immersive technologies to replicate disaster sites as a means of establishing a decedent recovery zone as well as use the technology to proactively assist government agencies to recognize the scope and breadth of DVI operations before a disaster occurs (Little Hoover Commission 2018).

Furthermore, ME/Cs will experience the advancement of computing networks. Network maturation and the ability to secure and compile information using blockchain, quantum computing, and cognitive automation will occur (Gordon 2009). Siwicki (2017) proffered these developments lead to a new field called cognitive artificial intelligence, which ME/Cs can use to transform their DVI case management system and seamlessly link their information to other agency stakeholders. No more manual cross-linking different network systems between postmortem, antemortem, missing persons, medical and dental charts, vital records, and legal systems. Blockchain, a technology that many are becoming more familiar with, offers a distributed decentralized platform known for being "immutable," a characteristic ME/Cs require when forming a permanent, tamper-proof case file for each decedent (Kastelein 2018). Such technology will allow for more security, less disruption, and greater transparency of data with specific end-users. Even improvements in the "Internet of Things" will transform interaction, enabling access to test results, reducing laboratory turnaround time, improving tracking, and more effectively compiling a comparative decedent manifest, a key component of DVI (Rueda-Sabater et al. 2010).

Finally, smart space technology will completely change how humans interact, connect, and coordinate with each other (Moore 2019). Such technology will shift how ME/Cs structure their office operations and how their people will interact. DVI aspects that were once centralized can be decentralized, outsourced, and become mobile. ME/C offices, known for being small and often lacking in resources, will likely not be as constrained in the future.

11.2.4 Megatrend #4: Social Media and Social Expectations

Although those outside the field may have no idea that many ME/C offices are not "up-to-date" and some are even considered highly dysfunctional, social media and social expectations propagate the notion "everything is possible now," which ultimately impacts the next of kin's DVI expectations (Stirling and Sullivan 2017; Thompson 2011). Certainly, social expectations based on media reporting and Hollywood movies already impact the forensic community, so much so that the Committee on Identifying the Needs of the Forensic Sciences Community, National Research Council (NRC) (2009) reported on the effect of the television show Crime Scene Investigation (CSI). They called it the "CSI Effect," having stated:

> Jurists and crime laboratory directors anecdotally report that jurors have come to expect the presentation of forensic evidence in every case, and they expect it to be conclusive. In short, CSI viewers were more critical of the forensic evidence presented at the trial and expressed more confidence in their verdicts than did nonviewers when forensic evidence was used. (NRC 2009)

Specific to disasters, even officials believe ME/Cs can swiftly and accurately obtain decedent information within hours or days of the incident. For example, in 2004, during the Madrid train bombing, when 191 people died as a result of 10 simultaneous improvised explosive device explosions, 80% of the decedents were identified within five days of the disaster (Adserias et al. 2014). This response was a staggeringly quick; however, those identifications were not made using confirmatory methods. Following the 2007 Virginia Tech University shooting, where the ME did use confirmatory decedent identification evidence for all 32 cases, sadly, family, media, and elected officials believed the ME's response was too slow (TriData Division 2009). And even though the Clark County Coroner's Office had all 58 victims identified using confirmatory analysis, within three days of the 2018 Route 91 Harvest Music Festival Shooting, many elected officials were calling the Coroner on the day of the disaster asking who perished

(Fudenberg 2018). Thus, the force of social expectations is real, driving public and elected official expectations about DVI operations.

Within the next century, other social changes will impact how citizens engage in disasters. Certainly, genetic profiling, which will become an $83.9 billion global market in 2024, suggests citizens may offer them as part of the standard antemortem data ME/Cs should gather (Giiresearch.com 2019). Yet, future disaster management practices will begin to engage citizens more directly, an idea that may incline ME/Cs to consider how they might direct citizens to gather and secure perishable decedent identification samples when they are shorthanded.

11.2.5 Megatrend #5: The Specialization of Ethics

Part and parcel to the social expectation trend is the practice and advancement of ethics. Certainly, for the medical community, the Hippocratic Oath to "first do no harm" cited as far back as 1595 has provided a foundation (Gaardner 2017). For the judicial community, previous ethics were based on "what is reasonable," and since 1992, the trend in many areas has been to use "evidence-based" decision-making. One of the best examples of applied ethics has manifested within the well-known 1992 Innocence Project. The Innocence Project has not only researched and identified wrongful convictions, but, according to LaPorte (2017), has identified "contributing causes," such as the inaccuracy of eyewitness accounts. Such efforts spotlight the importance of avoiding bias and implementing practices, such as unvalidated or improper forensic science because they negatively influence judicial outcomes.

Although the development of ethics is not new, sub-specialties within the body of knowledge are. For example, bioethics, the study of ethical issues resulting from emerging advances in biology and medicine, is now formalized, and other industries in business and technology deliberately employ ethical reviews as a regular practice (GlobalChange.com 2020; NIEHS 2019; Rouse 2020). Future jurisprudence areas, as stated by Ritter (2006) that will impact DVI, include:

- Using evidence-based models that are more realistic.
- Streamlining process of developing evidence and conducting evaluations.

- Devising methods for getting studies off the ground faster.
- Exploring which programs and practices do and do not work.

The NRC (2009) similarly reported a need to secure a more accurate interpretation of forensic evidence. The Committee recommended improvements are needed in the areas of research to establish limits and measures of performance, and those in the field must adhere to standardization, certification, and accreditation. All these elements would benefit from an ethical review.

Although most pundits focus on the relationship between ethics and the judicial system or medicine, the continued growth of ethics will create so much tension that ME/Cs will either see the need to formally develop DVI Ethics or continue to apply judicial, public health system, or funeral sector ethical bias when addressing MFIs. In the twenty-first century, ME/Cs that develop DVI Ethics would likely address: (1) what to do in a resource-constrained environment, (2) define principles when establishing disaster recovery site boundaries, (3) discuss how to balance DVI practices in extenuating circumstances, and (4) examine the need to perform analysis that helps reduce the number of fatalities.

11.2.6 Megatrend #6: A New Dynamic Disaster Management System

The establishment of a new disaster management system will also occur in the twenty-first century. FEMA's 2011 strategic foresight analysis implied the increased cost associated with disaster recovery would influence what the federal government will classify as a federal disaster. Certainly, the agency that has been around since 1979 will transition, as it has already undergone significant changes with the age of airline terrorism in the 1980s, the introduction of preparing the largest cities in America to mitigate the effects of weapons of mass destruction (WMD) in the mid-1990s, and the establishment of the Certified Emergency Manager and the formalization of local and state Emergency Management Agency responsibilities in the late 1990s. Future efforts will move away from a linear progression mindset where emergency workers prepare, respond, recover, and mitigate disasters to a future mindset that looks at disasters as part of a dynamic system (Gavin 2019) (see Figure 11.1). Within this Dynamic Disaster Management System

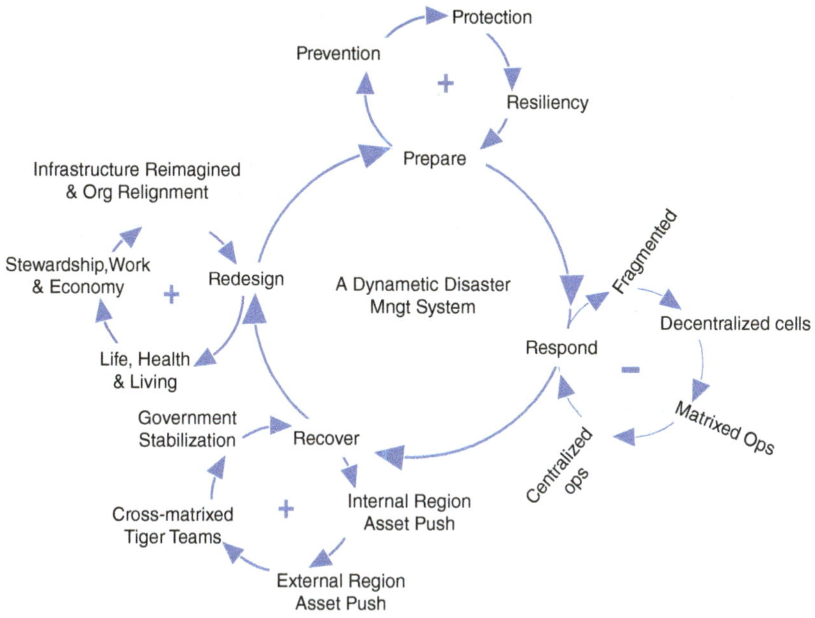

Figure 11.1 Dynamic disaster management system (Gavin 2019). As represented in NEXTGEN Leadership for managing disasters a future-oriented leadership model for local & state officials.

all stakeholders, both traditional responders (e.g., fire, police, hazmat, emergency medical services, and hospitals) and non-traditional stakeholders (e.g., Child Protective Services, Animal Control, Urban housing, private sector, and the public) will work to avoid, reduce, respond, and re-build communities using a future-oriented vision (Gavin 2019). Evidence that the current FEMA model is already in a state of decline is the ending of the federal Disaster Mortuary Operational Response Team (DMORT), which no longer maintains a standing WMD response capability (CDC 2019; DHHS 2019).

11.2.7 Megatrend #7: A New DVI Model

Housed within the broader disaster management system is the way ME/Cs conduct DVI operations. Many entities at the local, state, and federal levels have leveraged the DMORT model for years, which funeral directors and local ME/Cs developed in the late 1980s in response to airline disasters (US Army SBCCOM 2005). This model has used a multi-disciplined approach to determine a decedent's identification. Personnel move decedents from station to station where they employ all appropriate or applicable methods to gain as much information as possible to render a decedent's identification. Most stations focus on forensic dental, pathology, anthropology, latent print examination, and DNA testing (FEMA 2016). The international community, like Spain and Great Britain, employ a similar model where authorities set up a provisional "mortuary camp" that contains at least five identification disciplines such as fingerprint, a combination of dental and medical data, physical exam of unique marks such as tattoos, family testimony, and DNA analysis (Adserias et al. 2014).

Since September 11, 2001, however, the City of New York Office of Chief Medical Examiner (NYC OCME) broadened the DVI model, identifying fourteen operational fatality management components, of which the DMORT DVI process is one component (NYC OCME 2009). The fourteen components include missing persons, disaster site recovery, sifting operations, transport, storage, morgue operations, antemortem data collection, decedent manifest development, portion reassociation, family and faith coordination, hand-off to funeral directors and vital records, laboratory analysis, case management, and agency command that addresses field operations, morgue operations, and representation at the local Emergency Operations Center (NYC OCME 2009). In addition to this comprehensive model, the NYC OCME also created a different DVI approach for distributive events like a Pandemic Influenza Disaster that involves multiple, successive, and changing decedent recovery sites (NYC OCME 2008).

The US Department of Defense (DOD) Armed Forces Medical Examiner System comparably employs a DMORT-like model. What is noteworthy is the unique sharing and leveraging of DVI ideas between the US military and civilian DVI communities. For example, when the 1990–1991 Operations Desert Shield and Desert Storm took place, DOD Mortuary Affairs Companies focused on the decontamination methods personnel would employ if decedents were chemically contaminated. Approximately ten years later, the NYC OCME and DMORT also began to address the safe management of contaminated human remains, by initially focusing on decontamination of the body before it entered the morgue. Although DMORT no longer has a WMD team and the NYC OCME has not persisted in addressing chemical contamination, they have continued their efforts by addressing how to mitigate cross-contamination of biologically and radiologically contaminated human remains. Sharing ideas between the communities, the DOD has moved forward with developing a limited capability to handle chemically contaminated human remains safely. Since 2018, DOD has had the means to conduct recovery, reduction of chemical contamination, decedent identification processing, packaging, transport, and burial of a limited number of decedents contaminated by three types of chemical agents (US Army 2018).

During the twenty-first century, the DVI model will change. Perhaps prompted by new technology or an innovative way to consider the use of space, future DVI practices will become more field-oriented, simpler, and no longer warrant a large field morgue footprint that requires extensive logistical support. Instead, as people begin to wear biometric "smart" clothing, ME/Cs can use recorded information, just like airline authorities do to gather information from a black box, to document key characteristics just before one's demise. Also, with the development of handheld equipment like dental X-ray machines (e.g., a dental pantograph), other bio reporting technologies will become micro tools offering immediate data personnel can obtain upon decedent recovery. All this data can then be shared with remote experts. Ultimately, these technologies will change how ME/C will gather, employ, evaluate, and retain antemortem and postmortem data, significantly influencing DVI operations.

11.2.8 Megatrend #8: Healthcare and the National and International Privatization of Medicine

One of the most profound trends during the twenty-first century will be in healthcare. In the twenty-first century, there will be a rise in concierge medicine, and although large tertiary care centers will likely still exist in some form, the transition to customized medicine will take place (Lincoff 2015). Perhaps concierge medicine stems from the concept of personalized treatment, which cancer patients now receive based on their genetic profile; nevertheless, healthcare delivery and physician access will vary, providing even greater customization. In addition, hospitals will integrate robots into their system to reduce errors and handle time-consuming tasks, and other trends like 3D printing will tailor-make organs, thereby upsetting the existing organ transplant program doctors, donors, and hospitals currently employ (Siwicki 2017).

Destination medicine will not just involve travel to different countries but also include travel within the US anytime patients can obtain tailored surgeries more cost-effectively (ISTM 2020). Siwicki (2017) reported, instead of US citizens going to other countries, other countries will begin outsourcing rudimentary services such as healthcare accounting and specific types of surgeries to the US. Such a trend suggests forensic pathology could become one of those ultra-subspecialties, providing support to the international community following the occurrence of a disaster. Moreover, as healthcare becomes more privatized, ME/Cs may find themselves rethinking their view of jurisdictional authority and responsibility. No longer will it need to be tied to the geography where someone dies.

11.3 Forcefield Analysis

Following a review of megatrends, futuring involves a Forcefield Analysis to determine drivers and constrainers of change (Burnes and Cooke 2013). Certainly, the megatrends mentioned above will drive change, yet, ME/C should consider other more specific forces known to impact DVI efforts such as regulatory, legal, and political influencers, which have historically prompted a change. Aspects believed to constrain change include the pairing of DVI with other healthcare and law enforcement efforts; ME/Cs not being given a "seat at the table" at local, state, federal levels; the pending shortage of forensic pathologists; the lack of clarity regarding ME/Cs leadership position during disasters; and the ongoing Medical Examiner versus Coroner System Debate.

11.3.1 Drivers of Change: Regulation and Legal Factors

Historically, regulatory and legal trends in America are known to reduce the occurrence of death. For example, in 1942, 492 people died in the Rhode Island Cocoanut Grove Nightclub Fire, and in 2003, 97 deaths died in a similar incident in West Warwick, Rhode Island. Whereas there was no after-action report for the first event, the National Institute of Standards and Technology (NIST) published a

Table 11.1 Number of fire-related MFI

Year	Number of deaths	Location US and abroad
2015	64	Bucharest, Romania
2013	242	Santa Maria, Brazil
2009	156	Perm, Russia
2008	43	Shenzhen, China
2004	194	Buenos Aires, Argentina
2003	97	West Warwick, RI, US
2001	7	Belo Horizonte, Brazil
1942	492	Cocoanut Grove, RI, US

report following the second incident identifying the need to regulate facilities using more stringent building codes to prevent future incidents (NIST 2005). Table 11.1 identifies fire-related MFIs for the US and abroad, revealing regulations have resulted in a reduction in this cause of death in the US (CPRC 2015).

Other examples when legislation positively impacted DVI includes the 1974 establishment of the National Transportation Safety Board (NTSB) (NTSB 2019). Although the NTSB has no authority to regulate, fund, or be directly involved in the operation of any mode of transportation, their involvement in airline crash investigations as a means of identifying recommendations to prevent future accidents has been highly successful. The previously stated statistic provided by the Aviation Safety Network (2020) report again shows a significant drop in airline-related deaths since 2017.

A lesser-known area where regulation has prevented deaths is associated with mining disasters. ME/Cs' involvement in investigating mining fatalities has supplied needed evidence regarding safety practice violations as well as insight when authorities have needed to develop additional rules. Resultantly, the Federal Mine Safety and Health Act/Mine Safety and Health Administration have made several modifications to prevent the occurrence of future mining deaths (Krehbiel 2019).

11.3.2 Drivers and Constrainers of Change: Politics

What can make regulation and legal factors both a driver and a constrainer of change is the ME/Cs' involvement in the political debate to gain agenda priority and funding. To date, ME/Cs have experienced just as much traction as resistance.

In 1996, Congress added to NTSB's responsibility to coordinate federal assistance to support families of aviation accident victims. Fittingly, the NTSB created a Family Assistance Center model, which many ME/Cs use today to interact with the next of kin and gather antemortem data. Since then, the NTSB has expanded its Family Assistance Program to care for families of those that have died in all types of transportation accidents (NTSB 2019).

Following the September 11, 2001, terrorist attack on the World Trade Center, Mayor Rudolph Giuliani set in motion the political and financial support needed to develop the city's Forensic Biology Laboratory (Giuliani 2002). Scientists perform serology and DNA testing on nearly "40,000 items of evidence each year from nearly every category of crime including homicide, sexual assault, felony assault, robbery, burglary, hate crimes, and weapons possession" (NYC OCME 2020). Initially, this initiative was in response to family needs following the terrorist attack but has become pivotal in saving taxpayer money as the lab has processed their entire backlog of rape kits and helped reduce the burden for other components of the judicial system.

A third example of positive momentum occurred in 2011 when the Washington District of Columbia (DC) Medical Examiner Office transitioned to an independent agency. The agency, titled the Department of Forensic Sciences (DFS), was the direct result of the 2011 Department of Forensic Sciences Act (DC.gov 2019). Their mission has been to provide "high-quality, timely, accurate, and reliable forensic science services … [using] best practices and the best available technology, while ensuring unbiased science and providing transparency to enhance public safety" (DC.gov 2019). The DFS consolidated the Forensic Science Laboratory Division, the Public Health Laboratory Division, and the Crime Scene Sciences Division, and it includes the Office of the Medical Examiner.

One example where ME/Cs have not gained as much political traction as expected is related to the national Rape Kit Backlog issue.

Although this issue has been associated with the 2004 Justice for All Act, the 2005 DNA Fingerprint Act, the 2014 Debbie Smith Act, and the 2013 Violence Against Women Reauthorization Act, forensic science labs still do not receive the funding they need to process existing caseloads (RAINN 2020).

Another example where the ME/Cs have yet to gain a voice is related to mass fatality shootings. Despite the nation experiencing a significant increase in the number MFI-related shootings (see Table 11.2), political issues regarding gun control and mental health have not only consumed the debate but have drowned out the ME/Cs' and community's voice regarding DVI needs. This outcome is unfortunate because when considering Meng's (2009) definition of an Issue Life Cycle, the gun control debate has reached Phase 5 Dormancy (i.e., Phase 5 of 5). Little changes occur after this phase because once officials legislate an issue, the costs and public interest to change it would be exponential (Ashley and Morrison 1995). Thus, engaging in this debate offers the ME/C little positive momentum.

More recently, society has considered the MFI shooter's state of mental health. In 2013, the Central Florida Intelligence Exchange reported 79% of the 14 MFI that occurred between 2011 and 2013 were perpetrated by individuals that demonstrated signs of continuous behavioral and mental health illness (CFIE 2013). Only three of the 14 shooters did not have a mental health history. This issue, which is not galvanized like the gun control debate, is considered by Meng (2009) as an "emerging" one (e.g., Phase 2 of 5), which offers some opportunity for the ME/C to state their DVI needs.

The fourth indicator of constraint is that ME/Cs have not achieved an independent voice with their local and state officials. This lack of recognition has occurred following the September 11 2001, terrorist attack (NYC OCME 2012), the 2007 Virginia Tech shooting (TriData Division 2009), and the more recent 2017 Route 91 Harvest Music Festival (Fudenberg 2018). In each instance, local elected officials have not supported a closer inspection of DVI practices using the established Homeland Security Exercise and Evaluation Program After Action Review (AAR) approach (DHS 2013), like they have for their law enforcement counterparts. This lack of support is unfortunate, as AARs typically help agency leaders garner agenda priority and

Table 11.2 The rise in MFI-related shootings in the US. This represents information compiled from CNN Library (2018) and the Crime Prevention Research Center (CPRC 2015)

Year	Number killed	Location
2018	17	Broward County, FL
2017	58	Las Vegas, NV
2017	25	Sutherland Springs, TX
2016	49	Orlando, FL
2015	9	Oregon, WA
2015	9	Charleston, SC
2015	14	San Bernardino, CA
2015	5	Chattanooga, TN
2014	4	Springfield, MO
2014	4	Alturas, CA
2014	4	Marysville, WA
2013	12	Washington, DC
2013	4	Puerto Rico
2013	4	Herkimer, NY
2012	12	Aura, CO
2012	27	Newtown, CT
2012	6	Minneapolis, MN
2012	6	Oak Creek, WI
2012	5	Seattle, WA
2012	5	Oakland, CA
2011	8	Seal Beach, CA
2011	4	Carson City, NV
2011	6	Tucson, AZ
2010	8	Manchester, CT
2010	4	Hialeah, FL
2010	8	Appomattox, VA

(Continued)

Table 11.2 (Continued)

Year	Number killed	Location
2009	13	Fort Hood, TX
2009	4	Parkland, WA
2009	8	Carthage, NC
2009	13	Binghamton, NY
2009	10	Kinston, AL
2007	32	VA Tech, VA
2007	8	Omaha, NE
2005	9	Red Lake, MN
1999	13	Columbine, CO
1999	12	Atlanta, GA
1993	8	San Francisco, CA
1991	23	Killeen, TX
1991	9	Waddle, AZ
1990	9	Jacksonville, FL
1989	8	Louisville KY
1986	14	Edmond, OK
1984	21	San Ysidro, CA
1983	13	Seattle, WA
1982	13	Wilke-Barre, PA

funding once their agency has identified what worked, what did not, and what would be needed to close the capability gap.

One area the ME/C can gain political traction is related to the current opioid crisis. In 2017, President Donald J. Trump declared the opioid crisis a public health emergency, citing that in 2016 more than two million Americans had an addiction to prescription or illicit opioids (White House 2018). Subsequently, in 2018, Congress passed the Support Act, "the single largest legislative package addressing a single drug crisis in history" (White House 2018). Since then, eight states have declared the opioid crisis a state emergency (Pottorff 2018). Each opioid death involves an ME/C response, as it falls within the basic parameters of "unusual circumstances, suspicious circumstances, or when a person is not attended by a physician" (Md DH 2020). Deaths resulting from opioids present a different type of DVI scenario, however. Such incidents tend to occur at multiple incident sites, in singular instances; nevertheless, collectively, ME/Cs must investigate these deaths, obtain a victim identification, and determine cause and manner of death. Due to the totality of their response, they could choose to classify opioid-related deaths as a disaster. According to Meng's Issue Life Cycle concept, this crisis would be in Stage 3 of 5, where there is unconditional acceptance of an issue (Meng 2009). Thus, for ME/Cs, this leaves room for them to engage in the political debate and declare their DVI needs (Columbia Social Intervention Group 2020).

11.3.3 Constrainers of Change

Besides, the equal driving and restraining force of politics is an ME/C's constraining mindset that suggests DVI means implementing the "more business than usual plan" (Gruspier 2017). This mindset, coupled with four other aspects, restrains positive momentum.

Like the constant battle to achieve recognition when ME/C issues are discussed as part of the law enforcement mission, a similar constraint occurs when DVI needs are paired with public health and medical services. In disaster management, the federal government's disaster model coordinates state and local entities using Emergency Support Functions (ESF) (see Chapter 4). More specifically, fatality management is part of ESF #8, which focuses on "providing medical care and human services to those affected; reducing the public health and human service effects on the community; and enhancing community resiliency to respond to a disaster" (DHHS, ESF #8-1). What many may not realize is DVI is one of sixteen health and medical tasks, listed within ESF #8. For catastrophic events, such as pandemic outbreaks, the Department of Health and Human Services (DHHS) created Capability 5 to address fatality management. It declares public health entities must (DHHS 2019),

- Determine the role of public health fatality management.
- Activate public health fatality management operations.
- Assist in the collection and dissemination of antemortem data.

- Participate in survivor mental/behavioral health services.
- Participate in fatality processing and storage operations.

Although ESF 8 and Capability 5 may seem helpful, ME/Cs must always substantiate their DVI needs within the context of providing resources for the living.

While local and state emergency operations centers do not necessarily have to organize themselves in the same way as the federal government, DVI operations at the local and state levels traditionally follow suit. To consider the NYC OCME All Hazards Plan (2009) revealed there were fourteen components associated with fatality management alone, it is evident ESF #8 is overburdened and any discussion regarding DVI needs will naturally fall to the bottom of the priority list for most disasters (Gavin and Nesler 2014).

Part-n-parcel to the competition for resources issue is the follow-on consequence that ME/Cs often do not have a "seat at the table." One example of this is when FEMA revised the Incident Management System to incorporate an Intelligence and Investigation (IandI) Section. Several ME/Cs went to Washington DC to discuss how IandI was necessary but separate from Fatality Management Operations. ME/Cs lost their voice to law enforcement agencies that believed they should oversee their operations. In 2013 the Department of Homeland Security (DHS) published the IandI Functional Guidance and Field Operations Guide, suggesting it was appropriate for local law enforcement agencies to operationally control fatality management; however, they did leave the exact manner for structuring fatality management operations to the decision of local commanders (FEMA 2013).

Another example of the federal government not supporting DVI needs was when several ME/Cs in 2015 presented a National Call Center Initiative to the National Commission on Forensic Science. Having documented several instances when local, state, and federal entities were bombarded with 10–100 calls per victim and providing data regarding the lack of information sharing between 911 Call Centers, Missing Persons Reporting, American Red Cross Reunification Centers, 311 Information Centers, individual hospitals, Family Assistance Centers, and ME/C offices (DePaolo 2015), the ME/C community initially believed it would gain support. In 2017, the US

Attorney General even approved the recommendation, but subsequently, Congress only supported the measure as a means of caring for and reunifying missing children during a disaster (CDC 2019).

A third example of ME/Cs not having a seat at the table was when the federal government chose not to support the National Research Council's recommendation, brought forward by the 2009 Committee on Identifying the Needs of the Forensic Science Community, to establish a National Institute of Forensic Science (NIFS). This 72-person committee comprehensively researched and documented the forensic science community's needs over three years, carefully constructing 13 recommendations (NRC 2009), of which the NIFS proposal would work to address the other recommendations. Despite broad community support for this initiative, nothing has occurred to date.

Another prominent constrainer of change is the existing shortage of forensic pathologists. According to Elinson (2015), there are approximately 500 practicing board-certified forensic pathologists in the US, which constitutes less than half the number needed. The National Association of Medical Examiners (NAME) provided a baseline, purporting the annual caseload for one forensic pathologist should not exceed 250 cases, thereby providing a measure for estimating future needs (NRC 2009). Although the shortage of forensic pathologists has been a long-standing problem, as there have only been 1,300 certified forensic pathologists since 1959, the forecasted shortage will become more staggering when accounting for the average age of the forensic pathologist, which is 55 (Elinson 2015; NRC 2009). In less than ten years, there will be a large and simultaneous retirement of forensic pathologists, which will not only contribute to the existing backlog of autopsies but will also affect court cases directly, impacting how government officials execute justice and maintain social order.

Further, some states do not have any forensic pathologists, which means ME/C systems already routinely share resources. Plus, these shortages exist in other countries, such as Canada, as officials have reported, "As the crime rate and new diseases steadily increase, the additional demand for forensic pathologists follows" (Weebly.com 2019). Thus, the forensic pathologist shortage will impact society daily in addition to how ME/Cs will execute all future DVI operations.

The fourth constrainer of change is the continued discussion among ME/Cs regarding their role in a disaster. The City of New York OCME regularly demonstrates ME/Cs should be fully involved, leading their people at the disaster site, within their agency, and at every location where DVI operations take place (e.g., recovery and sifting operations) (DePaolo 2015). When contending with catastrophic disasters, such as ten-kiloton nuclear explosions, multiple and simultaneous explosion attacks, earthquakes, flooding, and biological outbreaks, the New Jersey, Pennsylvania, and Connecticut ME/C offices advocated similarly (RCPGP 2010). Yet, the reality is many ME/Cs stay housed within their organizational walls (Associated Press 2010), as was the case during the 2014 Washington Mudslides that killed 43 people (History.com 2014). Whether it is an individual or agency decision, or the resulting mindset associated with a Federal Incident Management System Command Structure that confuses where ME/Cs should engage, there is a continued lack of clarity regarding the ME/C's role and responsibilities before, during, and after a disaster; and this confusion permeates the mindset of other responding agencies and the community regarding the ME/C's importance.

Since 1928, those in the US have debated the difference between Medical Examiner and Coroner Systems. The most predominant recommendation has been for "the office of the Coroner to be abolished" (NRC 2009). Where other recommendations identify the need for scientifically trained and competent pathologists, and that both systems should include toxicology, bacteriology, and other sciences that support the scientific investigation the consistent message for ten decades has been that Coroner Systems should transition to Medical Examiner Systems. In 1954, the National Conference of Commissioners on Uniform State Laws issued the Model Post-Mortem Examinations Act (i.e., the Model Act) stating in part, "elected coroners are not well trained in the field of pathology and that each state office should be headed by a trained pathologist, that would have jurisdiction over post-mortem examinations for criminal purposes" (NRC 2009). By 1979, 12 states converted from a Coroner Systems to a Medical Examiner System; however, in 2015, the Centers for Disease Control and Prevention (CDC) identified of the 2,342 ME/C offices in the US, 14 states had county/district/

parish-based Coroner Systems, 14 states had a mixture of Coroner and Medical Examiner Systems, and only 25 states had Medical Examiner Systems (CDC 2015). More recently, in 2009, the National Research Council's Committee on Identifying the Needs of the Forensic Sciences Community again recommended that Corner

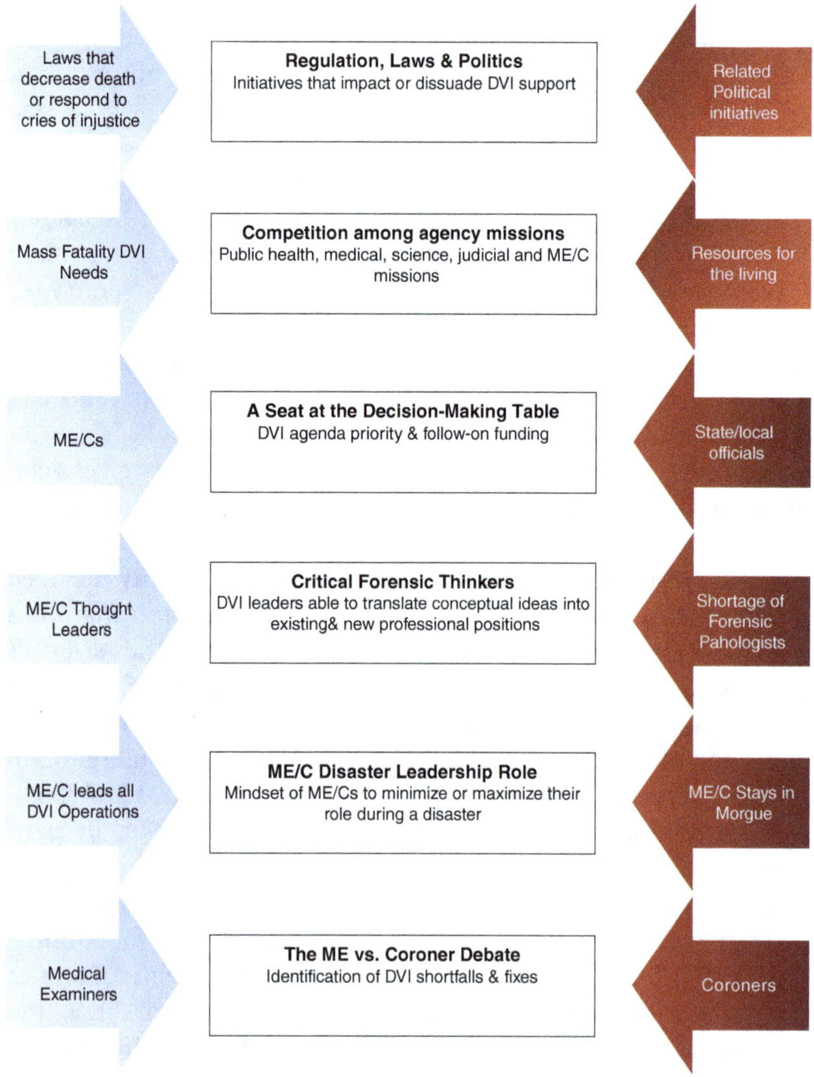

Figure 11.2 A neutral context to gain insight regarding driving and restraining forces.

Systems convert to Medical Examiner Systems. Yet, despite these continued discussions and national promptings, Coroner Systems continue to exist, suggesting that additional discussion will not only not result in a change but may also be a constrainer of change.

11.3.4 A Neutral Context to Gain Insight regarding Driving and Constraining Forces

To recap, ME/Cs experience numerous forces that prompt or restrain DVI change. When framing the issues within a neutral context, leaders can gain a better understanding of how these forces work. Figure 11.2 translates the issues mentioned above into a diagram, depicting the tension within a neutral context. In most instances, ME/Cs are contending with external forces, but in other cases, ME/Cs are either contending against themselves or not taking advantage of their societal position to gain DVI support. Following this figure is a discussion regarding "areas of uncertainty," meaning those areas that are harder to predict but will certainly influence DVI operations in the future.

By understanding the megatrends and driving and constraining forces, it is easier to recognize "areas of uncertainty," meaning those areas that are not so predictable but will influence the ME/C's future. These areas include: (1) the ME/Cs adoption rate of new technology, (2) the ME/C's role in disasters, (3) the level of support ME/Cs will receive from the local and state officials, and (4) the DVI management construct ME/Cs will employ (Figure 11.3).

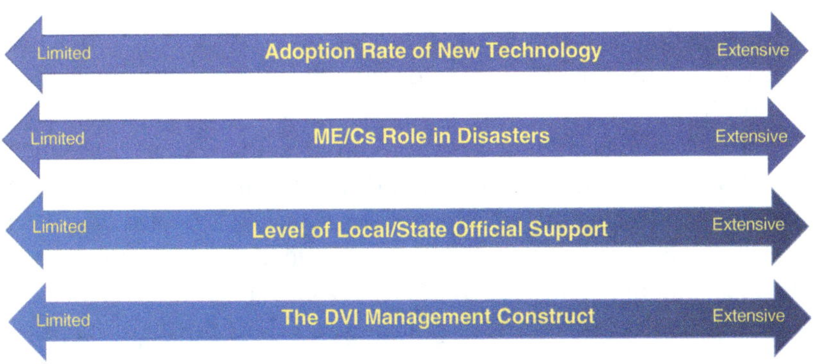

Figure 11.3 DVI areas of uncertainty.

The adoption rate of new technology will significantly influence DVI strategies, technical practices, and operations. So influential is this aspect, it will include both the ability of personnel to integrate new technologies into their daily practice, as well as the sophistication of the technology itself. In addition, as the world around ME/Cs begins to integrate new technologies into their medical, scientific, and judicial practices, ME/Cs will either be a "lagger, late-middle-early adopter, or innovator/inventor" regarding technological advancement and integration (Gordon 2009).

The role of ME/Cs in disasters conveys ME/Cs will take a prominent leadership role during disaster events, or they will minimize it, allowing other agencies to oversee and manage many components associated with DVI operations. This aspect addresses user behavior, team management, development of incident-specific strategies, requesting and coordinating support, as well as engaging professionals in critical thinking to develop incident-specific procedures. According to Carter (2019), future leaders must not just be complex problem solvers able to coordinate others, but also possess the cognitive flexibility, emotional intelligence, and negotiation skills to derive positive outcomes. As Einstein famously said, "The level of thinking required to solve a problem is different than the level of thinking that created it" (Carter 2019).

Support from local and state officials conveys the extent to which ME/C gain local and state official support to make changes to their organization. With support comes a recognition that the ME/C has a relevant voice, independent from their law enforcement, medical, public health, scientific, and judicial colleagues. When ME/Cs portray their independence, they will demonstrate how DVI serves and benefits society in broader terms, gaining agenda priority, and associated follow-on funding.

The DVI Management Construct conveys the extent to which ME/C position themselves within the disaster management structure as well as the extent to which they execute DVI operations. DVI management structures can be loose, inclusive of the 14 components, or flexible depending on the type of disaster. This aspect will also include the ability of ME/Cs to put alternate DVI practices in place based on resource-constrained circumstances.

11.4 DVI Futures in the Twenty-first Century

Using these Areas of Uncertainty, ME/Cs can forecast probable *DVI Futures in the Twenty-first Century*, denoting characteristics to describe the working environment. Titling the probable futures also helps, as it conveys a broader idea regarding the success of DVI efforts. According to Chermack (2009), using future scenario development not only helps the end-user identify "sign-posts" of change, but it is a way to convey a relevant, challenging, and plausible future that presents information in a consistent, yet compelling, manner (Chermack 2011). The more information ME/Cs develop for each future, the more insight they will gain regarding how DVI operations will work. The following provides a summary description of four ME/C future scenarios, named The Quantum Forensics World, The Modern Crowners World, The Launch-Resistant Forensics World, and The Hey Buddy Innovator World (Figure 11.4).

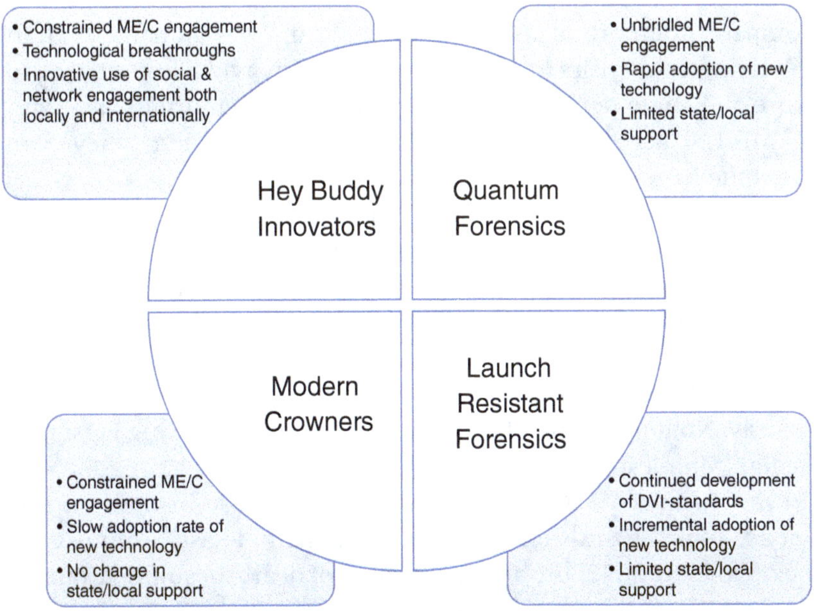

Figure 11.4 DVI futures in the twenty-first century.

11.4.1 The Quantum Forensics World

In this world, ME/Cs experience a rapid rate of technological adoption. "The future will be characterized by smart devices delivering increasingly insightful digital services everywhere you turn" (Moore 2019). ME/C will use augmented analytics, testing, and code generation to empower a wide range of users to develop forensic applications. Digital twin technology and immersive technology will help ME/Cs evaluate disaster events both before and after they occur. Technology will improve so much ME/Cs will get information faster, and systems will automatically share data between Missing Person Call Centers, hospitals, law enforcement, the Department of Vital Records, and any agency the ME/C grants access. Moreover, ME/Cs will no longer be tied to the lab or office, and the Family Assistance Centers, where ME/C collect antemortem data, will take on a truly virtual presence.

What is more, ME/Cs will use genetic technologies such as forensic DNA phenotyping and genealogy as well as non-genetic and underutilized technologies such a radiocarbon date and craniofacial reconstruction. Future smartphone capabilities will allow for 3-D modeling of the person's headshot image, and computer algorithms will be able to compare antemortem and postmortem findings (Pullman 2017). In the Quantum Forensics Future, new technology will allow citizens to capture and share perishable postmortem and antemortem data with the ME/C, becoming a valuable resource when they are short-staffed.

Blockchain technology will enable ME/Cs during disasters to expand the chronology of events, cross-level data to create an irrevocable transactional case file for each decedent as well as create an entire manifest of those who perished providing an exact timeline (Moore 2019). ME/Cs will use quantum computing to find anomalies because technology will be able to assess multiple points of data simultaneously. No longer will it be an issue to compile a Missing Person or Decedent Manifest.

In this future, ME/Cs will experience a decrease in their annual caseload, making the shortage of forensic pathologists a non-issue. For example, by 2022, the annual number of deaths resulting from US motor vehicle accidents will fall by 16%, which is a 6,000-incident decrease nationwide in the death toll in comparison to 2017. With the additional introduction of self-driving cars and new cities being designed for people, not cars, the overall number of vehicle accident-related deaths will become non-existent (McFarland 2017; World Resources Institute 2017).

The impact of these advancements will allow ME/C to take on an extended DVI role, which in turn will gain some local and state official recognition regarding their position in society. DVI management constructs will significantly change, decreasing the operational footprint overall.

11.4.2 The Modern Crowners World

In this world, ME/Cs lag behind their judicial, public health, and medical colleagues. The result will be most agencies will consider ME/Cs of limited value. Forensic pathology remains a subspecialty of medicine despite ME/Cs performing "investigation and physical examination of persons who died a sudden, unexpected, suspicious, or violent death" (NRC 2009).

Having little increased role, ME/Cs will cobble together other specialties, when needed, and when possible, to employ the existing DMORT DVI operation. ME/Cs will not be overly part of field investigations, and there will be little integration between them and law enforcement, medical, and judicial agencies. Labs will continue to use older DNA technology because the infrastructure will not have been improved, and wait times to receive information from regional labs become significantly protracted. Only when the judicial system starts making demands of local and state officials do ME/Cs receive limited DVI support.

ME/Cs prefer to stay within their known "cognitive and physical environment" during disasters, meaning their focus will only be on those things they can address from the autopsy table. For 80% of the disasters, which will be non-criminal, ME/C will get the resources officials believe they need, based on legitimatized standards of practice or the input of external experts. Although the role of the ME/C will remain connected to its historical forensic pathologists roots, to communicate (i.e., the meaning of forensics), and provide compassion or pity (i.e., the meaning of pathos) in response to suffering (NRC

2009), the ME/C will have a "quiet voice," creating an opportunity for other technical forensic specialties to replace them.

11.4.3 The Launch-Resistant Forensics World

In this world, ME/Cs experience moderate infrastructure build-out, but there will always be a concern regarding how advantageous these technologies will be. The ME/C's voice at the table focuses on addressing standards, certifications, and office practices in the strictest sense, and many ME/Cs believe they will not be adequately prepared for court cases, at least for certain types of crimes.

Both individual ME/Cs and their offices will be scared away from intensive reliance on technology, as some believe they will experience nefarious cyber-attacks. Social media automatically talks against court cases not justified by science, leveraging Innocence Project findings, and turning it into a dividing discussion that does not result in any positive changes for ME/Cs. More funding will go to laboratories directly to meet demands; nonetheless, case backlogs will continue (NRC 2009). Despite this resistance, some leaders within the forensic field will continue to establish new standards for analyzing evidence patterns.

In this world, disasters will put a strain on the ME/C's ability to respond. ME/Cs believe they need to take a more deliberate leadership role in DVI operation, operationalizing the 14-component model. Special interest groups will offer their capabilities to process decedents, and ME/Cs will establish "fee for service" contracts, paying exorbitant amounts so they can respond to their elected officials that say, "Make this problem go away! I don't want to get one more phone call from an angry family member!"

11.4.4 The Hey Buddy Innovator World

In this world, ME/Cs experience various types of non-uniform technological build-out. ME/Cs find creative ways to obtain and share resources, for both annual and disaster caseloads. Technology improves but ME/Cs must figure out how to creatively connect and share information among stakeholders during a disaster using the "hey buddy" can-you-help-me-out approach (Urban Dictionary 2009). Although demands for perfect evidence lead to rejection of some samples (e.g., partial or incomplete fingerprints or common donors in DNA mixtures), several ME/Cs gain a voice, able to persuade local and state officials to provide ad hoc support that will enable algorithm models to inform "random match probability" so the ME/Cs can demonstrate "a suspect could be one in 121,000 matches" (Madren 2013).

ME/Cs take on a unique role during disasters requesting the use of regionalized labs such as the Federal Bureau of Investigation (FBI) laboratory, US Secret Service Lab, Alcohol Tobacco and Firearms Labs, and those within the DOD Forensic Enterprise System based on the type of case or evidence. In this world, DVI associates become more supportive, allowing teams from the region and world to easily communicate and share. ME/Cs use hyper-tailored DVI management constructs for some cases and the traditional DMORT model for other cases.

11.5 Future DVI Strategy Performance

Unlike traditional analysis, the benefit of futuring is ME/Cs can "stress-test" DVI strategies to figure out if they will work in the twenty-first century. This insight will help leaders determine which strategies to support, as they will not perform equally in all futures. The following is a description of this analysis. We will look at specific DVI strategies, some known and some not. As a means of gaining clarity, we will recap the findings as a strength, weakness, opportunity, or threat.

11.5.1 DVI Strategies

ME/Cs have developed several DVI strategies, initiatives, or concepts. Professionals know about some of them, such as the National Call Center Initiative, and others may only be known by a few, such as the Field Expedient Forensic Approach. In this section, a summary of each is provided. "Expand" is intended to denote ME/Cs would modify a known or previously developed concept, "breakthrough" denotes the ME/C will experience a significant transition, and "future" denotes a new idea or concept ME/Cs have yet to implement or consider.

- ***EXPANSION of the National Call Center Strategy***: ME/Cs gain support to develop a National Call Center to synchronize Missing Person inquiries with DVI operations during a disaster.

- ***EXPANSION of Comprehensive DVI Standards and Credentials Strategy***: ME/Cs continue to expand their efforts to establish DVI standards, credentials, and institutional regulations to achieve consistency throughout the forensic science industry.
- ***BREAKTHROUGH Creation of a Separate Federal Emergency Support Function (ESF) For Fatality Management***: ME/Cs gain support to develop a new federal ESF focused on Fatality Management Operations.
- ***BREAKTHROUGH Transition as ME/C Maximize Their Disaster Role***: ME/Cs take on the broadest role during a disaster providing leadership in the field, within their office, and every location where DVI operations take place.
- ***FUTURE-Oriented Development of an Independent Regional Forensic Science System***: ME/Cs reorganize regionally, creating a combined office that addresses field operations, postmortem and antemortem data collection, and laboratory analysis for all aspects of forensic science, supporting the needs of multiple states.
- ***FUTURE-Oriented Creation of a Field Expedient Forensic Approach***: ME/Cs use technology to gather most, if not all, DVI information upon decedent recovery operations. Smart-clothing, smart-human remains pouches, and handheld and virtual devices diminish the need to centralize ante and postmortem data gathering.

11.5.2 Stress-Testing Strategies Against DVI Futures

In light of four possible futures, ME/Cs can generally determine the functionality of each DVI strategy. Figure 11.5 uses a color-coded matrix depicting each strategy's performance. Green suggests the strategy will perform well, yellow suggests the strategy will perform marginally, and red suggests the strategy will perform poorly.

Overall, DVI strategies will perform well or marginally in most future scenarios; however, this statement is predicated on the basic assumption ME/Cs fight to maintain their role in society. Whereas most DVI strategies will not perform well in the Modern Crowners World, the Quantum Forensics and Hey Buddy Innovator Worlds offer the most growth and expansion.

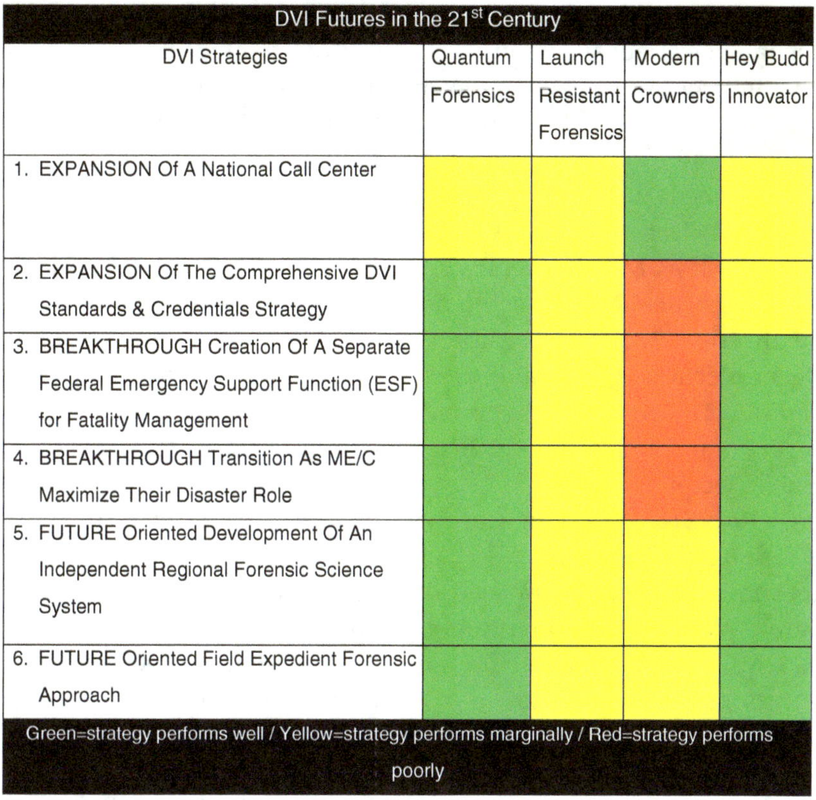

Figure 11.5 Stress test matrix of future DVI strategy performance.

#1 EXPANSION of the National Call Center Strategy

This strategy will perform marginally in most futures except the Modern Crowner's World, where it will perform well. Perhaps this is best explained, knowing implementing today's technology may not function optimally several decades from now when technological advancements redistribute responsibilities to citizens during disaster incidents.

- In the Quantum Forensics World, technological advancement, greater connectivity, and affordable device applications are likely to synergize DVI operations. Overall strategy performance may wane if the Call Center Concept is not based on future disasters, future technological advancement, and a future-oriented disaster model that incorporates citizen involvement in new and different ways.

- In the Launch-Resistant Forensic World, the National Call Center will only perform marginally, particularly if the concept is based on today's needs instead of future needs.
- In the Modern Crowners World, the National Call Center will perform well, as ME/C offices will experience an immediate positive impact, particularly if they do not have an existing capability.
- In the Hey Buddy Innovator World, ME/Cs will integrate other agency technologies, quilting together a capability at the time of the disaster. Depending on when a call center is needed, ME/Cs will leverage technological advancement from the private or external public sectors.

#2 EXPANSION of the Comprehensive DVI Standards and Credentials Strategy

This strategy will perform well or marginally in three of the four futures. What is interesting to note is that it is not likely to perform well if ME/Cs lose their voice or position of influence in society. Many futurists believe if you are not growing, then you are devolving (Gordon 2009).

- In the Quantum Forensics World, technological advancement, greater connectivity, and affordable device applications will make it easier for ME/C to synchronize their level of expertise and leverage algorithms and programs to check data previously done by hand. During a disaster, ME/Cs can learn new ways to engage and support one another, possibly decentralizing the disaster caseload among national ME/C registrants possessing up-to-date credentials.
- In the Launch-Resistant Forensic World, Comprehensive DVI Standards and Credentials will only perform marginally, particularly if ME/Cs are not funded to keep pace with recognized mandates. ME/C offices will still look to perform their disaster caseload, likely using the DMORT DVI model.
- In the Modern Crowners World, ME/C offices will probably not be able to keep pace with mandated practices. They will struggle, particularly when processing disaster caseloads.

- In the Hey Buddy Innovator World, ME/Cs will seek to apply alternate standards based on resource availability. ME/Cs may be able to leverage the technological advancement of other agencies to compensate for existing shortfalls.

#3 BREAKTHROUGH Creation of a Separate Federal Emergency Support Function (ESF) For Fatality Management

This strategy will perform well or marginally in all futures except for the Modern Crowners World. ME/Cs not able to provide an Emergency Operations Center representative under the current ESF model will not gain much improvement if the federal government establishes a separate Fatality Management ESF.

- In the Quantum Forensics World, ME/C will be able to engage and synchronize their involvement in local, state, regional, and federal disaster response planning. Connectivity will allow ME/Cs to access information remotely engaging subject matter experts that know how to leverage emergency operations center operations to improve the request for resources.
- In the Launch-Resistant Forensic World, a separate ESF on fatality management will incline ME/Cs to put a representative at the emergency operations center to address their concerns. Over time these representatives will likely learn how to interact with other ESF representatives to obtain needed DVI resources.
- In the Modern Crowners World, ME/C offices will not likely be able to keep pace with disaster requirements any more effectively than they are currently. Having a separate ESF focused on fatality management does not guarantee improved coordination among resource holders.
- In the Hey Buddy Innovator World, ME/Cs will see filling this position as essential for obtaining needed DVI resources, as it provides a means to creatively identify resources and network with others that possess resources originally intended for different use.

#4 BREAKTHROUGH Transition as ME/Cs Maximize Their Disaster Role

This strategy will perform well or marginally in all futures except for the Modern Crowners World, as ME/Cs that do not currently maximize their role in disasters today will not likely be able to fulfill a broader leadership role tomorrow.

- In the Quantum Forensics World, ME/C will take a leadership role in all DVI operations. Technology will lessen the operational footprint and simplify information exchange. Connectivity will allow local ME/Cs to engage other professionals to help them with their disaster caseload, as many decedent case report reviews can occur remotely.
- In the Launch-Resistant Forensic World, some, if not most, ME/Cs will begin to maximize their role in disasters. Those that do will find they can state their needs, set the pace for their organizations, and not allow outsiders to dictate DVI operations.
- In the Modern Crowners World, ME/Cs that do not currently maximize their role in disasters today, will not likely be able to fulfill this leadership role in the future. Local and state officials will heavily influence DVI decisions and operations, possibly pushing for the integration of outside support, based on false expectations.
- In the Hey Buddy Innovator World, ME/Cs will understand filling this position is essential for DVI success. ME/Cs able to take a leadership role will be able to make unique requests, obtaining resources from private and international sectors without an incident being declared a federal disaster.

#5 FUTURE Creation of an Independent Regional Forensic Science System

This strategy will perform well or marginally in all futures. Instead of trying to modernize at the local level, ME/C offices will experience growth and positive change when sharing resources at the regional level. Although everyone will experience a shift in their role and responsibilities, ME/Cs that put good leaders in place will help their followers transition to a future-oriented forensic model able to support annual and disaster caseloads.

- In the Quantum Forensics World, ME/Cs working within a regional system share infrastructure, technological advancement, and maintenance expenses, much like the advanced healthcare delivery model. ME/Cs begin to think about the management of annual and disaster caseloads like hospitals that are sanctioned as tertiary locations, employing 24-7 access to experts, and community locations that deliberately provide decentralized capabilities.

- In the Launch-Resistant Forensic World, ME/Cs start to engage in DVI operations with greater flexibility, while at the same time, working toward maintaining uniform practices.
- In the Modern Crowners World, the burden is lifted, at least in part, as local ME/C offices no longer need to justify their needs on their own. People who are minimizers are assigned focused positions.
- In the Hey Buddy Innovator World, an independent regional office allows for an exchange of ideas with experts from various fields on a more interactive level. Also, ME/Cs will be able to network remotely.

#6 FUTURE-Oriented Field Expedient Forensic Approach

This strategy will perform well or marginally in all futures. The management of DVI caseloads runs more quickly, with the removal of constraining constructs that demand a one-size-fits-all DVI approach.

- In the Quantum Forensics World, ME/Cs grow accustomed to fieldwork, not having offices, and gathering all needed data upon decedent recovery. With the ME/C and their staff working in the field, they immediately get a better understanding of the incident. Handheld devices and smart clothing and human remain pouches decrease the strain associated with handling decomposed bodies and body portions multiple times, and hoverboard drone devices move bodies to cold storage facilities. ME/Cs only perform physical exams using 2020 methods for atypical cases.
- In the Launch-Resistant Forensic World, ME/Cs start to engage in DVI operations differently. Some ME/Cs set up field morgues using 3D technology and begin sorting their cases using new methods that save time and effort. Other ME/Cs continue to use 2020 disaster plans, waiting for counterpart agencies (e.g., law enforcement volunteers) to bring decedents to their morgue.
- In the Modern Crowners World, many burdens are reduced as DVI processes become simpler. No longer is there a need to set up a large morgue footprint to accommodate DVI operations.
- In the Hey Buddy Innovator World, the field expedient approach invites the integration and use of cutting-edge commercial off the shelf technology. ME/C innovators prefer to "not have it all figured out" so that they can remain flexible, creating incident-specific

plans based on their immediate access to technology and subject matter experts.

11.6 SWOT Analysis

Figure 11.6 reframes the Future DVI Strategy Performance findings as a strength, weakness, opportunity, or threat (SWOT). The advantage of grouping the findings into SWOT categories is that it simplifies the content and helps leaders recognize issues of greatest concern (Chermack 2011).

11.6.1 Strengths

All strategies will perform well or marginally in the Quantum Forensics and Hey Buddy Innovator Worlds, where user behavior is unbridled, technological breakthrough occurs, and networks provide secure case files. These types of conditions enable the greatest DVI thinking, as ME/Cs envision future infrastructure using smart space constructs.

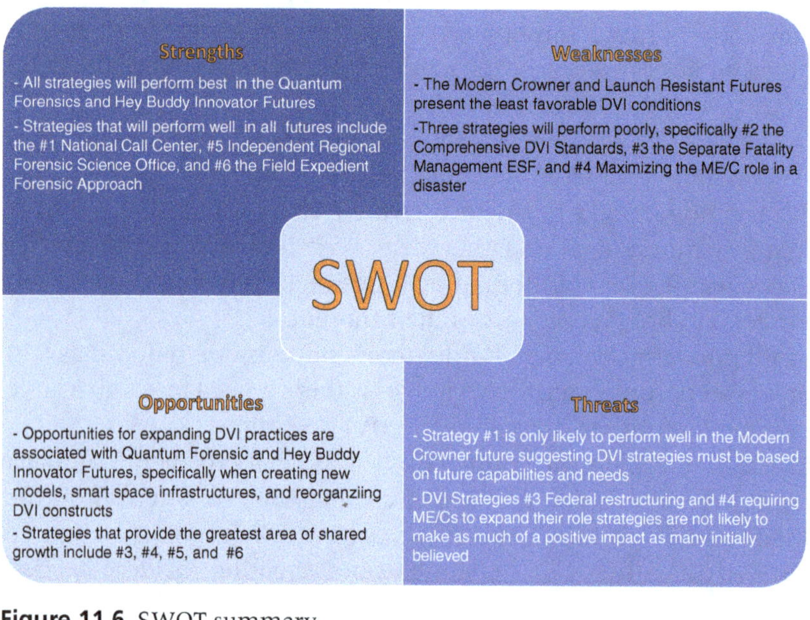

Figure 11.6 SWOT summary.

Innovation and creating things as needed becomes an advantage instead of a setback. With this understanding, ME/Cs start to think about the way they can mature their DVI technological advancements so that there is a more deliberate layering of old, new, and future technologies to support DVI operations. Concepts like the Regional ME/C Mass Fatality Management System morph and grow, based on future disaster types and resource needs. The tiered manner in obtaining DVI support used in 2020 (i.e., local, state, federal) significantly changes, as ME/Cs become more flexible asking any national ME/C and private or international entity for support without having to have a federal disaster declaration in place.

11.6.2 Weaknesses

The Modern Crowner and Launch Resistant Forensic Worlds offer the least amount of DVI growth and change. Efforts intended to stabilize DVI operations become a hindrance when responding to future disasters. For example, establishing a separate ESF for Fatality Management will likely provide some clarity and prompt some ME/Cs to put a person at the local or state emergency operations center; yet, requesting resources, integrating assets, and innovating new ways to meet needs is not a guaranteed outcome. Ultimately, when ME/Cs become too burdened, they will refrain from taking a leadership role during a disaster. They will let law enforcement, public health, emergency management, or medical authorities figure out how to respond and support DVI operations. For ME/C offices that modernize to some extent, they will still experience constraints when they are called to support international DVI operations. DVI strategies that are too American-centric will impose an unnecessary burden on their international counterparts.

11.6.3 Opportunities

Most opportunity for growth is associated with developing future-oriented DVI strategies. The two DVI strategies stress-tested included establishing an Independent Regional Forensic Science System and creating a Field Expedient Forensic Approach. This analysis suggests the DVI field is on the brink of change, waiting for ME/C to envision a future ability to keep up with twenty-first-century megatrends.

Instead of trying to layer existing concepts and technologies onto an old infrastructure, ME/Cs have the advantage of "starting from scratch" and developing "White Paper" concepts geared toward the future.

11.6.4 Threats

The results associated with the Modern Crowner World reveal the greatest DVI threats. Only the National Call Center Strategy performed well in this future, whereas all other DVI strategies performed marginally or poorly. Gordon (2009) proffered, nano, bio, artificial intelligence, and quantum innovations are economic forces that create jobs, industries, growth, and trade. This analysis means ME/Cs that do no incorporate how these aspects will impact forensic analysis, personnel, the breakdown of labor, and different ways to combine specialties will not survive. Simply continuing to do what we have been doing or putting in place what we think we need based on past disasters will not be enough.

11.7 Actionable Recommendations

11.7.1 Refresh the ME/C Mission Statement

Many ME/Cs may already think their mission statement is sufficient. These mission statements, however, were not created with the future in mind, and in most instances, they were derived from the ME/C's association with other agencies such as law enforcement, the broader judicial system, funeral directors, medicine, or public health agencies. From its origin, ME/Cs have been overly associated with other agency interests. For example, in Colonial America, ME/Cs were concerned with the king's interest in taxation when providing an official decree of death (NRC 2009). Since then, ME/Cs have incorporated aspects of science and medicine, when performing a death investigation. And even the NRC (2009) overly emphasized the ME/Cs association with the justice system when they stated the ME/C mission was "the development and application of the forensic science disciplines to support intelligence, investigations, and operations aimed at the prevention, interdiction, disruption, attribution, and prosecution of terrorism" (NRC 2009). Although these associations are important, they fail to address how ME/Cs can and should be serving society in all instances, including disasters, which may or may not be connected to a crime or only loosely associated with a public health emergency.

As such, the mission and role of ME/Cs must expand, not contract. The futuring scenarios demonstrate instead of ME/Cs only being the person to perform the internal exam or autopsy, they must become leaders possessing a specialized critical thinking ability to balance science, medicine, jurisprudence, public safety, forensics, technology, and leadership.

To develop a statement that can parlay the ME/C's unique missional complexity requires a little back-casting. The idea being we must identify tried and true concepts that have stood the test of time, as they offer a more grounded foundation upon which to sustain future purpose. Examples include Plato's, Aristotle's, and Saint Thomas Aquinas's four key virtues (i.e., righteousness, justice, courage, and comportment (Richert 2019)). ME/Cs that recreate their mission statement with these transcendent virtues in mind will be in a better position to meet the changing needs of the twenty-first century.

A mission statement grounded on righteousness, justice, courage, and comportment will broaden the ME/C's role and prompt them to communicate how they serve the society in broader terms. For instance, the ME/C's mission regarding justice would continue, but by incorporating righteousness, ME/Cs would address the need for accurate decedent identification, which substantiates human existence (NRC 2009). Next, when addressing courage, the ME/C must be able to do their work without bias or the influence of outside interests. Also, courage would expand the ME/Cs focus from death to protecting life, recognizing one of their responsibilities is to identify index cases for all types of situations, not just biological outbreaks. Specific to comportment or temperance, ME/Cs would be the first place where broken-hearted citizens could experience societal stability, which is particularly needed following a disaster. Consequently, ME/Cs must model the way for others to overcome fear, helping society remain emotionally and mentally "steady" when facing terrible obstacles. Although ME/Cs traditionally do this by adhering to reason, this virtue points out the need for ME/Cs to develop and adhere to a DVI

Ethics practice, in addition to operationalizing a well-thought-out approach, not one cobbled together with mediocre resources.

The impact of recreating the ME/C mission would be significant. First, ME/Cs would begin to change their cognitive environment, which has suffered from "bounded awareness" for decades (Bazerman and Tenbrunsel 2011). Instead of ME/Cs only looking at the past, gathering and analyzing evidence, and finding a cause of death, they would shift their perspective toward serving society more directly and comprehensively. Second, as the ME/C's mindset shifts, so would the perspective of others. As Willard (2006) said regarding each person's profession, "the Soldier's is to defend, the Pastor's is to teach, the Physician's is to keep health, the Lawyer's is to enforce justice, and the Merchant's to provide for those serving society." This conviction leaves room for the ME/C to fill the need to protect the value of human life.

More importantly, a new mission statement would enable ME/Cs to redesign how they think about their entire forensic field. Not only would new specialties become possible, but ME/C could invent a future-oriented multi-disciplinary profession. Instead of forensic pathology merely being a subset within the broader medical occupation, it could become an entity of its own. With this classification, ME/Cs could attract unique individuals interested in applying scientific thought to reveal patterns using careful comparison and systematic study. As a highly regarded critical thinking professional, they could construct explanations by developing and applying new methods, balancing the existing and future DVI practices using all manner of medicine, science, law, forensics, technology, and leadership.

11.7.2 Create an Enduring DVI Vision

To date, state and local officials have not developed a vision statement specific to disaster response. Since 1961, emergency workers and disaster response planners have established their mission statements, objectives, roles, and responsibilities using a definition of preparedness (Gavin 2019). Although this type of definition has some merit, it fails to provide leaders, followers, and citizens a vision of success. In basic leadership terms, without a vision, people get confused. This need for clarity is particularly true when catastrophic disasters result in a devolution of government, which was the case in 2005 when Hurricane Katrina struck. The City of New Orleans and many surrounding parishes were non-existent, leaving responders within the DOD with no civilian counterpart from which to garner the proper authority to execute lifesaving tasks (an important constitutional element) (Wise 2006).

Despite this lack of a broader disaster response vision, ME/C must not fall into the same trap by not having a DVI vision to direct their actions when all other mission statements, pre-scripted mission assignments, and operational cycle objectives become irrelevant due to experiencing an unthought-of disaster (e.g., disasters related to Russia's hypersonic weaponry or China's dark side of the moon project). Many may not see the value of a vision statement until they reflect on the mindset people had before September 11, 2001, when no one thought it possible the US could experience a disaster that would result in more fatalities than casualties. Yet, Dr. Charles Hirsch, the City of New York Chief Medical Examiner, following the incident, declared, "we will not be done until every decedent is identified" (NYC OCME 2012). This vision provided his agency, the mayor, and the federal government the clarity needed to engage in an insurmountable volume of work addressing more than 20,000 decedent cases (i.e., each fragmented portion was treated as a separate case) (DePaolo 2015). Nearly two decades later, that vision has prompted new DNA identification methods, formalized forensic anthropology as a key part of fatality management, created a sophisticated case management system, advanced antemortem victim identification practices, and established unique partnerships among national ME/Cs, Interpol, the private sector, and the US military (Gavin 2019). By 2007, the City of New York opened the world's largest DNA lab (NYC OCME 2020), all of which occurred when a vision helped others realize their purpose in a very chaotic situation.

Ideally, each community should create a disaster response vision statement first. This action would demonstrate the importance each agency has when their representatives take their "seat at the table." Moreover, such an effort not only confers buy-in but helps influence everyone's perspective regarding how they serve society. Gavin (2019) proffered communities should review and modify the following vision statement to meet their needs:

> We will always survive the disaster. We will never grow weary of caring for our fellow citizens. Together, we will strive to avoid what knowingly will devolve our sense of unity as we conduct our respective missions. As individuals, we will choose to act as a collective, knowing we must endure past this incident and in the end, we will become more cognizant of our humanity, our need for each other, and we will more deeply value the gift of human life, which sometimes can only be realized when we experience tragedy together. (Gavin 2019).

Even if the broader community works slowly toward developing their disaster response vision, ME/Cs can and should develop a befitting DVI vision. Such a statement should provide clarity so that when volatile, uncertain, ambiguous, or complex situations occur (Kraaijenbring 2018), leaders can communicate a trajectory of thought, action, and purpose that helps everyone move toward their future state of normal with a sense of hope.

11.7.3 Envision a Future Smart Independent Regional Forensic Science System and Move Toward Implementing This Model

Instead of continuing the debate between Medical Examiner and Corner Systems, ME/Cs must envision a future smart, independent regional forensic science system that serves local, state, and regional needs. Such a system would address both annual and disaster caseloads, developing capabilities that go beyond singular ideas like the National Call Center. Considering the future will be filled with change, ME/Cs that leverage strategic foresight concepts like the new Dynamic Disaster Management System that compliments both emergency and non-emergency groups, ME/Cs can similarly use this model to develop a future smart forensic system (Gavin 2019). Such a system would be better oriented to respond to distributive, transnational, and mega-regional disaster incidents like the New Madrid Faultline Earthquake and a simultaneous enemy border invasion.

Leveraging the work professionals have done as part of the NRC 2009 report, ME/Cs can put that analysis in the context of the future forecasting how an "integrated governance" approach would work

(NRC 2009). Instead of the focus being on public health or law enforcement, the regional system would become independent. Much like the 1974 legislation that mandated the NTSB was to become an independent agency, it and others had to recognize "their quasi-governmental status was intended to reveal the truth about what occurred, emphasizing actions that would prompt a better future society" (NTSB 2019).

As the Fourth Industrial Revolution unfolds, so too will the mental model for understanding how technology will redistribute economic and social sub-systems. Advanced robotics, drones, virtual and augmented reality systems, biotechnologies, and new multidimensional printing will create ways to generate energy and storage (Samans and Davis 2019). This transition leaves room for incorporating privatized functions, technological development, and yet-developed services.

Considering there will be so much technological advancement in the twenty-first century, ME/Cs that create a regional forensic system will be in a better position to pre-schedule advancements so that as one office's cutting-edge technology fades, another office's technology comes to fruition. Samans and Davis (2019) recommended there are four key principles planners should consider:

- Focus on the impact on systems, rather than simply the capability of technologies.
- Find ways to empower citizens and stakeholders rather than controlling them.
- Be conscious of design principles at the heart of evolving systems and shift these to being more human-centered.
- Make positive values a feature of technological systems rather than viewing ethical issues as matters of compliance, cost, or mere unintended consequences.

Within an Independent Regional Forensic System, ME/Cs can grow their profession. For example, Logan (2019) stated there would be a need for interpretive toxicology, and Geradts (2019) stated there would be a future need for digital and multi-media forensic analysts capable of extracting digital evidence from cameras, wearable biometrics, drones, and sensors. With critical thinking and strategic foresight, ME/Cs can learn to lead others toward their future, no longer waiting for the federal government to substantiate their relevancy.

Letting today's ME/C model end and moving toward an independent future smart system, others will adapt. Many of the issues previously discussed regarding the Incident Command System, Emergency Support Functions, and Emergency Operations Center representation will become inconsequential. With a regional forensic system in place, ME/C leaders and emergency planners will already have their subsystems in place, achieving alignment of key DVI stakeholders and resources before a disaster even occurs.

11.7.4 Develop Alternate DVI Standards

Specific to disasters, ME/Cs will need to regularly consider new DVI strategies versus thinking past strategies will work. If the one thing the futuring scenarios demonstrated, strategy performance varied based on ME/C infrastructure. Certainly, ME/Cs can start by characterizing each of the future disasters in Mass Fatality Management terms, yet, as technology influences disaster practices, so will how we characterize DVI needs. For example, if ME/Cs begin designing and using biotech 3D printing capable or recreating decedents after they are placed in Human Remains Pouches, smartphone body scanning, field DNA gathering and fingerprinting, and a hoverboard conveyance drones to move decedents, this type of DVI strategy may work for more than 80% of disaster cases, completely changing DVI operations.

In addition to regularly challenging DVI strategies, ME/Cs must consider what to do in a resource-constrained or resource-scarce environment. As the American Academy of Forensic Science and NIST diligently continue their work to create official DVI standards, there have been very few in the US and abroad that agree on overarching Mass Fatality Management (MFM) practices (Morgan et al. 2006) (e.g., management approaches like the NY-NJ-CT-PA Regional MFM Response System that describes the 14 components). This void will make it difficult for leaders to address alternate DVI standards, yet future disasters will overwhelm not only the government's ability to respond but also the private sector, thereby inclining ME/Cs to do this work now.

What preliminary DOD efforts have revealed regarding alternate standards is the need to identify the desired end state. Their team in

2015 proffered, "alternate standards or practices must demonstrate a compassionate, thoughtful phased degradation of services and execution of operations based on recognized triggers associated with specific resource-scarce conditions. Such a phased degradation should be associated with the occurrence of catastrophic events involving numerous decedents or require complex decedent management operations" (Gavin et al. 2015).

ME/C leaders can leverage this end state with the Institute of Medicine's 2009 effort to develop national guidelines that would establish and implement crisis standards of care. That year the Assistant Secretary of Preparedness and Response's Committee on *Guidance for Establishing Standards of Care for Use in Disaster Situations* defined key planning assumptions, revealing alternate practices would require (1) a substantial change when employing healthcare operations, (2) justifiable circumstances, (3) formal declaration by a State government/ authority, and (4) identification of the resource-scarce conditions (TRACIE 2020).

Next, the committee defined "bounding concepts" that would help them develop the crisis standards of care. They identified the need for:

- A strong ethical basis that enabled a process deemed equitable based on transparency, consistency, proportionality, and accountability.
- An integrated and ongoing community and provider engagement, education, and communication practice.
- The necessary legal authority and legal environment in which healthcare professionals would implement crisis standards.
- Clear indicators, triggers, and lines of responsibility.
- Leveraging evidence-based clinical processes and operations.

Following this groundwork, the committee developed a framework. This framework was to examine the impacts by end-user, develop templates for organizations responsible for planning and implementing the crisis standards, identify metrics associated with protocols, and develop tools for engaging the public (TRACIE 2020).

Specific to ME/Cs and DVI, DOD planners recognized several critical issues. These included but were not limited to the following:

- The complexity involved in harmonizing multiple perspectives (e.g., legal, cultural, political, and forensic).

- The limitation of existing case management processes that were not developed with degraded decision making in mind.
- The limitation of appropriate scientific data, as much of what exists, would not apply in extreme conditions.
- The lack of acceptance to revitalize low-tech solutions.
- The reality that DVI operations would be delayed due to their own or other agency technical or operational constraints.

That leaders and followers would experience a high degree of operational failure if fatality management operations were defined too narrowly or too extensively (Gavin et al. 2015).

- Despite these issues, ME/Cs must develop alternate DVI standards suitable for resource-scarce conditions that go beyond the default practice of instituting the long-term temporary interment concept (US Army SBCCOM 2005). Instead, as ME/Cs engage in the alternate standards discussion, they will challenge former concepts, realizing they are not as constrained as they might have been at the beginning of the twenty-first century.

11.8 Closing Thoughts

As ME/Cs, we must consider our future more than our past. Certainly, the past informs us regarding specific drivers and constrainers of change, yet it is by understanding how the megatrends will impact ME/Cs and DVI that we will gain insight regarding the changes we will need to make in the twenty-first century. Using the force field analysis method, our perspectives shifted regarding what aspects have been holding us back. In some cases, it was external forces, and in other instances, it had been ourselves. Arrested by this realization and the power of a futuring mindset, ME/Cs can accept our failures have now become a gateway to success. Failures such as the National Call Center and NIFS were just embryonic ideas revealing ME/Cs needed to think bigger, broader, and with the future in mind.

With an abundant amount of research and analysis already complete, ME/Cs no longer need to wait for the federal government to enable them to attain positional influence. Instead, they can work within their local and state offices to move toward an independent regional forensic system oriented toward addressing annual and disaster caseloads based on future trends. Perhaps the words written within the 2009 NRC report were correct but we misinterpreted them when it said,

> The forensic science community needs strong governance to adopt and promote an aggressive, long-term agenda to help strengthen forensic science. Governance must be strong enough and independent enough to identify the limitations of forensic science methodologies and must be well connected with the Nation's scientific research base in order to affect meaningful advances in forensic science practices. (NRC 2009)

as this edict is something ME/C can employ now by recreating their mission statement. As ME/Cs redefine who they are and how they serve society, they and others will recognize they must be free from bias, political agendas, and other mission interests.

With this foundation, ME/C can then branch out, engaging emergency management agencies to help them realize DVI is a fundamental means by which to cultivate societal resilience. Not only will ME/Cs be pivotal indirectly providing community resiliency, but also, they can spearhead efforts to create a "vision" to help everyone understand their purpose when a disaster occurs. With such a vision, ME/Cs will not be relegated to the smallest operational element. They will have a "seat at the table" during all cycles (i.e., preparedness, response, mitigation, and redesign) that comprise a Dynamic Disaster Management System.

When designing a future smart forensic science capability, ME/C can engage in professional forecasting to meet the needs associated with future MFIs. Working within a Dynamic Disaster Management Model and characterizing DVI needs based on future events, real issues will surface, enabling leaders to let go of old arguments and past approaches. Instead, DVI will take on new meaning, particularly when addressing the most extreme conditions like the New Madrid Earthquake, transnational terrorism, and multi-simultaneous and distributive enemy border invasion.

The development of alternate standards will be taxing, and it may even have us guessing if DVI is still the right term to use. Nevertheless, when leaders focus on "what is success in these conditions?" and "what is our desired strategic end state?" they can keep moving toward the future instead of living in the past. Such a mindset will broaden the ME/C's role, responsibilities, use of technology, and assessment methods. The purpose of the investigation will go way beyond knowing who died, and the cause and manner of death, prompting a different type of investigation that will help society live more fully. Yes, the challenges in the twenty-first century will be many, but society will become more resilient when their vigilant guardian whose job it is to protect the value of human life stands ready no matter how devastating the disaster.

References

Adalga, A.A., Watson, M., Toner, E.S., Cicero, A. and Inglesby, T.V. (2018). *The Characteristics of Pandemic Pathogens*. Baltimore: Johns Hopkins Bloomberg School of Public Health.

Adserias, J., Zapico, S.C. and Prieto, J.L. (2014). Management of mass disasters in Spain: The March Madrid train bombing. In: *66th Annual Meeting of the American Academy of Forensic Sciences* 21 February. Seattle: American Academy of Forensic Sciences.

Ashley, W. and Morrison, J. (1995). *Anticipatory Management 10 Power Tools for Achieving Excellence into the 21st Century*. Leesburg: Issue Action Publications.

Associated Press (2010). Death toll in Washington mudslide rises to 30, while 17 still reported missing [online]. Available at: https://www.nydailynews.com/news/national/death-toll-washington-mudslide-rises-30-17-reported-missing-article-1.1744327 (Accessed 17 January 2020).

Aviation Safety Network (2020). Statistics [online]. Available at: https://aviation-safety.net/statistics/period/stats.php?cat=A1 (Accessed 4 January 2020).

Bazerman, M.H. and Tenbrunsel, A.E. (2011). *Blind Spots*. New Jersey: Princeton University Press.

Bolwell, D. (2018). 3D printing is transforming these industries. [online]. Available at: https://hpmegatrends.com/3d-printing-is-transforming-these-industries-f94661c6b1b3 (Accessed 12 December 2019).

Burnes, B. and Cooke, B. (2013). Kurt Lewin's field theory: A review and re-evaluation. *International Journal of Management Reviews* 15: 408–425.

Carter, J. (2019). Why leaders today will become laggers of tomorrow [online]. Available at: https://www.rapportleadership.com.au/leadership/leaders-today-will-become-laggers-tomorrow (Accessed 19 January 2020).

CDC (2015). Death investigation systems [online]. Available at: https://www.cdc.gov/phlp/publications/coroner/death.html (Accessed 17 January 2020).

CDC (2019). Reunification: reuniting with children in emergencies [online]. Available at: https://www.cdc.gov/childrenindisasters/reunification.html (Accessed 12 January 2020).

CFIE (2013). Fusion center study finds 79% of recent mass shootings from 2011-2013 attributable to history of mental illness [online]. Available at: https://publicintelligence.net/mass-shootings-mental-illness (Accessed 6 September 2020).

Chermack, T. (2009). *Scenario Planning as a Strategic Learning System, in Legend Services Part III*. Seoul Korea: global HR forum 2009 [online]. Available at: http://www.youtube.com/watch?v=VxPsrHwhxzw (accessed 6 September 2020).

Chermack, T.J. (2011). *Scenario Planning in Organizations How to Create, Use, and Assess Scenarios*. San Francisco: Berrett-Koehler.

CNN Library (2018). Deadliest mass shooting in modern US history fast facts [online]. Available at: https://www.cnn.com/2013/09/16/us/20-deadliest-mass-shootings-in-u-s-history-fast-facts/index.html (Accessed25 September 2018).

Columbia Social Intervention Group (2020). Events: The opioid crisis: medical examiner roles and strategic innovations [online]. Available at: https://sig.columbia.edu/events/opioid-crisis-medical-examiner-roles-and-strategic-innovations (Accessed 17 January 2020).

CPRC (2015). Public shootings and mass public violence in the US and Europe [online]. Available at: https://crimeresearch.org/2015/06/comparing-death-rates-from-mass-public-shootings-in-the-us-and-europe (Accessed 25 September 2018).

DC.gov (2019). Department of forensic sciences [online]. Available at: https://dfs.dc.gov/page/about-dfs (Accessed 22 December 2019).

Dedaj, P. (2018). Hundreds of Hondurans head for the US border in mass migration 'march': Report [online]. Available at: https://www.foxnews.com/us/over-1000-hondurans-head-for-us-border-in-mass-migration-march-report (Accessed 7 January 2020).

DePaolo, F. (2015). *The Role of Forensic Science in Mass Fatality Management*. Washington DC: National Commission on Forensic Science Meeting.

DHHS (2019). *Public Health Preparedness Capabilities National Standards for State and Local Planning: Capability 5: Fatality Management*. Washington DC: United States Department of Health and Human Services.

DHS (2013). Homeland security exercise and evaluation program (HSEEP), District of Columbia: United States Department of Homeland Security. 109th Congress (2005-2006), 2006. S.3721 – Post-Katrina Emergency Management Reform Act of 2006 [online]. Available at: https://www.congress.gov/bill/109th-congress/senate-bill/3721 (Accessed 18 December 2019).

Duncan, I. (2019). Baltimore estimates cost of ransomware attack at $18.2 million as the government begins to restore email accounts [online].

Available at: https://www.baltimoresun.com/maryland/baltimore-city/bs-md-ci-ransomware-email-20190529-story.html (Accessed 4 January 2020).

Elinson, Z. (2015). States' shortage of forensic pathologists displays autopsies [online]. Available at: https://www.wsj.com/articles/states-shortage-of-forensic-pathologists-delays-autopsies-1444689715 (Accessed 17 January 2020).

Facty.com (2020). How many people have pacemakers? [online]. Available at: https://www.reference.com/world-view/many-people-pacemakers-ad932529c8ba04dd (Accessed 4 January 2020).

FEMA (2011). *Strategic Foresight Initiative "Getting Urgent about the Future.* Washington DC: United States Department of Homeland Security.

FEMA (2013). National incident management system: Intelligence/investigations function guidance and field operations guide [online]. Available at: https://publicintelligence.net/dhs-nims-intel-guide (Accessed 12 January 2020).

FEMA (2016). *Resource Typing Definition for Public Health, Healthcare, and Emergency Medical Services Fatality Management Disaster Portable Morgue Unit.* Washington DC: United States Federal Emergency Management Agency.

Fudenberg, J. (2018). *Interview of the Clark County Coroner following the 1 October 2017 Shooting.* Las Vegas: Gavin.

Gaardner, J. (2017). The ethics of the future [online]. Available at: https://www.huffpost.com/entry/ethics-future_b_8576266 (Accessed 12 January 2020).

Gavin, C. (2019). *NEXTGEN Leadership for Managing Disasters, a Future-oriented Leadership Model for Local and State Officials.* Baltimore: Uptown Press.

Gavin, C. and Nesler, J. (2014). *Complex Mass Fatality Management (CMFM) Thought Leadership Position Paper: The Field of Fatality Management Requires Its Own Emergency Support Function (ESF) within the National Response Framework.* Columbus: Battelle Memorial Institute.

Gavin, C., Nesler, J. and Wilt, D. (2015). *Mass Fatality Management Standards of Practice in a Resource Scarce Environment.* Arlington: Department of Defense Joint Staff J4.

Geradts, Z. (2019). Digital and multimedia sciences. In: *Forensic Science in Focus: The Future of Forensic Science.* (ed. D. Martell), 31–47. Hoboken: Wiley.

Giiresearch.com (2017). Digital forensics market global scenario, market size, outlook, trend, and forecast, 2015-20124 [online]. Available at: https://www.giiresearch.com/report/var508286-digital-forensics-market-by-type-network-forensics.html (Accessed 12 December 2019).

Giiresearch.com (2019). Human identification: forensics, geneaology and security applications [online]. Available at: https://www.giiresearch.com/report/bc906078-human-identification-forensics-genealogy-security.html (Accessed 12 December 2019).

Giuliani, R.W. (2002). *Leadership.* New York: Miramax Books.

GlobalChange.com (2020). Future of business ethics [online]. Available at: https://www.globalchange.com/businessethics.htm (Accessed 12 January 2020).

Gordon, A. (2009). *Future Savvy*. New York: AMACOM.

Gruspier, K. (2017). A multiple fatality response to nine indigenous deaths in a burned house in Pikangikum, Ontario. In: *69th Annual Meeting of the American Academy of Forensic Sciences* 16 February. New Orleans: American Academy of Forensic Sciences.

History.com (2014). This day in history March 22 2014 mudslide in Washington State kills more than 40 people [online]. Available at: https://www.history.com/this-day-in-history/mudslide-in-washington-state-kills-more-than-40-people (Accessed 17 January 2020).

ISTM (2020). International society of travel medicine mission [online]. Available at: https://www.istm.org (Accessed 12 January 2020).

Kanter, R.M. (2011). The blog of Beth Kerr [online]. Available at: https://bethkerrblog.wordpress.com/2011/04/12/change-is-disturbing-when-done-to-us-exhilarating-when-done-by-us-rosabeth-moss-kanter (Accessed 25 September 2018).

Kastelein, R. (2018). PwC survey: 84% of companies now using blockchain, so what does the future hold? [online]. Available at: https://www.the-blockchain.com/2018/08/28/pwc-survey-84-of-companies-now-using-blockchain-so-what-does-the-future-hold (Accessed 12 December 2019).

Kraaijenbring, J. (2018). What does VUCA really mean? [online]. Available at: https://www.forbes.com/sites/jeroenkraaijenbrink/2018/12/19/what-does-vuca-really-mean/#47401d017d62 (Accessed 28 January 2020).

Krehbiel, K. (2019). A death investigation of mining fatalities: The Utah experience. In: *71st Annual Meeting of the American Academy of Forensic Sciences* 21 February. Baltimore: American Academy of Forensic Sciences.

Langreth, R. and Cortez, M. (2020). US readies for coronavirus pandemic some experts now see as likely this is about mitigation at this point [online]. Available at: https://www.bloomberg.com/news/articles/2020-02-05/coronavirus-update-governments-prepare-for-pandemic (Accessed 6 September 2020).

LaPorte, G. (2017). Wrongful convictions and DNA exonerations: Understanding the role of forensic science [online]. Available at: https://nij.ojp.gov/topics/articles/wrongful-convictions-and-dna-exonerations-understanding-role-forensic-science (Accessed 19 November 2019).

Latham, K.E., O'Daniel, A. and Spradley, K. (2018). Humanitarian science in the Texas borderlands: Incorporating a sociopolitical perspective to the forensic investigation of migrant identification. In: *70th Annual Meeting of the American Academy of Forensic Sciences* 21 February. Seattle: American Academy of Forensic Sciences.

Lincoff, N. (2015). The future of healthcare could be in concierge medicine [online]. Available at: https://www.healthline.com/health-news/

the-future-of-healthcare-could-be-in-concierge-medicine-063015 (Accessed 12 January 2020).

Little Hoover Commission (2018). *Artificial Intelligence: A Roadmap for California*. Sacramento: Milton Marks Commission on California State Government Organization and Economy.

Logan, B. (2019). Past perspectives and future directions in forensic toxicology. In: *Forensic Science in Focus: The Future of Forensic Science*. (ed. D. Martell), 159–174. Hoboken: Wiley.

Lu, J. (2018) Jeannie Mai: Fight against human trafficking [online]. Available at: https://www.digitalistmag.com/improving-lives/2018/03/12/jeannie-mai-fight-against-human-trafficking-05964308 (Accessed 12 December 2019).

Madren, C. (2013). Investigating the future of forensics [online]. Available at: https://www.aaas.org/investigating-future-forensics (Accessed 5 December 2019).

Martell, D. (2019). Preface. In: *Forensic Science in Focus: The Future of Forensic Science*. (ed. D. Martell), xxi–xxii. Hoboken: Wiley.

Md DH (2020). Office of the chief medical examiner [online]. Available at: https://health.maryland.gov/ocme/Pages/Home.aspx (Accessed 17 January 2020).

McFarland, M. (2017). US roads keep getting more dangerous [online]. Available at: https://money.cnn.com/2017/01/13/technology/traffic-deaths-2016/index.html?sr=twCNN011517traffic-deaths-20160207PMVODtopLinkandlinkId=33373507 (Accessed 2019 December 2019).

Meng, M. (2009) Issue life cycle clarifies the difference between "issues management" and "crisis management" [online]. Available at: http://alexanderps.com/blog/blog-issuelifecycle.html (Accessed 17 January 2020).

Moore, S. (2019). Gartner top 10 strategic technology trends for 2020 [online]. Available at: https://www.gartner.com/smarterwithgartner/top-trends-from-gartner-hype-cycle-for-digital-government-technology-2019 (Accessed 5 December 2019).

Morgan, O., Sribanditmongkol, P., Perera, C., Sulasmi, Y., Van Alphen, D. and Sondorp, E. (2006). Mass fatality management following the South Asian tsunami disaster: Case studies in Thailand, Indonesia, and Sri Lanka. *PLOS Medicine* 3: 809–815. [online]. Available at: https://journals.plos.org/plosmedicine/article?id=10.1371/journal.pmed.0030195 (Accessed 7 September 2020).

Morgan, S. (2017). Cybercrime damages $6 trillion by 2021 [online]. Available at: https://cybersecurityventures.com/hackerpocalypse-cybercrime-report-2016 (Accessed 12 December 2019).

NIEHS (2019). Bioethics [online]. Available at: https://www.niehs.nih.gov/research/resources/bioethics/index.cfm (Accessed 12 January 2020).

NIST (2005). *Report of the Technical Investigation of the Station Nightclub Fire NCSTAR 2: Vol. 1*. Washington: National Institute of Standards and Technology.

NRC (2009). *Strengthening Forensic Science in the United States a Path Forward*. Washington DC: The National Academies Press.

NTSB (2019). History of the national transportation safety board [online]. Available at: https://www.ntsb.gov/about/history/Pages/default.aspx (Accessed 22 December 2019).

NYC OCME (2008). *City of New York Office of Chief Medical Examiner Pandemic Influenza Surge Plan to Manage in and Out of Hospital Deaths*. New York: Gavin Emergency Management Consultants.

NYC OCME (2009). *City of New York Office of Chief Medical Examiner All-hazards Mass Fatality Management Plan*. New York: Gavin Emergency Management Consultants.

NYC OCME (2012). International mass fatality management conference and workshop [online]. Available at: http://www.nyc.gov/html/ocme/downloads/pdf/International%20Mass%20Fatality%20Workshop%20April%2025-27%202012.pdf (Accessed 12 January 2020).

NYC OCME (2020). City of New York office of chief medical examiner department of forensic biology [online]. Available at: https://www1.nyc.gov/site/ocme/services/department-of-forensic-biology.page (Accessed 7 September 2020).

Pottorff, A. (2018). Should the opioid crisis be declared a state emergency? [online]. Available at: https://www.richlandsource.com/oped/should-the-opioid-crisis-be-declared-a-state-emergency/article_adbc3ed2-6b52-11e8-9593-67b31a22b622.html (Accessed 17 January 2020).

Pullman, G. (2017). Top 10 cutting-edge innovations in the future of forensic science [online]. Available at: https://listverse.com/2017/06/12/top-10-cutting-edge-innovations-in-the-future-of-forensic-science (Accessed 5 December 2019).

RAINN (2020). Addressing the rape kit backlog [online]. Available at: https://www.rainn.org/articles/addressing-rape-kit-backlog (Accessed 12 January 2020).

Ralston, B. and Wilson, I. (2006). Annex D. In: *Scan. Radar for Signals of Change. The Scenario-planning Handbook* 245–257. Mason: South-Western Educational.

RCPGP (2010). Regional mass fatality management response system [online]. Available at: https://info.publicintelligence.net/RCPT-Fatality.pdf (Accessed 17 January 2020).

Richert, S. (2019). What are the 4 cardinal virtues? [online]. Available at: https://www.learnreligions.com/the-cardinal-virtues-542142 (Accessed 19 November 2019).

Ritter, N. (2006). What will criminal justice look like in 2040? [online]. Available at: http://nij.ojp.gov/topics/articles/preparing-future-criminal-justice-2040 (Accessed 12 December 2019).

Rouse, M. (2020). Definition of technology ethics [online]. Available at: https://searchcio.techtarget.com/definition/Technology-Ethics (Accessed 12 January 2020).

Rueda-Sabater, E., Derosby, D., Johnston, J. and Murphy, N. (2010). *The Evolving Internet: Driving Forces, Uncertainties, and Four Scenarios to 2025*. San Francisco: CISCO and Global Business Network.

Samans, R. and Davis, N. (2019). *G20 Insights: Advancing Human-centered Economic Industrial Revolution: A Leadership*. Germany: G20.

Siwicki, B. (2017). 10 health IT predictions for 2018: AI, blockchain, robotics, and a $100 million class-action suit [online]. Available at: https://www.healthcareitnews.com/news/10-health-it-predictions-2018-al-blockchain-robotics-and-100-million-class-action-suit (Accessed 5 December 2019).

Stirling, S. and Sullivan, S.P. (2017). Death and dysfunction how N.J. fails the dead, betrays the living and is a national disgrace [online]. Available at: http://death.nj.com (Accessed 7 September 2020).

Thompson, A. (2011). Medical examiners in America: A dysfunctional system [online]. Available at: https://www.huffingtonpost.com/2011/02/02/the-real-csi-how-americas_n_816842.html (Accessed7 September 2020).

Tkacik, C. (2018). Remembering the Baltimore riots after Freddie Gray's death, 3 years later [online]. Available at: https://www.baltimoresun.com/maryland/baltimore-city/bs-md-ci-riots-three-years-later-20180426-story.html (Accessed 7 January 2020).

TRACIE (2020). Topic collection: crisis standards of care [online]. Available at: https://asprtracie.hhs.gov/technical-resources/63/crisis-standards-of-care/0 (Accessed 31 January 2020).

TriData Division (2009). *Mass Shootings at Virginia Tech Addendum to the Report of the Review Panel*. Arlington: System Planning Corporation.

Ubelaker, D. (2019). New directions in forensic anthropology. In: *Forensic Science in Focus: The Future of Forensic Science*. (ed. D. Martell), 1–18. Hoboken: Wiley.

Urban Dictionary (2009). Hey buddy [online]. Available at: https://www.urbandictionary.com/define.php?term=hey%20buddy (Accessed 22 December 2019).

US Army SBCCOM (2005). Mass fatality management capstone document [online]. Available at: http://www.ecbc.army.mil/hld/dl/MFM_Capstone_August_2005.pdf (Accessed 12 September 2020)

US Army (2018). *The US Army's Recommendation in Response to the US Central Command's Joint Urgent Operational Needs Statement-0559*. Arlington: US Army.

Weebly.com (2019). Future demand [online]. Available at: https://forensicpathologistcareer.weebly.com/future-demand.html (Accessed 17 January 2020).

White House (2018). Ending America's opioid crisis [online]. Available at: https://www.whitehouse.gov/opioids (Accessed 17 January 2020).

WHP (2020). April 19 1861 the Baltimore riot of 1861 [online]. Available at: https://worldhistoryproject.org/1861/4/19/the-baltimore-riot-of-1861 (Accessed 7 January 2020).

Willard, D. (2006). The business of business. *Provocation* (11 October), pp. 103–105.

Wise, C.R. (2006). Organizing for homeland security after Katrina: Is adaptive management what's missing?. In: *Public Administration Review* 302–318.

World Resources Institute (2017). RELEASE: World resources institute: Ross Center wins prestigious prince Michael International Road Safety Award [online]. Available at: https://www.wri.org/news/2017/12/release-wri-ross-center-wins-prestigious-prince-michael-international-road-safety-award (Accessed 19 December 2019).

Index

Disaster Victim Identification in the 21st Century: A US Perspective, First Edition.
Edited by John A Williams and Victor W Weedn.

www.ingramcontent.com/pod-product-compliance
Lightning Source LLC
LaVergne TN
LVHW011517200926
848484LV00001B/60
9781119652786